MILADY'S STANDARD SYSTEM OF SALON SKILLS:

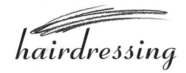

hairdressing

Student Course Book

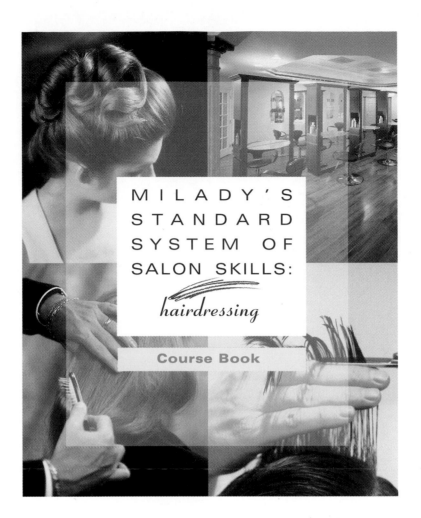

MILADY'S STANDARD SYSTEM OF SALON SKILLS: *hairdressing*

Course Book

▶ **Contributing Authors**

MARYBETH JANSSEN

DWIGHT MILLER

FLOYD KENYATTA

CHARLENE CARROLL

DAVID RACCUGLIA

COLLEEN HENNESSEY

JOEL MOORE

LOUANN WERKSMA

EXCEL, INC.

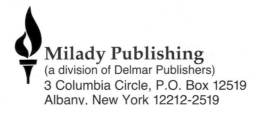

Milady Publishing
(a division of Delmar Publishers)
3 Columbia Circle, P.O. Box 12519
Albany, New York 12212-2519

Publisher does not warrant or guarantee any of the products described herein or perform any independent analysis in connection with any of the product information contained herein. Publisher does not assume, and expressly disclaims, any obligation to obtain and include information other than that provided to it by the manufacturer.

The reader is expressly warned to consider and adopt all safety precautions that might be indicated by the activities herein and to avoid all potential hazards. By following the instructions contained herein, the reader willingly assumes all risks in connection with such instructions.

The publisher makes no representation or warranties of any kind, including but not limited to, the warranties of fitness for particular purpose or merchantability, nor are any such representations implied with respect to the material set forth herein, and the publisher takes no responsibility with respect to such material. The publisher shall not be liable for any special, consequential, or exemplary damages resulting, in whole or part, from the readers' use of, or reliance upon, this material.

Milady Staff

Acquisitions Editor: Pamela Lappies
Project Editor: Nancy Jean Downey
Editorial Assistant: Elizabeth Keller
Production Manager: Karen Leet
Art and Design Coordinator: Suzanne Nelson
Marketing Manager: Donna Lewis
Marketing Assistant: Tammy Race-Holmes
Team Assistant: Lisa Borkowski

Cover Design: Delgado Design, Inc.
Interior Design and Production: Delgado Design, Inc
Illustrations: Paul Colin/Cezanne Studio

Copyright © 1999
Milady Publishing
(a division of Delmar Publishing)
an International Thomson Publishing company I(T)P®

Printed in the United States of America
Printed and distributed simultaneously in Canada

For more information, contact:
Milady Publishing
3 Columbia Circle, Box 12519
Albany, New York 12212-2519

6 7 8 9 10 XXX 03

Library of Congress Cataloging-in-Publication Data
Milady's standard system of salon skills: hairdressing.
p. cm.
Includes index.
ISBN 1-56253-398-3
1. Hairdressing. I. Milady Publishing Company.
TT972.M55 1998
646.7'24–dc21
                              98-7543
                              CIP

Contents

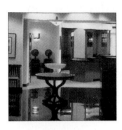

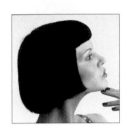

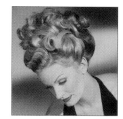

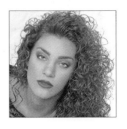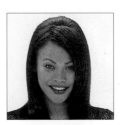

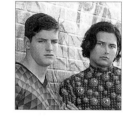

Preface

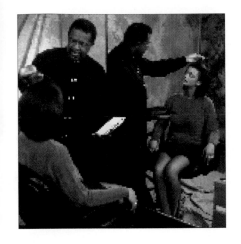

THE NEED FOR CHANGE

We at Milady have been listening to what our customers—students, instructors, and salons—have been saying, and we heard you say that you needed something more than what was available for use in the classroom and clinic. We learned that you needed a different kind of program to complement *Milady's Standard Textbook of Cosmetology*, a program that would pick up where that book leaves off to provide students entering the professional field with practical skills that would serve them well in the salon. Salon owners spoke of the need for graduates who are savvy in business and communications skills as well as experienced in technical abilities. School owners spoke of the need for better programs to teach students more than the basics needed for licensure. Graduates beginning employment in the salon voiced their frustration over being expected to know skills that had never been taught. We at Milady heard those concerns voiced repeatedly, and so we took action.

Through market research, surveys, formal inquiries, and numerous one-on-one discussions, we learned what needed to be covered to provide the most thorough package available, a package that when integrated into the curriculum would revolutionize cosmetology education. Carlos Valenzuela, a respected cosmetology educator and former school owner, conducted the market research through telephone and written surveys to determine what salons and schools said needed to change in order for students to be better prepared after graduation. Those surveys formed the basis of what you'll find in this program.

CONTENT BY EXPERTS

To present the technical skills in this program, we went to the best artists in the field, the seven talented professionals featured on these pages and in the accompanying Video Library. They will show you, step-by-step, how to create the most desired cuts, styles, texture services, and color services—the technical skills needed to succeed.

You will meet our authors on pages xvi and xvii, "About the Authors," but in addition to that, each author is interviewed in the section that he or she wrote. There you will learn how each expert got his or her start as a cosmetologist and what turns the road to success has taken.

BUSINESS AND COMMUNICATION SKILLS

But technical skills don't guarantee success. Salon owners surveyed said that the most sought-after characteristics in new stylists are not necessarily technical abilities. They are instead:

▸ The ability to communicate well to clients and to coworkers and employers

▸ An understanding of the business of hairdressing

That's why you'll find throughout our program short essays on business and communications skills, the tools that will unlock the doors to success. These "Business Bits," as they're called, are interspersed with the technical training to emphasize the importance of learning the skills they address as well as the technical skills.

ACCOUNTING FOR LEARNING STYLES

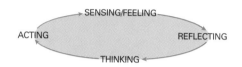

But we didn't stop with what to cover; we also researched how to cover it. And for that we went to the best in the education field. EXCEL, Inc., one of the most respected educational design companies in the world, partnered with us to fashion the content of our program through their 4MAT™ System for Teaching and Learning, which presents information in a manner that all learner types can easily access and understand. Based on a model for teaching rooted in the natural cycle of learning, the 4MAT™ System uses four quadrants of a circle to illustrate the four basic ways of learning. *

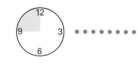

▸ The twelve o'clock position represents the **sensing/feeling** aspect of learning. It comprises all the personal experiences a learner has had that can relate to the new material about to be studied. These experiences provide the learner with a personal connection to the subject matter–**why** it is important.

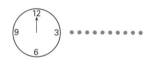

▸ The learner moves through the first quadrant to the three o'clock position, which involves **reflecting** upon these life experiences in light of the subject matter. Here the learner moves from percept to concept–**what** it is that will be studied.

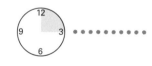

▸ The six o'clock position is characterized by **thinking**, where the learner applies intellectual and organizational abilities to the subject being learned. This launches the learner into the third quadrant–the **how** stage.

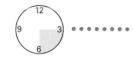

▸ In the third quadrant the learner moves from thinking to **doing**, represented by the nine o'clock position, which begins the fourth quadrant. Here the learner acts and reacts to the subject, ultimately finding personal uses for it. The learner tinkers with the concept, exploring the possibilities — the **what if** phase of learning.

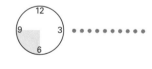

▸ At the end of the fourth quadrant, the learner is approaching the sensing/feeling stage once again, this time having experienced the subject matter throughout all the quadrants and having come full circle. The learning cycle never really ends but spirals on, continuing through various stages of development.

The *Standard System of Salon Skills* has been developed to link with the four quadrants, providing students who tend to learn primarily in one quadrant the same opportunity to grasp the material as students in others.

* The model is taken from the *4MAT System: Teaching to Learning Styles with Right/Left Mode Techniques*, by Bernice McCarthy, ©1980, 1987 by Excel, Inc. and *About Learning*, by Bernice McCarthy, ©1996 by Excel, Inc. Portions of the text are derived from these books and are used with permission. Those desiring a copy of the complete works may acquire them from the publisher, Excel, Inc., 23385 Old Barrington Road, Barrington, IL 60010, 847-382-7272 or 800-822-4MAT, www.excelcorp.com.

Features
of this Program

Milady's Standard System of Salon Skills: Hairdressing contains two student books. The first, *this* book, is designed for use in the classroom. The accompanying volume, the *Clinic Success Journal*, is much more portable, so that you can easily carry it with you into the clinic and throughout your day.

STUDENT COURSE BOOK

Salon Exploration. Part One of the Student Course Book is "Salon Exploration," which provides an overview of the kinds of salons you may choose to work in as well as a "tour" of the various parts of a full-service salon.

Fundamentals of Hairdressing. Part Two, "Fundamentals of Hairdressing," is the heart of the program. In it you will learn the step-by-step techniques for Women's Haircutting, Hairstyling, Texture Services, Haircoloring, and Men's Haircutting.

The technicals in the "Fundamentals of Hairdressing" feature all or most of the following categories:

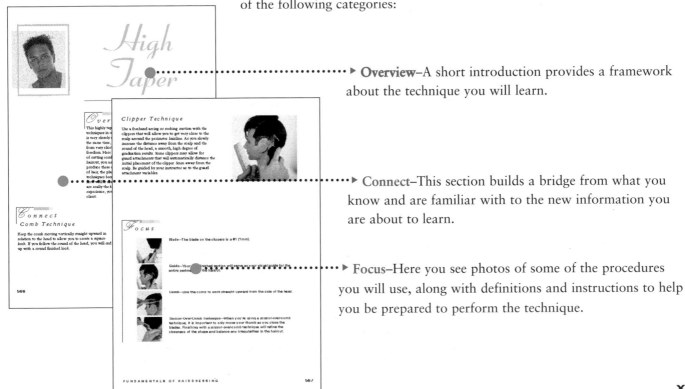

▶ **Overview**–A short introduction provides a framework about the technique you will learn.

▶ **Connect**–This section builds a bridge from what you know and are familiar with to the new information you are about to learn.

▶ **Focus**–Here you see photos of some of the procedures you will use, along with definitions and instructions to help you be prepared to perform the technique.

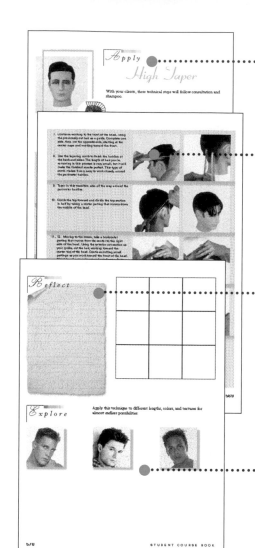

▶ **Apply**–This is the step-by-step part of the technique. You will follow the steps through photos and accompanying text.

▶ **Reflect**–Use the note page to record anything you want to remember about the technique and a windowpane in which you will draw the key features of focus points from the Focus section. Your instructor will guide you about how to use this section.

▶ **Explore**–Finally, you will see photos of the same technique performed on different hair length, color, and texture to help ignite your imagination. This will help you consider different ways to put what you've learned to work in many creative ways.

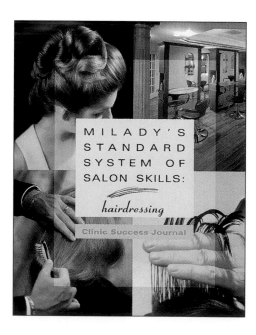

CLINIC SUCCESS JOURNAL

The *Clinic Success Journal* contains sections for scheduling and planning, games and activities, and exercises that build communication and business skills.

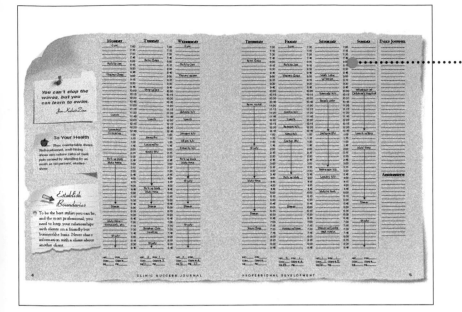

Part One, "Professional Development," contains a 50-week **Appointment Journal** to help you schedule classes and appointments, as well as organize your personal life. Keep your *Clinic Success Journal* with you throughout the day. Every weekly spread features a motivational quote, a Wellness Tip, and a Professional Development idea, followed by lined spaces for every quarter hour of all seven days.

After the Appointment Journal come the **Professional Development Activities**, featuring exercises and assignments that relate to the Business Bits in the Student Course Book, puzzles, and practical exercises to perform on your mannequin.

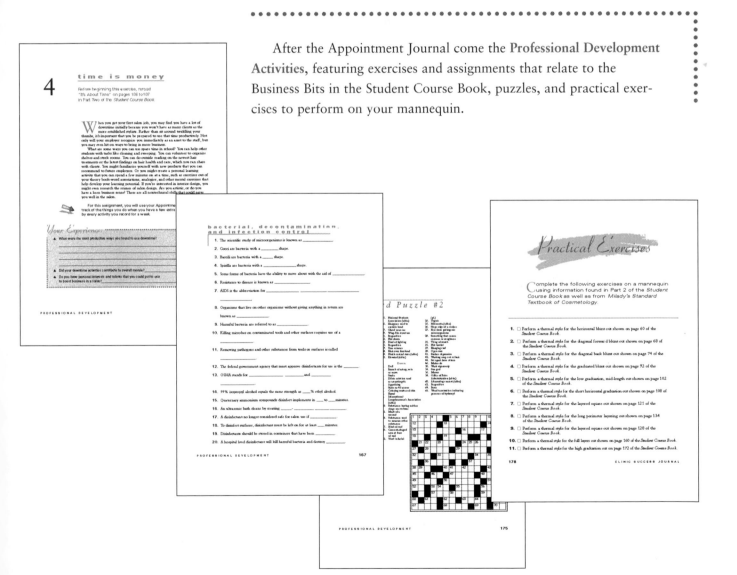

Part Two of the *Clinic Success Journal*, "Get Set to Style," contains helpful how-to material for making the transition from school to salon. Writing resumes, responding to help-wanted ads, and making those important first contacts are all included, as well as tips for following up, beginning your first job, and continuing your education as your career progresses.

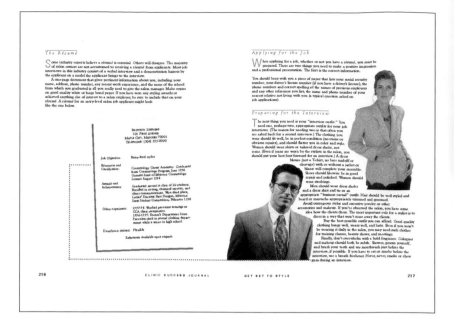

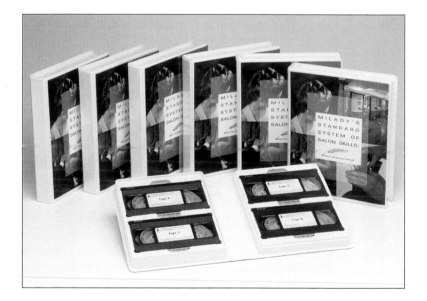

VIDEO LIBRARY

The 20-tape video library will become the part of this program you will rely on again and again. Every step-by-step technical presented in the *Student Course Book* is included in the video library, along with additional technicals not represented in the book. The video library follows the order of the technicals in the Student Course Book, with brief versions of most of the Business Bits interspersed throughout. Viewing the video as you study a technical in the book will help you to see exactly how each technique is done by the featured expert and will answer any questions not addressed in the still photos.

LEADER'S MANUAL

The *Leader's Manual for Milady's Standard System of Salon Skills: Hairdressing* provides full instructor support for the student materials. Reproduced at a smaller size is the Student Course Book in its entirety, with teaching instruction and pedagogical information provided in the surrounding margins. Before the beginning of the *Student Course Book* reproduction is valuable information for educators on how to use the program, along with information about the educational theory. Implementation of the program is assisted through the separately packaged lesson plans, which are three-hole punched to allow the instructor to place wherever it is most convenient in the *Leader's Manual*. Curriculum planning cards and instructions are also supplied with the detailed lesson plans, which provide activities, games, and motivational material.

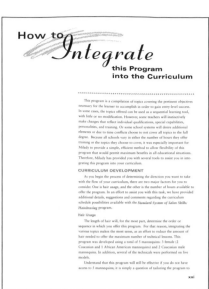

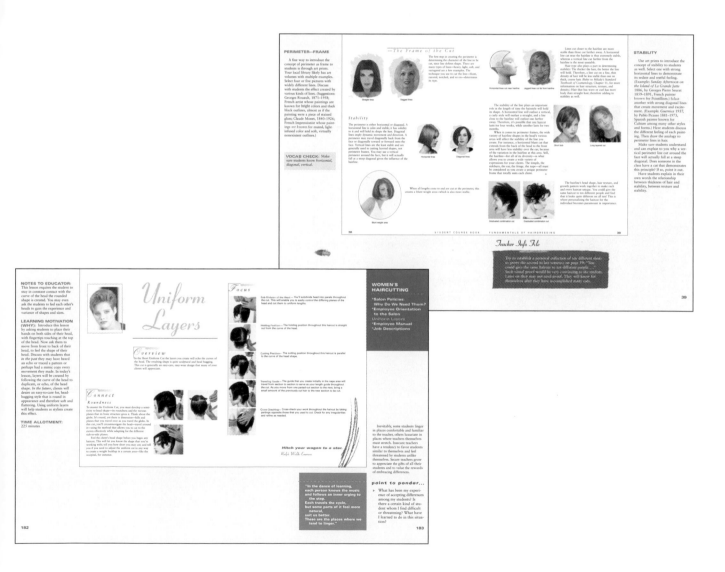

About the Authors

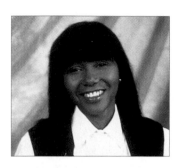

CHARLENE CARROLL

Charlene Carroll has been in the world of hair design for 25 years and continues to break new ground. She is a member of the current NCA Design Team. She is a motivator, educator and highly competitive in her quest for excellence. Carroll has been a salon owner for over 19 years and works as a consultant to companies such as Revlon, American Beauty Products, and Soft Sheen. She has been featured in national publications such as *Black Hair*, *Shop Talk*, and *Black Enterprise*. Carroll's skills in multicultural services are illustrated in the Women's Haircutting, Hairstyling, and Texture Services.

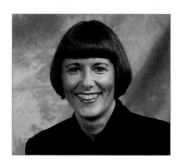

COLLEEN HENNESSEY

Colleen Hennessey is recognized nationally as a master haircolorist, platform artist and educator. Formally Clairol Professional's exclusive color designer and Senior Manager of Clairol Professionalís Education, she works actively as a salon educator, and also writes a professional advice column, which reaches thousands of stylists nationwide. Hennessey is currently a master colorist at the respected salon Adam Broderick Salon and Day Spa in Ridgefield, Connecticut. As an established platform artist, Hennessey performs throughout the US and brings her expertise to trade shows such as Haircolor USA, Long Beach, IBS, and Midwest Beauty Show. Her mastery of color services and unique abilities are exemplified in the Haircoloring technicals in the program.

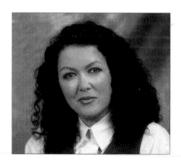

MARY BETH JANSSEN

Mary Beth Janssen is the creative director of Innovated Styling Options (ISO). Formerly the International Artistic Director for Pivot Point International, she is the recipient of the 1996 *Rocco Bellino* award (given at the Midwest Beauty Show) for outstanding contributions in education. A hairstylist and cosmetology educator, Janssen has been a guest artist throughout the world and is renowned in the salon industry for her creative and motivational talents. Her work has appeared in leading trade and consumer publications. She has coordinated the hair and makeup for television shows and commercials, and she continues to be one of the most well-known women in the salon industry today. Janssen brings her expertise to the project through the presentation of Texture Services.

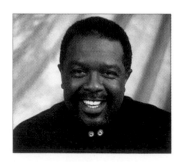

FLOYD KENYATTA

Floyd Kenyatta is the Global Ambassador for John Paul Mitchell Systems, President of Nu-Age Distributors, Founder of the USA Black Hair Olympic Team and Chairman of the US Council of Black Salon Owners. With over 30 years in the professional beauty industry, Kenyatta has played a role in virtually every modern cutting and styling technique currently used on black hair. Respected worldwide for his unique and innovative approaches to black hair design and styling, Kenyatta is credited with the development of specialized techniques for chemically relaxed hair. He brings his considerable talents and expertise to the Women's Haircutting and Texture Services sections of this program.

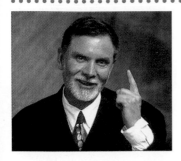

DWIGHT MILLER

Dwight Miller is among the most respected American hairdressers in the international community. He has created dozens of influential trends, such as the Stack Perm in the 70s, the 60s look in the 80s, and the High Roller phenomenon in the 90s. Miller has helped in the development of numerous product lines, such as Bain de Terre, Systeme Biolage, and Anasazi. He developed the first comprehensive system of scalp manipulations. Miller's work graces the covers of international hair magazines, and he continues to be one of the strongest underlying influences in the industry today. He lends his considerable expertise and artistry to the Women's Haircutting portion of the program.

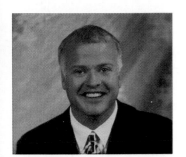

JOEL MOORE

Joel Moore has been a salon and school owner in Savannah, Georgia, for the past eighteen years. He formerly worked with Revlon as Artistic Director and as chairman of the University of Georgia's School of Continuing Cosmetology Education. Joel is also the recipient of the NCA's Charles award. Most recently he headed the creative effort as trainer of the USA Hairstyling Team that competed at Hair World '96 and ultimately placed 4th in the world. His strong foundation in styling basics, combined with a focus on contemporary teachings, makes him the ideal contributor for our Hairstyling section.

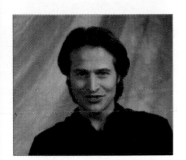

DAVID RACCUGLIA

David Raccuglia is the President and founder of American Crew. He was selected top men's artist in the world by *American Salon*. He is an internationally renowned educator and artist whose creative styles have been published in major hair and fashion magazines worldwide. Raccuglia has appeared as a platform artist in major trade shows throughout the US, Europe, and Asia. He has created hair imagery ads, product brochures, and packaging for several major product companies. He has also created the styles for national television commercials for various manufacturers. Raccuglia's talents make him the natural choice to lead the Men's Haircutting section of this new program.

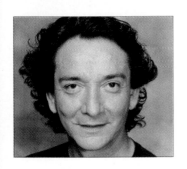

CARLOS VALENZUELA

Carlos Valenzuela has taken the beauty industry by storm as an award-winning designer, international educator, and manufacturer's spokesperson. He founded the Carlos Valenzuela Academy in 1983 and built it into one of the most successful schools ever in the US. He is the author/producer of many industry educational programs and a popular presenter the world over. Named "Business Star of Tomorrow" at the International Beauty Show in 1996, Valenzuela's insightful, knowledgeable, and passionate presentations have received rave reviews from audiences all over the US and in 15 countries. His ongoing work with salons gives him the edge to help focus this program squarely on the entry level job skills needed for today's job market. He was specifically chosen as a consultant on this project to represent the industry voice from salons and to coordinate the market research.

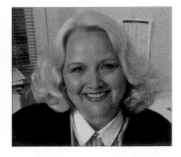

LOUANN WERKSMA

Louann Werksma combines a corporate sales and marketing background with a communications degree and experience in advertising, reporting, feature writing, and book editing for the salon industry. She has served as a public relations coordinator, news reporter, magazine editor, and director of educational services. She was editor of *Cutter* magazine and helped develop a program of communication skills for an internationally known school. Werksma brings her twenty years of in-depth experience to this program via the short, "Business Bit" essays found in the Student Coursebook, as well as in other parts of the program.

Acknowledgments

Without the assistance of a great number of people and organizations, this program would not have been possible. Milady Publishing and the authors wish to thank the following people, companies, and institutions for their immeasurable help in creating this book.

Contributing authors:
PAUL COLE
PORTER SHIMER
ELIZABETH TINSLEY
VICTORIA WURDINGER

Furniture and equipment for photo and video shoots:
TAKARA BELMONT DESIGN CENTER
DOWNERS GROVE, ILLINOIS

Mannequins:
BURMAX COMPANY, INC.
HOLTSVILLE, NEW YORK

Mannequin makeup:
SCOTT AMENT

Photo and video shoot locations:
ZANOS SALON
CHICAGO, ILLINOIS

Photo research:
LYNN MAESTRO

Special thanks to our subject matter experts, who reviewed parts of this program:

Louis Atkins
DIRECTOR OF EDUCATION
GENE JUAREZ SALONS AND SPAS, GENE JUAREZ ACADEMY
BAINBRIDGE ISLAND, WA

Olivia Barr
ADMINISTRATIVE DIRECTOR OF EDUCATION
SOFT SHEEN PRODUCTS INC.
CHICAGO, IL

Nicole Buschong
DIRECTOR OF EDUCATION
COSMETOLOGY EDUCATION CENTER
GLOUCESTER CITY, NJ

Rick Butler
SALES REPRESENTATIVE
MARIANNA INC.
AMES, IOWA

Introduction

Congratulations! You are about to begin an exciting new adventure that can change your life and impact the lives of others in a very positive way. You've made the giant step of beginning a process to change your life and create a world of new opportunities. By signing up for this course and beginning to use this program, you have elected to set out to become a stylist who will be in demand by salons and by clients, for you will have learned the skills that both are looking for.

SKILLS FOR BUSINESS AND COMMUNICATION

You'll learn that the word "skills" means much more than haircutting abilities or haircolor applications. Those are your technical skills, and they are important–a good part of this program is devoted to learning them from some of the most successful people in the industry! But your success will depend on more than that. You'll also need to have the skills to help you communicate–with your clients, with your coworkers, and with your employer. Communication is the key to success, both professionally and financially. That's why this program goes far beyond the teaching of technical skills to include short essays, "Business Bits" on communications, and business skills. You need many kinds of skills to succeed, and with this program you can be sure you have a good head start on them all.

ADAPTING FOR DIFFERENT LEARNING STYLES

This program is designed to teach you the technical skills you need to know from several approaches, to make it easy for all types of learners. We understand that not all students learn in the same way. Some of you learn best from analogy–describing a technique or skill by comparing it to something you've already experienced–while some of you need to reflect on something new before you can really absorb it. Many of you need to actually experience what is being taught, and some of you need to analyze it. Most of us, though, learn by using a little bit of all these methods and more. That's why we've enlisted the aid of Excel, Inc., one of the top educational design firms, to help us present each haircut, style, perm, or color service in several ways, to make it easy for each of you to understand the ideas and techniques.

You will be learning these skills and techniques not only in ways that make them easy to understand but from people who have become masters in their fields. Be sure to read about the authors involved, both in the front of

• •

this book and through their interviews in the Fundamentals of Hairdressing section, to learn their amazing stories of how they climbed to the top. They will inspire and motivate you to be the best you can be and to keep working toward your dreams, no matter what obstacles you encounter.

ATTITUDE IS KEY

That leads us to another part of this program that runs through all sections. It's the attitude needed to succeed, whether in hairdressing or any other aspect of life. We've offered you all the tools you'll need, but what you bring to it is just as important. To remain cheerful when things go wrong, to pitch in and help your coworkers, to stay late when it will help your employer–these are all the results of maintaining an attitude of cooperation and optimism. Your willingness to do more than what is required, to be the first to welcome someone into the salon, to send a note thanking a client for a referral will make or break your career. Start today to be the best you can be by developing a positive attitude at school with your fellows students and your instructor. Start now to develop good grooming and work habits, such as being on time. Start today to change the little things that can affect the way you look and feel, such as getting enough sleep and eating the right foods. Nothing will change in a day, but as the days mount up and the weeks and months go by, you'll see big changes in your work and in your life!

Today, the cosmetology industry holds many, many opportunities for those who are willing to put into practice all the skills we've included in this program, both technical and personal. The demand for stylists far exceeds the number available. As you begin this extensive program, keep in mind that we at Milady believe that students like you can achieve great heights in this environment, if you're willing to learn and to practice all that you're about to be taught. We believe that you can succeed, and we will be there beside you, now and in the future, to provide you with the education and encouragement you'll need to get there.

—MILADY/SALONOVATIONS PUBLISHING

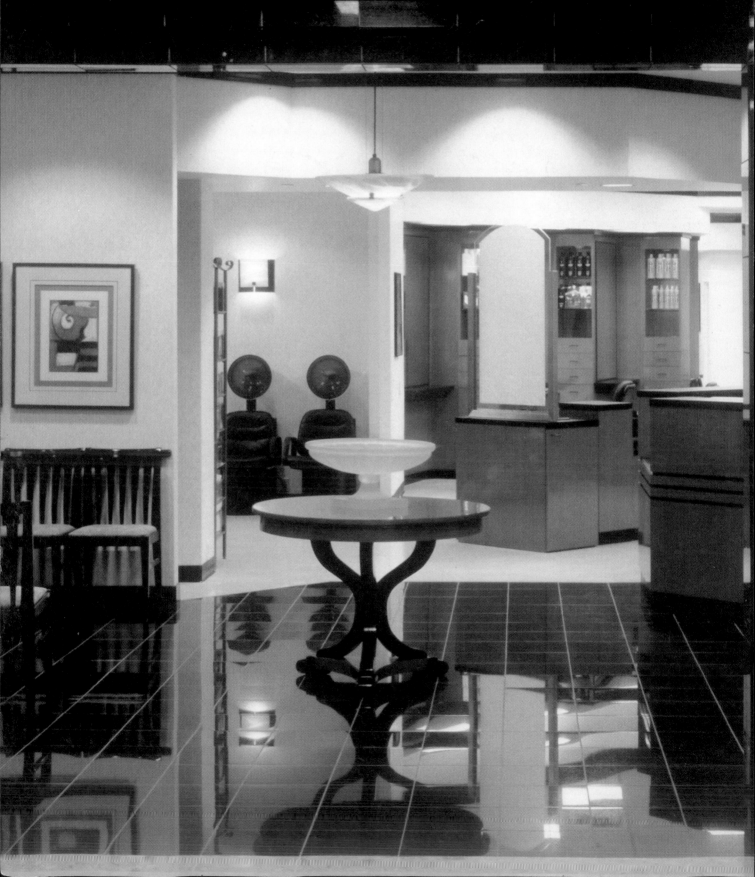

STYLING SALON
DAY SPA

part one

Salon Exploration

Congratulations and Welcome!

Congratulations and welcome to the wonderful world of hairdressing! This is an important moment for you. You've made the decision that you want a life of your own making. You've decided that you want more than a job—you want a rich and rewarding career. You want to elevate yourself, to grow into a respected professional in a respected profession.

You are about to join the tens of thousands of women and men entering this exciting profession each year. By enrolling in this program you've taken a big first step toward a career that will give you a chance to show the world who you are and what you can do. You've chosen a path, a new direction, and you may feel exhilarated—and maybe just a little scared. That's understandable. Even the biggest names in this business were once where you are right now. You may be comforted to know you're not alone. You'll have lots of companions on this journey, and many will become valued friends and colleagues.

What led you here? Your reasons are as individual as you are, but you'll probably find that you have a lot in common with others who've made the same choice.

You may be fresh out of school and looking around, wondering about the rest of your life, asking yourself, "What's the next step? What do I really want to do?"

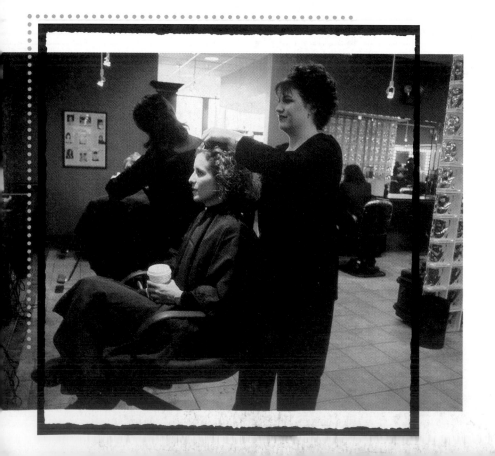

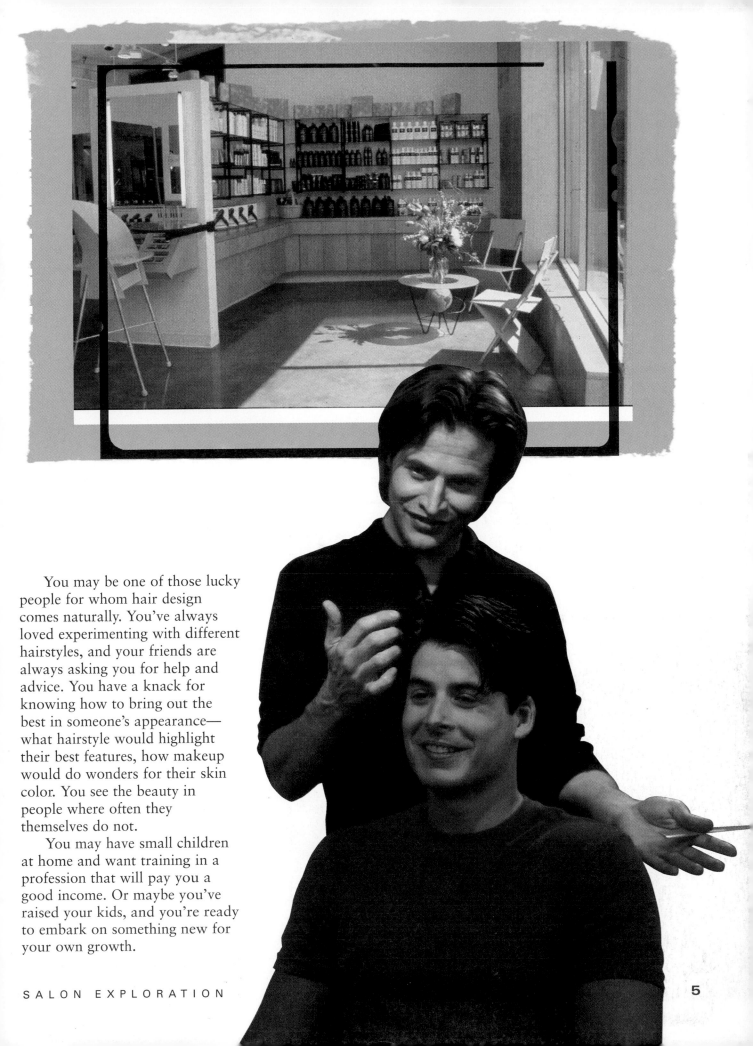

You may be one of those lucky people for whom hair design comes naturally. You've always loved experimenting with different hairstyles, and your friends are always asking you for help and advice. You have a knack for knowing how to bring out the best in someone's appearance— what hairstyle would highlight their best features, how makeup would do wonders for their skin color. You see the beauty in people where often they themselves do not.

You may have small children at home and want training in a profession that will pay you a good income. Or maybe you've raised your kids, and you're ready to embark on something new for your own growth.

You may be a "people person." Maybe you've tried your hand at other kinds of work and decided you want a career in which you provide an important service for a wide variety of people every day.

What's your story? Do you recognize yourself already? Yes or no, today, with this course, you are starting your own story within this time-honored profession. What are some of the reasons this program is tailor-made for you? You're joining an honorable and respected calling with great traditions in every world culture. But as ancient as the profession is, it is also ever new and growing. Trends, fashions, styles change. You change and grow with them as you build your skills and experience. Career options open up before you. Your work is fulfilling, rewarding, and financially sustaining.

You touch people, literally, and you touch their lives. You have the privilege of helping others look and feel better. In becoming a professional hairdresser, you're making a contribution to the beauty, order, and harmony of the world around you.

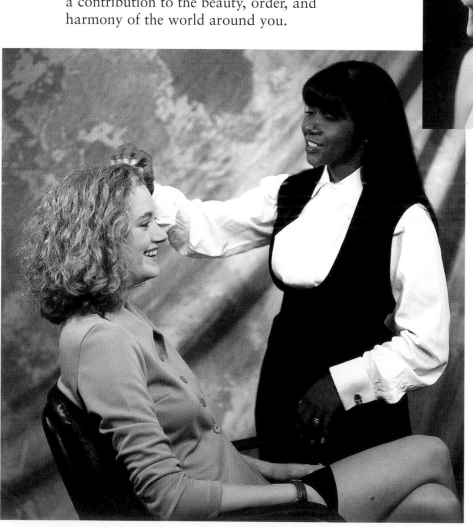

preparing for Opportunity

How do you get the job you want? Read the interviews in Part 2 and learn how the authors of this book made the most of the opportunities they encountered. You will see that the key ingredients are:

- Motivation
- Integrity
- Good technical and communications skills
- Strong work ethic
- Enthusiasm for learning, growing, and expanding skills and knowledge

In this program we provide you with the basic tools you'll need to learn your trade. If you're willing to challenge yourself and ready to work hard, you've already taken the first important step toward lifelong professional success.

focus on the *Salon*

Inside the big, wide world of the hair and beauty industry is another large and influential world: the professional salon business. There are over 250,000 licensed professional salons in the United States and more than 1 million active cosmetologists. Every year, tens of thousands of students enroll in cosmetology school. Not all graduate, but of those who do, the vast majority will find their first jobs in one of the types of salons described below.

small independent salons ▼

Small independent salons are owned by one person or two or more partners and make up the majority of professional salons. The average independent has one to three styling chairs. Usually the owner or owners are hairstylists who maintain their own clientele while managing the business and hiring and training other stylists. There are nearly as many different kinds of independent salons as there are owners; image, decor, services, prices, and clientele all reflect the owner's experience and taste. Depending on the owner's willingness to help a newcomer learn and grow, a beginning stylist can learn a great deal and earn a good living in an independent salon.

independent salon chains ▼

These are chains of ten or fewer salons owned by one individual or two or more partners. There are approximately 250,000 independent salon chains in the U.S. Independents—both single and chain—range from basic hair salons to full-service salons to day spas, from low-priced to very high-priced. In the larger of these (ten or more styling stations and a minimum of ten full-time staff), stylists can advance to positions as specialists (in color, nail, skin care, or other chemical services). Some larger salons also employ education directors and styles directors, and stylists are often hired to manage the different locations.

Business

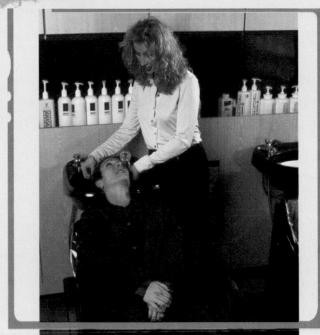

large national salon chains ▼

These companies operate salons throughout the country or large regions of the country. They can be budget- or value-priced haircut-only salons, or full-service, mid-price operations. Some salon chains operate within department store chains. Management and marketing professionals at corporate headquarters make all the decisions for each salon: size, decor, hours, services, prices, advertising, and profit targets.

Many cosmetology school graduates who find their first job in a national chain salon like the secure pay and benefits, additional paid training, management opportunities, and corporate advertising, which helps them attract a clientele. Because the chains are large and widespread, employees may have the advantage of being able to transfer from one location to another. If you like the idea of a businesslike workplace (job descriptions, policy manuals, employee evaluations) and you want a secure, regular paycheck and the opportunity to advance to a management position, this may be a perfect environment for you.

franchise salons ▼

This is another form of the chain salon organization, one with a national name and a consistent image and business formula throughout the chain. Franchises are owned by individuals who pay a fee to use the name, receive a business plan, and take advantage of the national marketing campaign. Such decisions as size, location, decor, and prices are determined in advance by the parent company. Franchises are generally not owned by hairstylists but rather by investors who seek a return on their profit. Franchise salons often offer employees the same benefits as corporate-owned chain salons.

Priced to Upscale

Within each form of ownership—independent, small chain, large chain, and franchise chain—are different salon types or "formulas." A formula is simply the whole package of salon image, decor, services, prices, and policies that work together to attract and retain a specific type of clientele. Let's look at some examples.

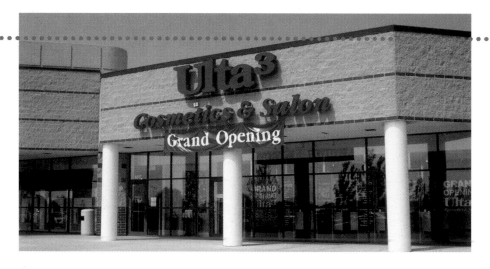

basic value-priced operations ▼

Often located in busy strip shopping centers, where rents are lower than in shopping malls and there's a supermarket or other business nearby, these outlets depend on lots of walk-in traffic. They hire recent grads and generally pay them by the hour, sometimes adding commission-style bonuses if their individual sales pass a certain level. They usually charge around $10, some even less, for a haircut, and they train stylists to do them fast, with no frills. Shampoo and conditioning services are available, usually for an additional charge. Perms or color services, if offered, are limited. These salons may have their own "private label" retail products, which also sell at budget prices. Men and children tend to be the most frequent clients. If you enjoy a busy schedule and an in-and-out flow of customers, if you like the challenge of giving a good haircut in 15 to 20 minutes, you'll feel right at home here.

Formula

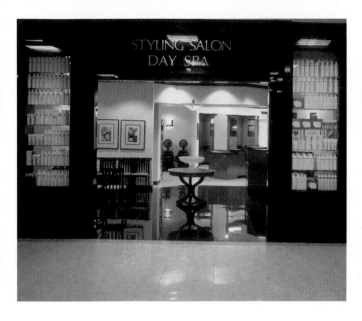

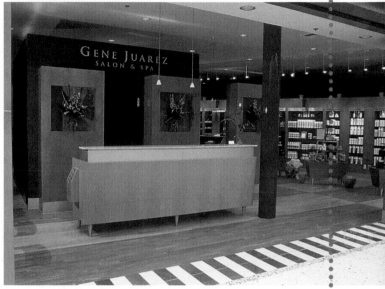

Mid-Priced Full-Service Salons ▼

These salons cater to men, women, and children with a complete menu of hair, nail, and skin services and retail products. Successful mid-priced salons promote their most profitable services and offer "service and retail packages" to entice haircut-only clients to purchase a wider range of services and products; they also have strong marketing programs that encourage client returns and referrals. These salons rely on a strong receptionist and train their professional styling team to be as productive and profitable as possible. If you're inclined to give more time to each client during the consultation, you may like working in a full-service salon. You'll have the opportunity here to build a relationship with clients that may extend over time and include a variety of services.

High-End "Image" Salons or Day Spas ▼

At the other end of the salon spectrum from the value-priced operation is the salon to which clients come to have their hair styled by a renowned stylist and/or to be pampered with luxurious, higher-priced services and treatments. Most high-end salons are located in trendy, upscale sections of large cities; others may be located in elegant, renovated mansions, in high-rent office and retail towers, or in luxury hotels and resorts. Clients expect a high level of personal service, and the salons hire proven stylists whose technical expertise, personal appearance, and communications skills meet their high standards. If you have a flair for fashion and style and are skilled at the demanding, more time-consuming hair services a high-end salon offers, this may be just the place for you.

Inside the Salon

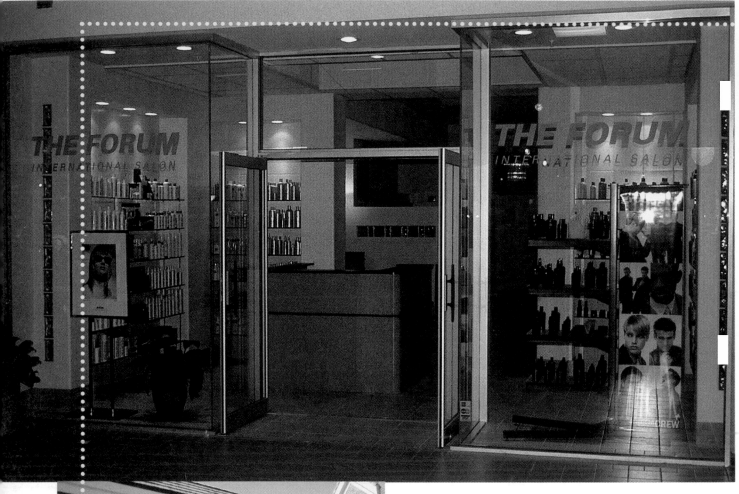

How does a salon "work"? The salon workplace is made up of many different elements, each of which is an important part of the whole. It's critical to your professional success to appreciate how each part of the salon supports you in your work and makes it possible for you to succeed. If any element is running less than smoothly, the entire operation suffers. If every part is running well, everyone benefits!

Come along as we take you inside a salon and give you a glimpse of its inner workings. We've selected a full-service salon in a midwestern city, one with prices somewhere in the middle of the range for that city.

Reception Area

Say hello to the receptionist—the link between the client and the salon staff. She impacts all parts of the business. Not only is she in charge of the salon's command center—answering the phone, keeping the appointment book, controlling the traffic, assigning walk-in clients, and keeping track of sales, expenses, and product inventory—she's usually the first face a client sees. By smiling and making eye contact, she makes clients feel welcome and at ease, and she's setting the stage for you, the stylist. She makes your job easier, because a client who's comfortable and relaxed will be more receptive to you and the services you provide. You can see how important the receptionist is to the salon: She can set the tone for each client's experience, and she can help you succeed at satisfying your customers and encouraging them to return. She's a key player on the salon team, and the more support you give each other, the more successful all of you will be.

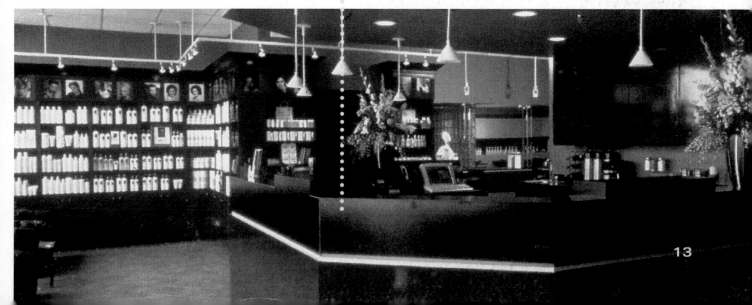

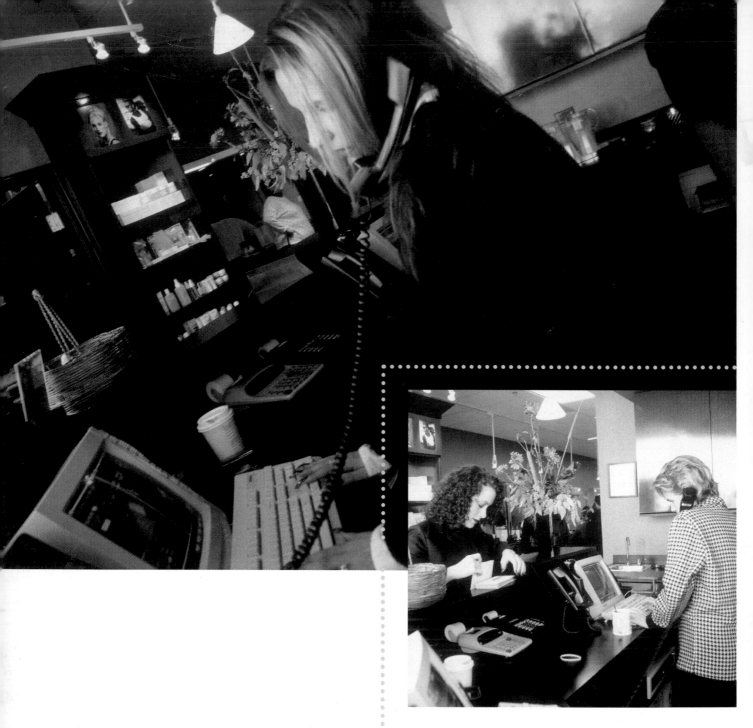

As a stylist you're in the business of helping people create a desired image. The salon should reflect that image. When clients walk in the door, the reception area is the first thing they see. Their first impression is based on how it looks.

You're a professional with high standards; those standards apply to your environment, too. It should be spotlessly clean, "well groomed," and comfortable—a place of beauty and style. You show respect for yourself and your clients when you make sure the reception and waiting area is neat and attractive, and they show their appreciation by returning again and again.

Retail Center

The retail display area or center is a vitally important part of the salon business. Smart salon professionals know that they don't finish with a client service, remove the client's cape, and say good-bye at the station. Instead, they escort their clients back to the reception area, help them schedule their next appointment, and suggest retail products for home hair care between salon visits.

Everyone benefits when your client purchases hair-care products from the salon. The client receives your professional guidance on the best products for her particular hair type and style. The salon owner gets a return on his or her investment in inventory, which can add substantially to profits. And you, the stylist, earn not only your clients' trust and appreciation but a higher income from sales commissions, too!

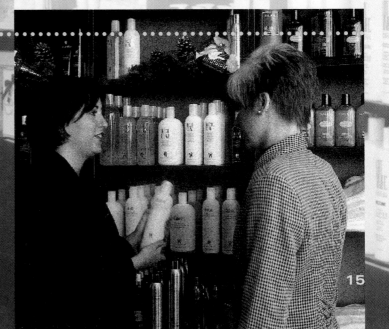

Shampoo Area

The shampoo procedure is usually the first time you touch your client. You've had your initial consultation and have begun to build rapport, but the shampoo bowl is where the client really puts herself in your hands. When you're attentive to her needs and alert to any signs of discomfort, she can relax and enjoy the shampoo and scalp massage. And you've set a positive, upbeat tone for the rest of her visit. If you're giving a shampoo to a first-time client, it's an opportunity to earn her trust and deepen the rapport; with a regular client you're giving her a pleasurable experience she looks forward to with every visit.

Styling Station

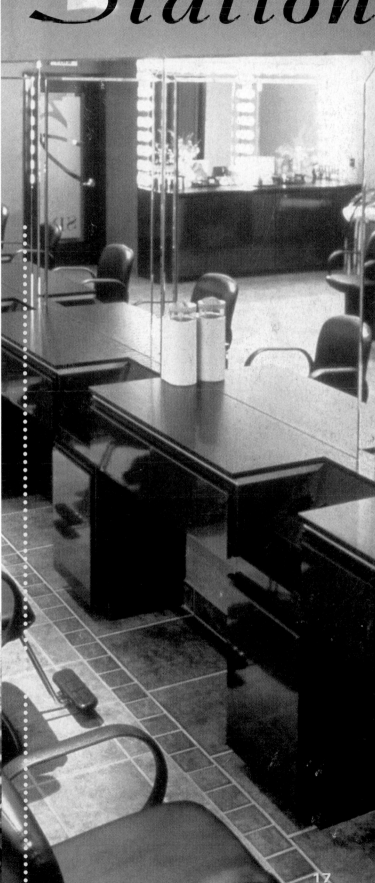

The styling station is the hairstylist's "command center." Notice how clean and attractive the stations in the photograph are. It's your job as a stylist to project an image of beauty, style, and professionalism as well as respect for each client. Your station is part of your image. A messy work surface is not a pretty sight, nor a welcoming one, and it doesn't speak well of you. On the other hand, a station that's clean, orderly, properly lit, and ready for business makes everyone look and feel good.

While you may think of your work station as just that—yours—it should be a pleasing, connected part of the whole salon picture. Personal photos and mementos should usually not be displayed because they invite discussion of your personal life when the focus needs to stay on the business at hand. By concentrating on the client's needs, not only do you provide the best service you can, you may even raise it to another level— turning a haircut into a haircut and color service, for instance.

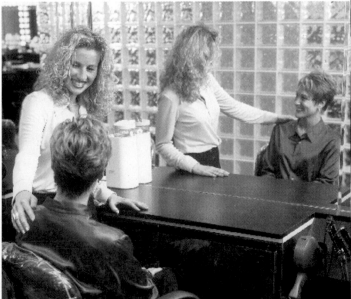

Dispensary

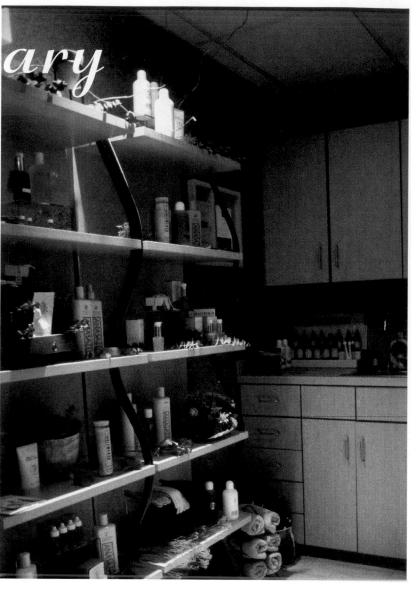

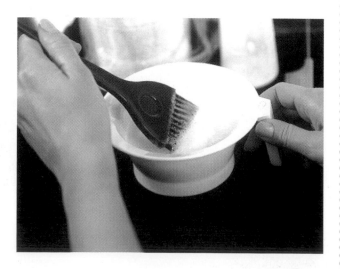

The dispensary is where the color solutions, permanent wave chemicals, rollers, shampoos, styling products, towels, capes, and a wide variety of other "tools of the trade" are stored. Although the dispensary may be hidden from public view, it plays an important role in the efficient operation of the salon. How well organized your workday is depends in large part on how well organized the dispensary is. If it's properly stocked and the items in it are handled and cleaned correctly, the products and equipment you need will always be there when you need them.

As a salon employee and team player, you'll be expected to help with stocking, arranging, and maintaining the dispensary. Remember, the better organized you are behind the scenes, the more successful you'll be "onstage."

Nail Stations

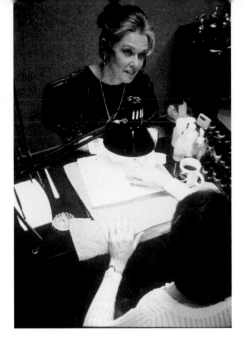

Nail technicians are essential to the success of a full-service salon. The more services a salon offers, the more types of clients it will attract. The larger and more varied the clientele, the more profitable the business is for everyone involved. The nail technician is an important team player. Like you, she helps clients create an image of beauty, style, and good grooming.

Other Service Areas

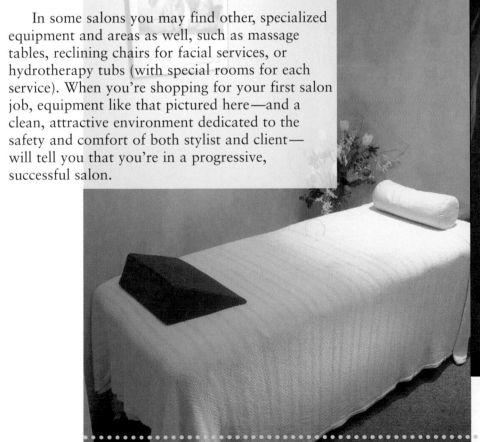

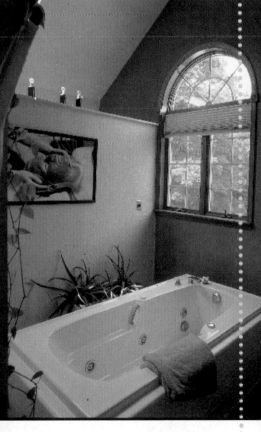

In some salons you may find other, specialized equipment and areas as well, such as massage tables, reclining chairs for facial services, or hydrotherapy tubs (with special rooms for each service). When you're shopping for your first salon job, equipment like that pictured here—and a clean, attractive environment dedicated to the safety and comfort of both stylist and client—will tell you that you're in a progressive, successful salon.

Job Opportunities

The U.S. Department of Labor lists "professional hairstylist" as one of the professions likely to experience rapid growth into the twenty-first century. While the majority of hairstylists work in salons, a large minority choose to make a living, often a very good living, in jobs outside the salon. Some of these options are listed below:

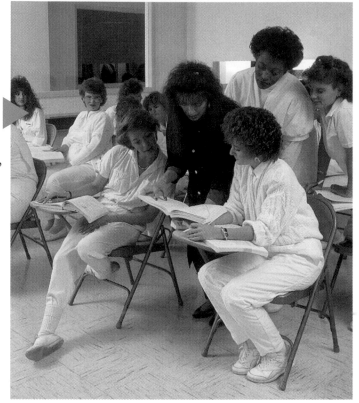

educator

▸ Primary location: Classrooms in schools and salons; workshops at hair shows, trade shows, and conventions around the U.S. and abroad.

▸ Primary function: Facilitate learning.

▸ Educational background: Cosmetology license. Additional training in an accredited school and a special teacher's certificate or license; 2 years' experience in some cases.

▸ Skills required: Public speaking experience, leadership ability, creativity, patience, passion for learning and teaching.

▸ Salary range: $15,000–$40,000

platform artist

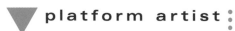

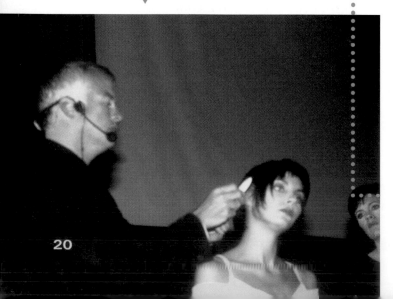

▸ Primary location: Hair shows and conventions.

▸ Primary function: Design hairstyles on live models and/or mannequins, usually before live audiences; promote products or equipment for manufacturers and distributors.

▸ Educational background: Cosmetology license.

▸ Skills required: Excellent technical and communications skills; knowledge of current fashion trends, products, and tools.

▸ Salary range: The sky's the limit!

20

Outside the Salon

photo stylist ▶

- Primary location: As a freelancer, you would travel to various photo shoot locations. Working full-time, you would be located at one magazine or company.

- Primary function: Style hair and/or apply makeup to models and celebrities being photographed for newspapers, magazines, and books. May be done part-time or full-time.

- Educational background: Cosmetology license.

- Skills required: Excellent hairstyling and makeup skills; familiarity with current trends and fashions; some knowledge of photographic lighting, how it affects color and clarity.

- Salary range: From $75-150/hour to $400–600/day (depending on your geographic location)

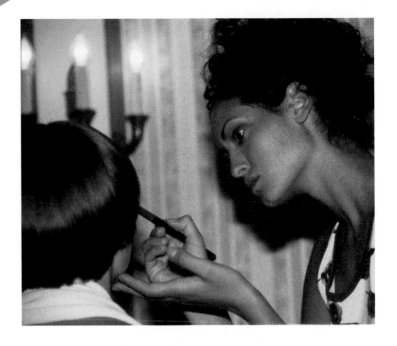

▼ styles director / artistic director

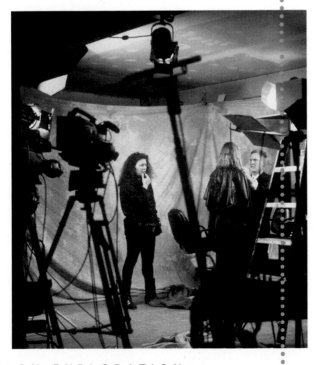

- Primary location: Salons, fashion magazines, product manufacturers, publishing companies, and education companies.

- Primary function: Hire and direct stylists, photographers, videographers, sound and lighting experts for magazine and book layouts; stage live fashion productions.

- Educational background: Cosmetology license.

- Skills required: Creativity, artistic talent, ability to manage crews, meet deadlines, and work within a budget.

- Salary range: A styles director in a salon would receive a raise in his or her current salary. As a corporate styles director, the pay would start at $40,000 and go up from there!

Journey to the
Center of the Industry:
Stylist

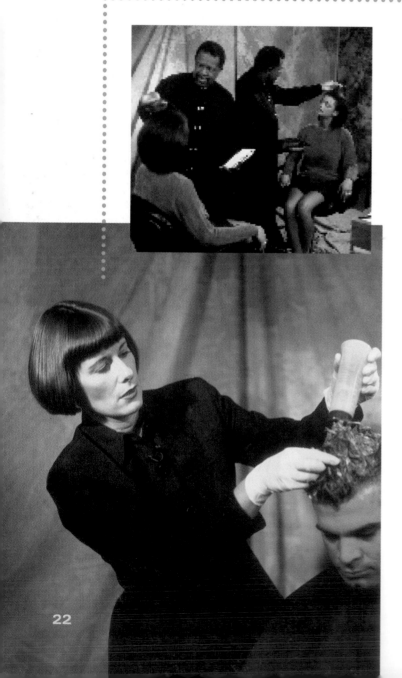

At the very heart of this big, wide, fascinating world of hair design and beauty is you, the salon professional. Without you, none of it would be possible. The robot hasn't been created that can understand a client's needs, communicate with a client, build a relationship, and provide both technical skills and personal service to help that client look and feel better.

We hope you read the stories in Part 2 about the "industry stars" who were involved in the creation of this course. The purpose of telling their stories is to show you, the new student, that they were once where you are right now. Not one of them started out wealthy or famous or got a lucky break. They all worked hard, educated themselves, and were ready to take advantage of opportunity when it presented itself. And you can be like them someday. This is one of the few professions in which where you went to college and what degrees you earned aren't as important as what you know and what you can do.

But that's not all. What does it take to make it in this or any profession? Good work habits. Cultivate a strong work ethic now, as you're starting out, and you can succeed at anything you put your mind to. Make a copy of the Connect with Success tips on the next page, and read them frequently to remind yourself of what you need to do to succeed. And now, let the learning, doing, and practicing begin. You're embarking on a wonderful journey—enjoy it!

Connect with Success

Follow these guidelines and you're sure to achieve your goals!

- Always be punctual. Go the extra mile if you can: arrive at school a little early and leave a little late.
- Dress like a professional. Come to class well groomed, making sure your clothes are clean and pressed.
- Keep your work station clean, neat, and orderly.
- Strive for 100% attendance.
- Be a team player.
- Take care of yourself. Work smart—follow all safety procedures.
- Be willing to learn. Study all you can. Practice.
- Once you've achieved success, do your part to help others. With each successful practitioner, the industry becomes stronger and more respected.

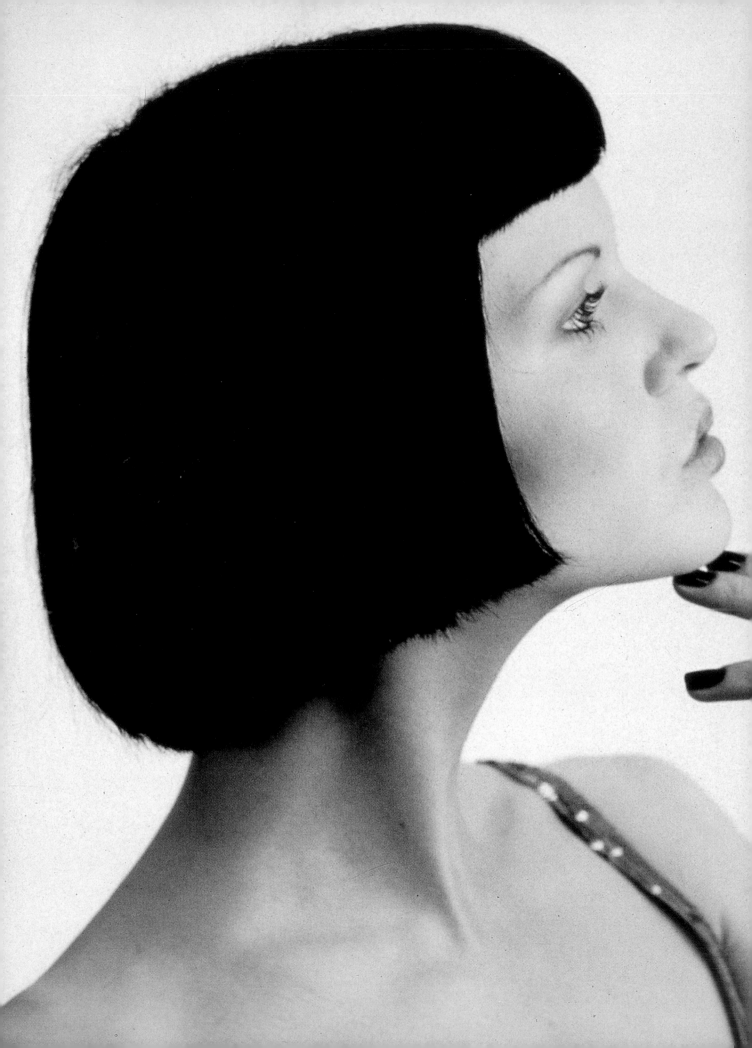

part two

Fundamentals of Hairdressing

Women's Haircutting

The Art and Craft of Cutting Hair

*Y*ou have chosen a profession in which working with hair, in all of its facets, will bring you tremendous creative and financial satisfaction. Hair is the material you will sculpt, mold, color, and texturize to meet your client's very individual needs—for functionality (the style must be easy to care for) and for aesthetic appeal (it must complement his or her facial features, head shape, bone structure, and body proportions). In fact, the right hairstyle can make your client feel

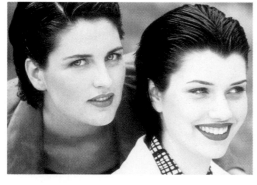

Classic cuts

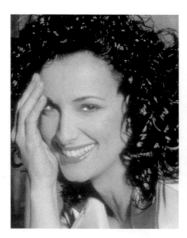

Trendy look

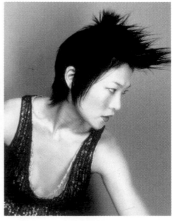

Cut with texture

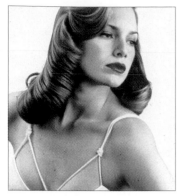

Romantic look

wonderful, because it captures her spirit and defines her sense of self—the image that she wants to project to the world. Is he or she a romantic, natural, modern, or classic type? In every case, you can create the feeling that will define and enliven your client's personality.

If this sounds like a tall order to fill, remember that your own intuitive sense will become highly developed as you consult with your clients on a daily basis. And because you're the individual and the hair designer that you are, you'll attract clients who appreciate your unique creativity and technical skill.

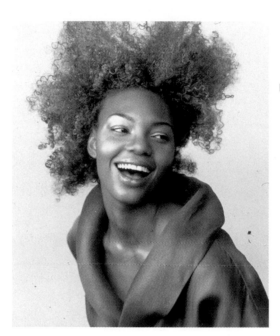

Modern look

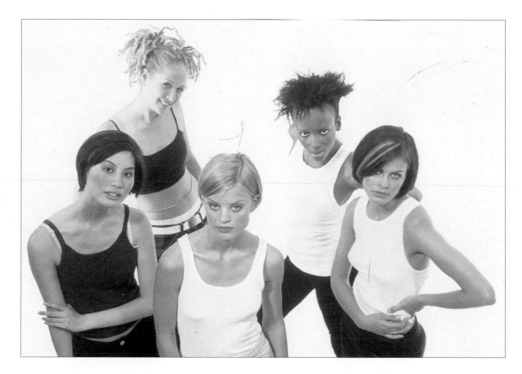

Natural look

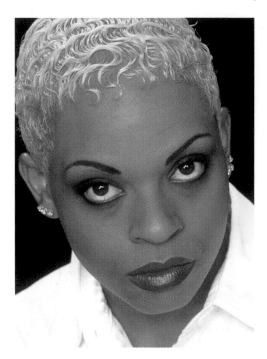

Marcel wave style

The world of hair has not always focused on creating the right style for the client. At the turn of the century, hair was highly ornamental. With a technique called the Marcel Wave, hair was tamed into place by being formed into artistic, labyrinthine shapes. In the Roaring Twenties, Antoine, of Paris, introduced the shingle haircut, a revolutionary short, bobbed hairstyle embellished with classical finger waving (waves molded into the hair and dried). Later, in the 1940s, the invention of the hollow roller sent hair fashion in a new direction. Guillaume of Paris—a genius at molding the hair—created fantastic and wearable styles that featured solid, voluminous shapes. Called the bouffant, this style saw its way into the 1950s with many variations. Hairdressers prided themselves on the artistry and complexity of their designs—which, of course, required frequent visits to the salon.

During the 1960s, however, a revolution was brewing in the vision of a man by the name of Vidal Sassoon. The shapes he created handled volume in dramatically different ways from the bouffant look of the times. The precise geometric haircut gave incredible freedom to its wearer; it was very modern and offered natural movement, yet always fell gracefully back in place.

This period changed our profession—precision haircutting technique and craftsmanship became essential. As we've evolved since then, haircuts have become softer in shape, yet are still based on

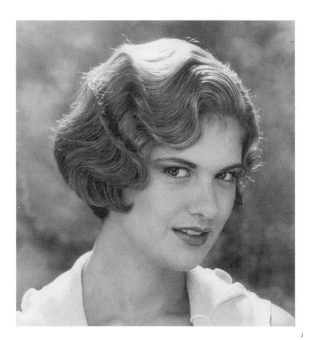

Finger wave

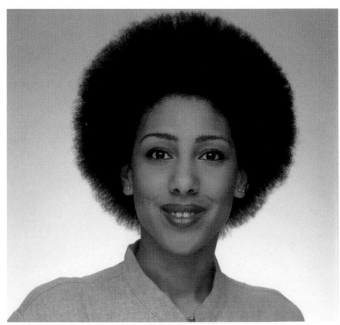

Afro hairstyle

the same premise: uncomplicated, natural, and easy-care silhouettes. Having experienced the simplicity and ease of these haircuts, clients will probably not go back to the old routine of frequent and time-consuming visits to the salon. Discipline and solid craftsmanship will, therefore, serve you well in your career.

Once you have this absolutely essential foundation of haircutting knowledge and skill, then you can add creative flair to it, to make every haircut an individual work of art. To bring out the unique character of each client's face—to create a style that suits her personality—you will need technical expertise, creativity, and sensitivity to human nature. Your hands and your creative intuition will indeed determine your success. And the haircuts you will learn in this program will spur your imagination to create many new looks that will harmonize with your client's lifestyle and appearance.

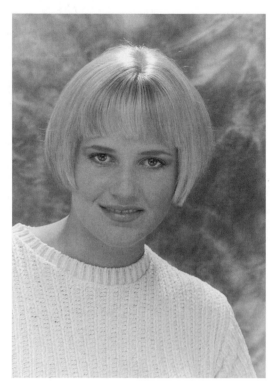

Sassoon cut

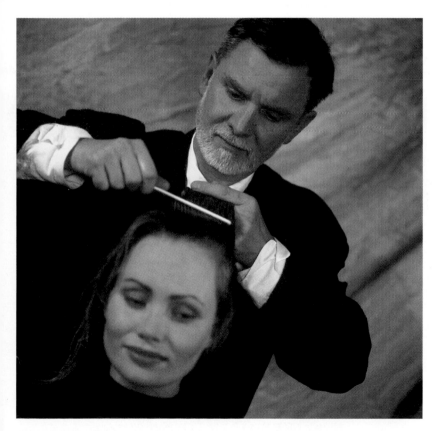

Successful stylist

What You'll Learn

During the women's and men's cutting, styling, and texture service parts of the program, the techniques you learn will progress from longer to shorter. In the cutting section, you will explore blunt, graduated, and long- and short-layered shapes. You will primarily be cutting with scissors, although you'll receive an introduction to razor and clipper cutting. And as you work through these haircuts, you'll also be able to integrate appropriate texture services, color services, and styling techniques. Understanding how to cut multicultural hair will be explored in this section as well.

The lengths you'll cut in this program reflect commercial salon lengths. Naturally, you must adapt them according to your clients' specific wishes and needs. You'll make these decisions based on thorough communication with each client.

Let's take a walk through some of the fundamental concepts you should be aware of as you begin your journey into the world of haircutting. All of these terms and ideas relate to three main concepts—shape, proportion, and position. These three central ideas form the foundation of the haircutting system presented in this text for both women's and men's cuts.

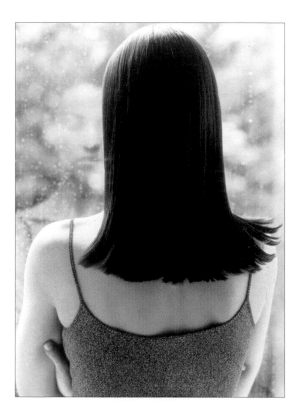

Long blunt style

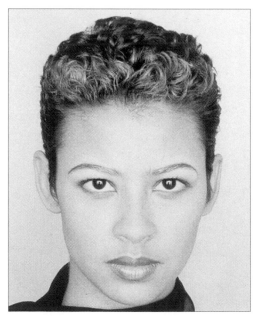

Short graduated cut

Shape

Just as an architect creates the structure of a building to fit within a designated space, so do we as haircutters create structure, or shape, in hair. Shape is defined by the outer boundary of the haircut or style, and it should enhance the client's facial shape and features as well as complement her head shape and body proportions. (See Chapter 9 in Milady's *Standard Textbook of Cosmetology* for more details.)

Face Shape

Guidelines on adapting hairstyles for different facial shapes are just that: guidelines. It has become more prevalent within fashion circles to accentuate and bring out strong features. For example, a round or square face might be played up to create a cherubic effect, or with a pear-shaped face, the hair around the jawline might be eliminated to accentuate the strong bone structure. The other approach is illusionary—for example, using hair to create an illusion of a narrower face. If the face is round or square, then you should accentuate volume in the top area of the design; if the face is oblong, you should minimize volume in the top and consider ways to widen the silhouette in your cutting and styling technique.

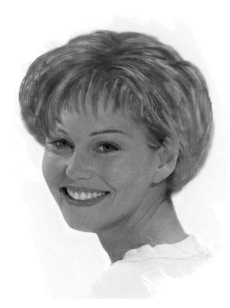

Wide face with round hairstyle

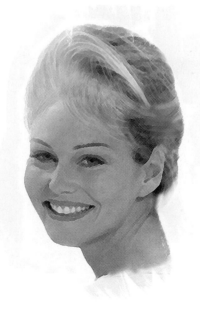

Wide face with volume in top

Body Shape

And how do you adapt haircuts to different body shapes? For large-bodied individuals, try not to cut the hair too short, which might diminish the head and make it look disproportionate to the body. Conversely, if the body is petite, the hair shape shouldn't be excessively long or large in its dimension; this can overwhelm the body, giving t he appearance of "all hair."

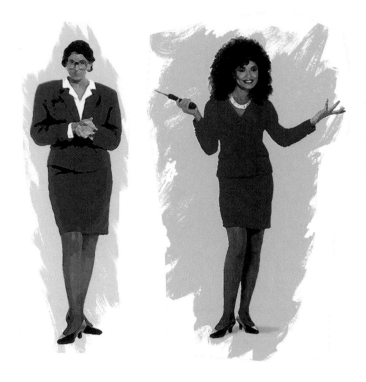

Shapes may be rounded, squared, triangular, rectangular, or oblong. Each shape creates a different look. Because you're cutting along the curved surface of the head, all shapes will be three-dimensional—they'll have length, width, and depth. Texture or styling techniques can then be used to accentuate the dimension and fullness of the cut. On the other hand, leaving the cut hair straight will give a smooth, sleek look that defines the head shape, rather than having more spatial dimension.

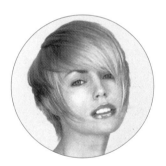

Round hairstyle

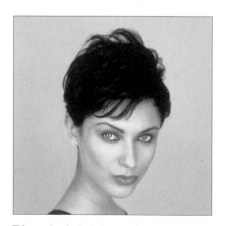

Triangular hairstyle

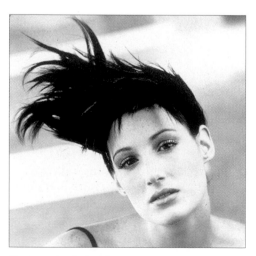

Rectangular hairstyle

Symmetry or Asymmetry

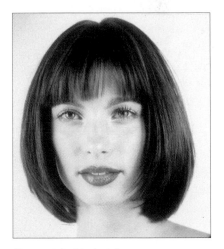

Symmetrical hairstyle

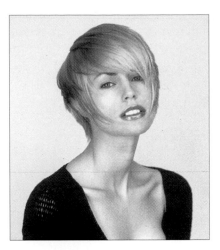

Asymmetrical hairstyle

In cutting, you may choose to create an evenly balanced, symmetric design, or you may choose an asymmetric style. Asymmetry can occur in the interior lengths, if you work off a side parting; or you can create an asymmetric line at the perimeter area of the haircut.

Cut Shape and Styled Shape

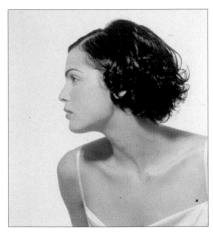

Blunt cut with texture

Cut shape is not the same as styled shape. For example, a three-inch length cut on straight hair throughout the top area of the head can become very dimensional and full if you apply a curling iron. And a sleek, shoulder-length blunt cut can stand on its own as a classic style, yet it takes on a totally different feeling when texture is introduced. This is where superb communication with your client is essential, to determine her expectations for the style, and your vision for how to create this.

The Basic Cut Shapes

There are three fundamental cut shapes—blunt, graduated, and layered shapes. Once you've mastered these, combining them is your natural next step.

Blunt—The blunt shape consists of lengths of hair that all come to one hanging level, forming a weight line or area. Depending on the length and the line you use to cut this shape, it can be square or oblong. Adding texture will expand the weight area, giving the finished style a more triangular shape.

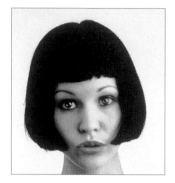

Blunt cut

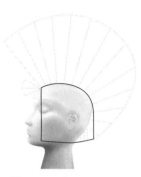

Blunt cut diagram

Graduated—The graduated shape, or wedge, has a stacked area around its exterior. This graduated or stacked effect is highly adaptable, depending on the technique you use to create it. Graduation is triangular in shape. This is subtle on straight or wavy hair, but becomes much more evident on highly textured hair.

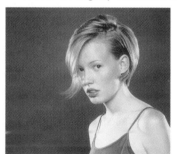

Graduated cut

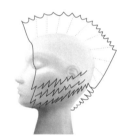

Graduated cut diagram

Layered—Layered shapes are incredibly diverse, from long to short. The long-layered shape that increases in length from its interior to its perimeter has a more oval character. In these layered shapes, distribution of length and weight generally moves from the interior toward the exterior of the head. Uniform layers reflect the curve of the head, creating a rounded, feminine silhouette. This shape is often combined with short graduation around the perimeter hairline area for a striking silhouette.

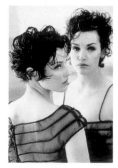

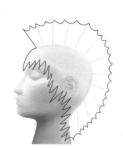

Layered cut   Layered cut diagram

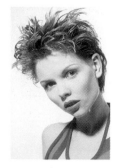

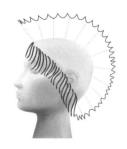

Uniformally layered cut   Uniformally ayered cut diagram

Proportion

Now that you know the basic shapes you can create, it is important that you realize that a large number of the cuts you perform on your clients will be combinations of these cut shapes. This is where it is essential to have an understanding of proportion, which is the relationship between the different areas and shapes within a single cut. A harmonious relationship between the lines, the shapes, and the dimensions or sizes within the haircut will make for a cut that is balanced, symmetrical, and, in essence, suitable for the client.

There is also proportion between the haircut you create and the client's facial features, facial and head shape, and body.

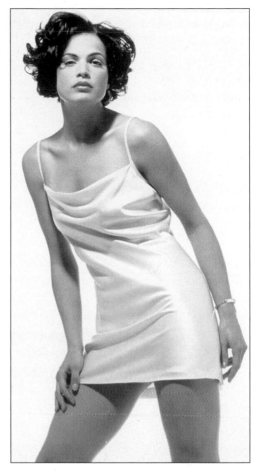

Equal proportion between hair and body

Blending

When combining line and shape from one area of the head to the next, it is important to cut sections between these areas to blend them. Whether connecting along the same line or moving into a new line, blending is an important part of the cutting process. As you blend, adjust your holding position to move seamlessly from one area to the other.

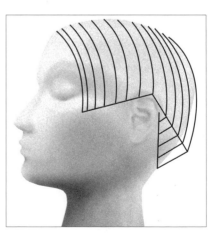

Blending

Areas of the Head

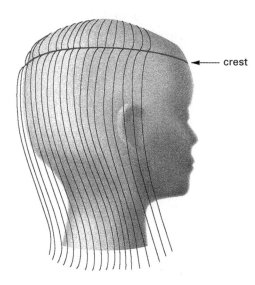

Crest area of head

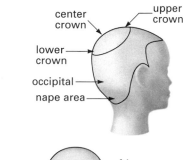

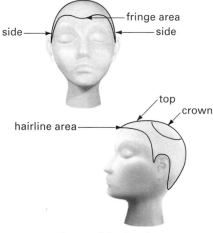

Areas of the head

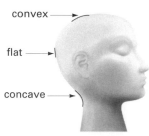

Surfaces of the head

Understanding the areas of the head ties directly into the proportion and blending concepts just discussed. These areas will help you understand how to structure and approach the cut. They can also serve as blending areas, where you combine shapes.

The *crest* area is the widest rounded area of the head. It divides the exterior area of the head from the interior. While falling freely with gravity from the crest area, hair simply lies on the top interior area of the head. (More on this later as we get into the actual cutting procedure.)

There are other areas of the head as well. The *hairline* is the line that travels around the edge of the growth of the hair around the face and neck. The *top* of the head is the uppermost front section of the head. The *sides* of the head are the areas above and in front of the ears. The *back* of the head is the area of the head behind the ears. The nape is the back part of the neck. The *occipital* is the bone that forms the back and lower part of the head. The *crown* is the topmost part of the skull or head. The *fringe* area is the area of the face near the hairline.

Each area of the head has its own plane or curved surface, and these vary from person to person. Some areas are definitely flat; others are *concave* (hollow and round or curving inward) or convex (curving outward like an exterior segment of a circle). As you progress in your training, you will become very sensitive to cutting these different areas. You'll need to adapt your technique to these changes in head shape when you want to create a certain weight distribution. For instance, if your client's head is flat through the back, she might require a weight buildup to be created at her occipital area, which will give her a more rounded head shape.

Special Challenges

When cutting hair in some areas of the head, such as the hairline and crown, you may be faced with interesting challenges—unusual growth patterns and cowlicks, for instance. Study the examples here. As you begin to work on clients, you will learn how to finesse your technique to handle these situations—whether you scissor these lengths away, cut into the growth pattern, or use minimal tension to create a more precise line.

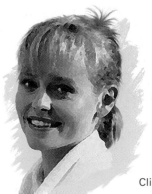

Client with a cowlick

Perimeter

The perimeter is the outer boundary of the hair shape, and, for this reason, it is the foundation of the haircut—it defines the look and contour of the shape, the framing around the face, and how the cut fits with the body. The line that you cut around the perimeter of the hair is a key to adapting the cut. In a blunt cut, the perimeter will serve as the guide to which you bring all the hair lengths; in a graduated cut, you'll graduate upward from the perimeter; and in a layered cut, you'll layer to or from it. In heavily layered shapes, the perimeter frame may be finalized after having layered internally.

In the consultation process, with the client standing, you may assess the perimeter of her cut and its adaptability to her body and face. Have her look in the mirror, so that you can observe her reactions during the discussion about the perimeter length and shape—in essence, the haircut she now has, and the one you'll give her.

Generally, the perimeter, or frame, is determined by the initial guideline that you cut around the hairline. In some instances you may want to cut the frame with your client standing, particularly on longer lengths. If she's sitting as you cut the frame area, make sure she's sitting up straight and that her legs are not crossed, because these factors can lead to an off-balance perimeter.

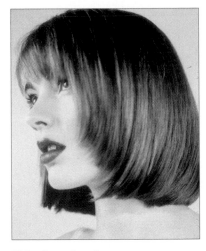

Side view of perimeter

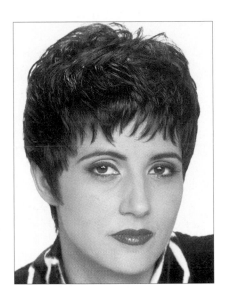

Front view of perimeter

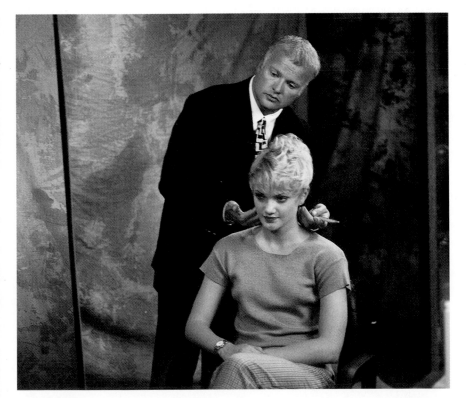

Consultation

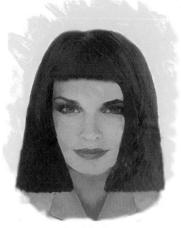

Straight lines

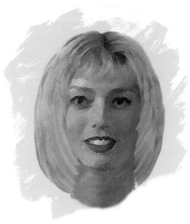

Sagged lines

The first step in creating the perimeter is determining the character of the line to be cut, since line defines shape. There are many types of lines—heavy, light, soft, and variegated are a few examples. The technique you use to cut the line—blunt, razored, notched, and so on—determines its type.

Stability

The perimeter is either horizontal or diagonal. A horizontal line is calm and stable; it has solidity to it and will hold its shape the best. Diagonal lines imply dynamic movement and direction. A perimeter may travel diagonally back from the face or diagonally toward or forward onto the face. Vertical lines are the least stable and are generally used in cutting layered shapes, not perimeter frames. You may use a vertical perimeter around the face, but it will actually fall at a steep diagonal given the influence of the hairline.

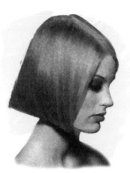

Horizontal lines

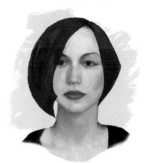

Diagonal lines

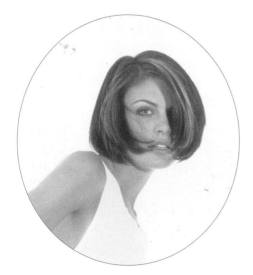

Blunt weight area

When all lengths come to and are cut at the perimeter, this creates a blunt weight area—which is also more stable.

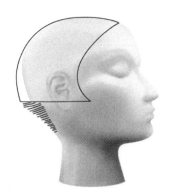

Horizontal lines cut near hairline

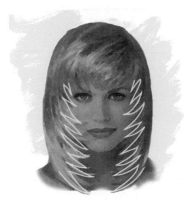

Jagged lines cut far from hairline

Lines cut closer to the hairline are more stable than those cut farther away. A horizontal line cut near the hairline is thus extremely stable, whereas a vertical line cut farther from the hairline is the most unstable.

Hair type also plays a part in determining stability: The thicker the hair, the better the line will hold. Therefore, a line cut on a fine, thin density of hair will be less stable than one on thick, coarse hair. (Refer to *Milady's Standard Textbook of Cosmetology,* Chapter 11, for more information on hair structure, texture, and density.) Hair that has wave or curl has more body than straight hair; therefore adding to stability as well.

The stability of the line plays an important role in the length of time the hairstyle will hold its shape. A horizontal line will outlast a vertical, a curly style will outlast a straight, and a line close to the hairline will outlast one farther away. Therefore, it's possible that one haircut lasts for four weeks, while another lasts for two months.

When it comes to perimeter frames, the wide variety of hairline shapes in the head's various areas will affect the stability of the line you create. For instance, a horizontal blunt cut that extends from the back of the head to the front area will have less stability over the ear, because of the variation in the hairline at this area. Still, the hairline—for all of its diversity—is what allows you to create a wide variety of expressions for your clients. The temple, the sideburn, the ear, the fringe, the nape—all must be considered as you create a unique perimeter frame that totally suits each client.

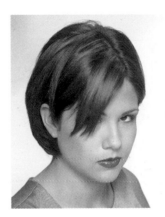

Short bob

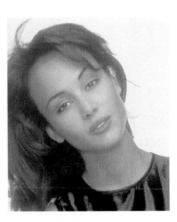

Long layered cut

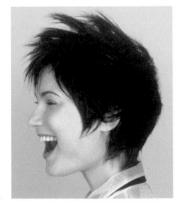

Graduated combination cut

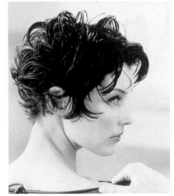

Graduated combination cut

The hairline's head shape, hair texture, and growth pattern work together to make each and every haircut unique. You could give the same haircut to ten different people and find that it looks quite different on all ten! This is where personalizing the haircut for the individual becomes paramount in importance.

Length Guides

An important way to achieve balance in a cut is to use areas of the body as length guides while you work around the head. You check balance points throughout the cut against the predetermined length that the client desires. This use of areas on the body to discuss length is also a very effective way to communicate with your client. Study the length guides illustrated here—the shoulder, jawline, lipline, tip and bridge of the nose, brow, ear, nape hairline, and so on. You can use these length guides to create the perimeter frame as well as to indicate where layers will fall. Perhaps the first layers in a long-layered cut will fall to the lipline, for example, or perhaps the ridge line (the top longest length in a stacked graduation) will fall to the browline.

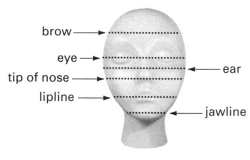

Length guides

Remember that when you cut wavy or curly hair that is damp, it will reduce in length when dry. Always take this into account when consulting with your client and determining length. You will want to cut with minimal tension and leave the hair subtly longer to allow for this length reduction. This is especially important on silhouettes that are midlength or longer.

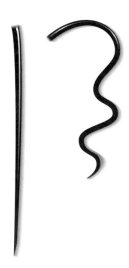

Same length curly hair—
wet and dry

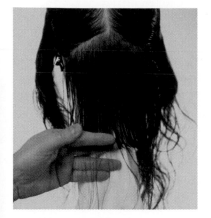
Established cutting guide

Cutting Guides

The cutting guide is the first section of hair within a given area that you cut. It will serve as a pattern for you to follow. This guide will be related to the desired perimeter or to the internal shape you're creating (horizontal, diagonal, or vertical). It will either be stable or traveling. Some advanced techniques call for freeform cutting and don't necessarily follow a guide; however, now is the time for you to master cutting to a precise guide line.

Stable guide—The guide is considered stable when you bring each new section of hair to your original guide, which does not change or move. Generally, stable guides are used to accentuate a buildup of weight or length, such as when you're cutting blunt, low graduation, and long– (light–) layered shapes.

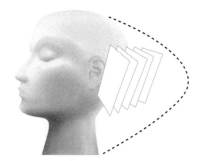
Stable guide

Traveling guide—A guide that moves from one parting to the next as you work through the haircut or through a given area is called a traveling guide. These guides are generally used to create high graduation or heavily layered shapes—whether progressive or uniform layers.

Whether you're using a stable or traveling guide, it should be visible at all times as you cut. If the guide is not visible as you cut, you have lost the pattern that will enable you to create a balanced, precise shape.

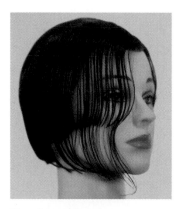
Traveling guide

Cross-checking—Cross-checking is done by using the opposite line that was used to cut the shape. You are cross-checking to ensure precision of line and shape, only removing any irregularities in the line edges. Remember that cross-checking is a control method to check your line only and not to recut the hair.

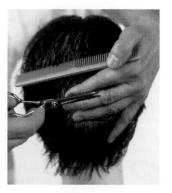
Cross-checking

Position

Three primary positions form the basis for this entire system of cutting—holding position, cutting position, and scissor position. Here we will explore them briefly, along with two other considerations involving the head position of the client and your body position in relation to the client. The technicals that introduce you to the different cuts will explain the three basic positions in more depth.

Holding Position

The holding position is the direction in which you comb and hold the hair from the head in preparation for cutting. The holding position determines how you build the structure of the cut, and thus the shape, that you're creating.

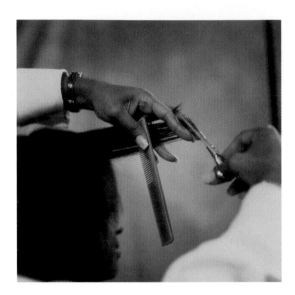

Stylist holding hair

Natural Fall

Natural fall is the direction that hair flows naturally around the curve of the head. Because of gravity, this direction is downward from the crest area. Natural fall is the holding position you'll use to create blunt shapes. (In this case, it can also be called zero degree, or zero rad.)

Natural fall is also the point of reference from which you elevate hair upward. In other words, you will consistently comb hair into natural fall within a given area to be cut, before you elevate it to the desired angle for cutting. This will allow for consistency and the proper perspective in picking up sections, thus ensuring precision.

If hair is combed or held away from natural fall in either direction, then it is being overdirected or shifted. This technique is most often used around the front hairline area for blending or off of diagonal parts when you're creating graduation.

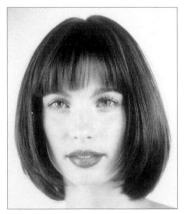

Hair in natural fall

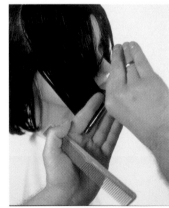

Hair being overdirected in front

Elevation

Elevation is the angle at which you hold the hair away from the head for cutting. This angle may be referred to as zero elevation, low elevation, medium elevation, or high elevation. Elevation may also be defined in terms of degrees (rad), from 0 to 90 (0 to 1.5).

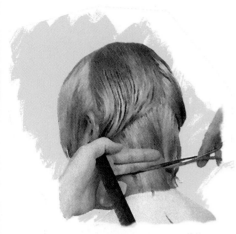

Hair held in elevation

Zero Elevation—The zero elevation holding position is used when creating blunt shapes. It can also be used to define the angle you'll use for holding the first guide when you're layering with a stable guide in the interior.

Low Elevation—This holding position is used to create a subtle amount of graduation along the perimeter frame area. One-finger elevation is a form of low elevation. Low elevation may also be used in positioning the stable guide for layered effects.

Medium Elevation—Medium elevation is generally used as the holding position for graduated shapes. It can also describe the angle you use for your stable guide in layered shapes.

High Elevation—High elevation. High elevation is used when creating high graduation and heavily layered effects. When this position is consistently used throughout the head, it is also referred to as the straight-out holding position—generally for creating uniform layers. You may also use this for elevating your stable guide in light-layered effects. In other words, bring all lengths to the guide, which you hold straight out from the curve of the head.

Directional Holding Position

We may also speak of the holding position in directional terms.

Horizontal or straight-cut—With this holding position, you hold the hair in a horizontal position, straight out from the side of the head and parallel to the ground. A horizontal holding position can be used to layer or graduate the hair. This may be used with a stable or traveling guide to create progressive layers or graduation.

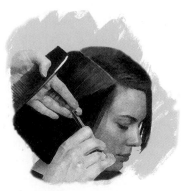

Hair held horizonally

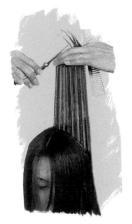

Hair held vertically

Vertical or straight-up—A vertical or straight-up holding position is used most often in creating layered shapes. When using a traveling guide, hold all hair vertically (straight) up from the top of the head. When using a stable guide, hold it straight up and bring all lengths to the guide to cut.

Diagonal—A diagonal holding position is most often used when creating graduated effects, especially when you're using vertical base partings to travel around the head, along with a traveling guide. You continually shift the hair into a downward diagonal position from the head.

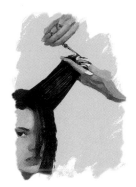

Hair held diagonally

Cutting Position

The cutting position is the angle at which you position your fingers along the hair where you'll cut. The cutting position determines the line you create at the perimeter of the cut as well as the internal shape. The placement of your fingers at a given line will also determine length. The cutting, or finger, position is described by direction, i.e. horizontal, vertical, diagonal.

Horizontal Cutting Position

This is used to create blunt, graduated, and layered effects. When you're using a horizontal cutting position in the interior, it is important that you be exact in your horizontal positioning, as you'll be directing hair off (not against) the head.

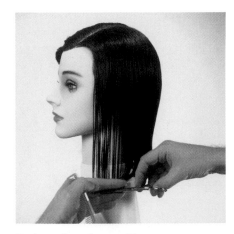

Horizontal cutting position

Vertical Cutting Position

A vertical cutting position is most often used when creating layered or graduated effects. Again, you must take great care to align your fingers consistently on a vertical line, as you will be cutting hair out from the head and not against the head shape.

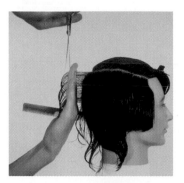

Vertical cutting position

Diagonal Cutting Position

The diagonal cutting position is used when cutting blunt, graduated, and layered effects. In blunt and graduated shapes, use the face as a point of reference to cut the diagonal. The diagonal travels back (from the face downward to the back of the head) or travels forward (downward toward the face from the back). In cutting internally with the diagonal line, you can use either a stable or a traveling guide.

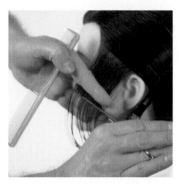

Diagonal cutting position

Cutting In and Cutting Out

Whenever you angle your fingers along a diagonal line in relation to the head, the length will travel from shorter to longer. This is where the concepts of cutting in and cutting out come in. Cutting in relates to a finger position that is angled at a diagonal, building length and weight from the exterior toward the interior (as in graduating). Cutting out relates to a finger position that is angled at a diagonal, building length and weight from the interior toward the exterior (as in layering).

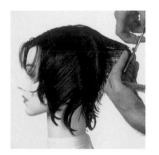
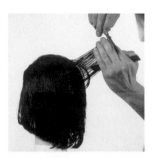

Cutting in   Cutting out

These concepts allow you far more flexibility as you work within the shape. Divide the head at the crest line, or round of the head. Above the round of the head you can use cutting in (producing length and weight upward) or cutting out (producing length and weight downward). This applies below the crest of the head as well: Cutting in produces length and weight upward, while cutting out produces length and weight downward.

Parallel to the Curve of the Head

In this cutting position, hold your fingers parallel to the curve of the head. It is most often used when creating uniform layers.

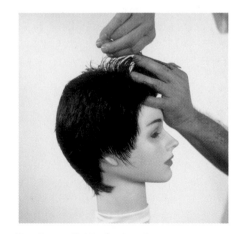

Hands parallel to the head

Scissor Position

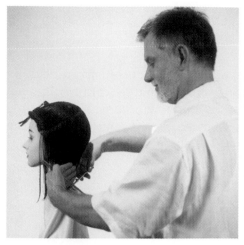

Scissor position

The third element of the cutting system is the scissor position. This is the position of your hand holding the scissors. You should always use the most comfortable position to cut. The position of the scissors that you use in cutting relates to how you position your palm.

Try to minimize holding the hands for long periods of time with the wrists hyperextended. The scissor position is very important from an ergonomic point of view. Ergonomics have become a very important consideration in our profession. The term actually means "the laws of work," and it refers to positioning your body in a way that minimizes strain. In other words, fit your job to your body, and not your body to your job!

Use the Correct Scissor Positions

When cutting hair, it is very easy to use hand positions that will over a period of time cause cumulative trauma disorders, or CTDs. These include tendonitis and carpal tunnel syndrome, a debilitative and painful condition involving the wrists.

It is most important that you do not make hyperextended—extremely angled or bent—wrist positions a routine. Try to keep your wrist as relaxed and straight as you can. Form the right habits of cutting, standing, and bending now, and you will limit fatigue. Having just as much energy for the last client in your day as you had for your first will ensure you enjoyable workdays and a long career.

Cutting with Zero Elevation

Two positions are used to cut with zero elevation. These allow you to cut in two different directions without having to move. In the palm-down position, cut toward the left of your body, below your fingers. In the palm-up position, cut toward the right of your body, below your fingers.

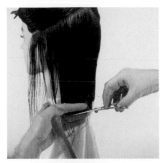

Palm-down position

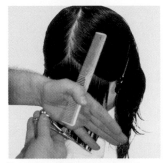

Palm-up position

Palm to Palm

This is the main position used for graduation with horizontal and diagonal lines, below the fingers. The palm of the hand holding the scissors faces the palm of the hand holding the hair.

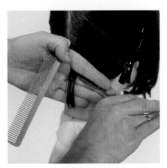

Palm to palm position

Palm Towards Knuckles

Use this position for layering when you're cutting above your fingers.

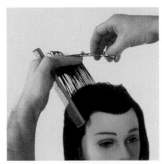

Palm toward knuckles
position

Palm Away or Toward

In these positions, your palm is away or toward your body (depending on the area that you are working on). The palm-away position maintains a straighter wrist. These positions are used when you're cutting in while graduating with a traveling guide along vertical partings. They're also used when you're notching, pointing, and trimming around the ears or hairline, above or below your fingers.

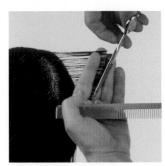

Palm away or toward
position

Other Position Considerations

While holding position, cutting position, and scissor position are the three basic positions you must be aware of when completing a cut, two other positions should be taken into consideration, the client's head position and your body's position in relation to the client.

Client's Head Position

Throughout the haircuts to come you will see references to the positioning of the client's head while you cut. Primarily, you should move his or her head into the position that will enable you to cut most efficiently within a given area. One guideline, however, is that you should maintain the head in the same position throughout a given area. Moving it around while you cut through an area may lessen your balance and precision. Also, when natural fall is the holding position you're using, it is best to maintain an upright head position.

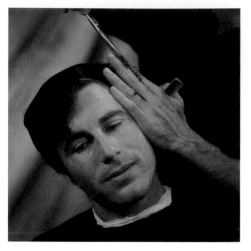

Head position

Stylist's Body Position

Here's another point related to ergonomics: It's important for you to stand facing your work. If your client is standing straight, then so are you. If she is sitting, it is very important that you place her chair high enough so that you are able to stand straight. Your arms should be in a natural position as far down as your cutting position will allow, and relaxed in form and appearance. Proper body position will prevent neck, shoulder, and back problems from arising. A current trend in the salon is for cutters to use cutting chairs.

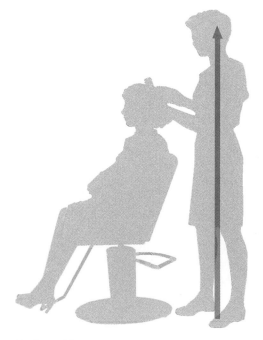

Body position

The Tools

As with any profession, the right tools can make all the difference in the execution of a technique. In cutting hair, you'll use some that have been around for centuries and some that are relative newcomers. Study the tools that follow and learn how to use each effectively.

All-purpose comb—The all-purpose cutting comb has both narrow and widely spaced teeth to allow for precision in distributing andsmoothing the hair when combing. The end of the comb is used for parting out sections.

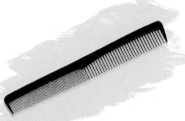

All-purpose comb

Large comb—Use a large wide-toothed comb when you want to cut longer lengths of hair or comb through wet or tangled hair. This comb is also used in scissor or clipper over comb work. It will allow for working through the hair with minimized tension.

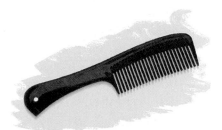

Large comb

Scissors (Shears)—Scissors may range from four to six inches (10 to 15 cm) in length. We work with 5.5-inch (13.75 cm) scissors in this program. The quality of scissors available to you is very wide ranging. You will ultimately want to use the highest-quality scissors that you can, to give you the most efficiency, precision, and comfort. This is the tool of your art and craft. Don't shortchange yourself. Most scissors are designed for right-handed people. However, left-handed scissors are available. (While this program was written with right-handedness in mind for simplicity's sake, you can easily adapt the instructions for left-handedness.)

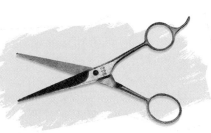

Scissors

Clipper, razor and tapering scissors—Use a clipper to trim, to create close clipper-over-comb effects, and to create the entire shape. The razor is an incredibly diverse tool that allows you to create soft, diffused effects. The tapering scissors will allow you to taper or texturize the shape, either creating variegation along the edges, or creating shorter lengths internally that will allow for more volume and expansion of the shape. (See Chapter 7 of Milady's Standard Textbook of Cosmetology for additional information.)

Don't Skimp on Tools

When you enter the salon, consider making an investment in the best tools that you can afford. You may be exposed to these tools at beauty supply distributor stores, by distributor salon consultants who visit the salon, or at shows and seminars.

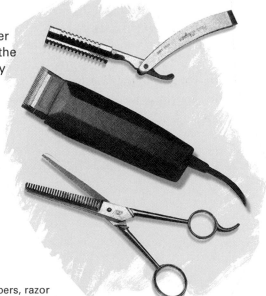

Clippers, razor
and tapering scissors

Caring for Tools

An appreciation for the tools of your art and craft—using them and taking care of them well—will allow for your comfort, as well as precision in your results. If dull scissors are forcing you to use forceful gripping motions, this will hinder both your work and your comfort. Take good care of your scissors. Place a drop of oil at the adjustable screw/pivot area at the end of every day's work. Use a small piece of chamois cloth or cotton to wipe away the excess. Sanitize all your tools in accordance with established industry regulations.

Practice with Your Scissors

Use of your scissors together with your comb will make for comfort and precision in technique. Practice this technique before you begin your first haircut.

Place your scissors across your palm, with your ring finger in one handle. Reach the tip of your thumb into the other handle. Do not extend your ring finger or thumb any farther than shown here (not past the first knuckle). This will allow you the most control when you cut your line with the tips of the scissors. When your fingers are extended farther into the handles, you'll experience a loss of control.

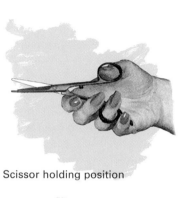

Scissor holding position

Practice removing your thumb from the one handle and placing the scissors inside the palm of your hand as you grasp the comb in preparation for parting and controlling the hair. Now transfer the comb to your opposite hand, as shown, in preparation for cutting. Reposition your thumb back into the handle and proceed to cut along the fingers you've positioned along the cutting line. This is the primary procedure that you will use to control your scissors and comb for cutting.

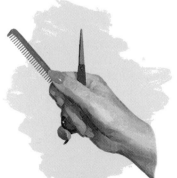

Scissor holding position

Handling the Comb

Practice manipulating the comb to flip from its wide- to its narrow-spaced teeth, holding it in one hand. The wider-spaced teeth are most often used to part and section hair, and to distribute hair neatly. They are also used when you want less tension on the hair or the hair is thick, curly, or coarse. The narrowly spaced teeth will give you your most precise distribution of hair with the most tension.

Cutting Textured Hair

When you're cutting textured hair that's damp, it's desirable to minimize tension and use a larger comb. Your other approach is to straighten the hair before you cut, then cut it dry. This will ensure the most precise shape. You will be exploring this concept in this chapter.

A Word on Tension

Tension may range from minimum to maximum. You can control tension with the back of your holding hand when you're cutting along the skin or with your fingers when you're holding the hair between them. Also, the spacing of the teeth of your comb can affect tension. The closer the teeth, the greater the tension on the hair.

When you're determining proper tension, consider the texture of hair that you're cutting as well as its growth patterns and cowlicks. Use maximum tension on straighter hair, where you want very precise lines. Use minimum tension when you're cutting highly textured hair or in growth pattern areas. (Too much tension on these hair types could cause irregularities in line or shape.) Tension should also be minimized around the ear area, so you don't cause a "hole" in the line.

Dwight Miller

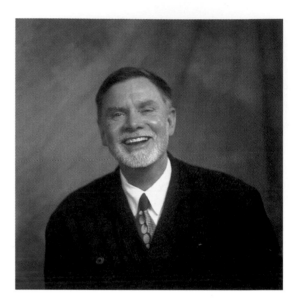

Dwight Miller, author of the Women's Haircutting education in this course, was set to re-enlist in the Marine Corps decades ago when he made a career move into cosmetology. Off duty one day, Dwight accompanied a friend who was going to a beauty school clinic for a haircut. While waiting, he was approached by a woman from the school, who spoke to him about becoming a cosmetologist.

"I'm not sure what she said to me that day, but she enticed me to make an immediate life change," remembered Dwight. Within weeks his enlistment ended and, instead of staying in military law enforcement, he enrolled in cosmetology school in San Diego, California and embarked on a career that has made him one of the most innovative and talented hairdressers ever to grace a stage or influence a trend. "It was a perfect fit. What I found was constant positive reinforcement. Each client brought a new opportunity to explore creatively, and I loved it," remarked Dwight.

An instinctive entrepreneur, Dwight started building his clientele and his reputation with persistence and passion. He printed his own business cards and, during his free time, handed them out to models, actors, and others he met. Of those days, he said, "You have to put yourself out there. You have to go out and build your career. If you try something and it doesn't work, try something else."

After graduation, Dwight took his first job as a designer in a salon in Del Mar, California, home of the famed horseracing arena. "It was the height of race season, and I was styling the hair of movie stars and millionaires," he reminisced. "It was an amazing way to start." Dwight not only kept up with cutting-edge fashion, he started creating it. His hallmark: "Don't just follow trends, start them."

Although he built a strong client following during his first year as a professional stylist, he wanted to know more. He headed for Hollywood, landed a salon job, and enrolled in an advanced training program to hone his craft. "It is good to have a solid skill base, but to gain expertise, you have to give yourself the opportunity to change perspectives. Education gives you a new angle to gain confidence, and once you have that you can go on to make up your own rules," commented Dwight.

Asked to start the first Vidal Sassoon educational centers in the United States, Dwight ventured to London, England, for training and ended up staying on for four years. His expertise and irreverent style were equally adored by the Europeans, and to this day his following includes international peers and clientele. Throughout all his endeavors, he remained the "hairdresser's hairdresser." He explained, "This industry will always be about what happens at the chair."

Dwight pursued his career with several major professional product manufacturers, graduating to increasingly influential roles at a rapid pace.

He launched new product lines, handling everything from product formulation to package design, advertising, and promotion campaigns. He became known throughout the world of fashion and beauty as an image and sales builder for every company he touched.

Then Dwight happened on a southwestern powwow and, again, his life changed. He quit his corporate job and founded Anasazi, the Sante Fe, New Mexico, company known for pioneering hair care treatments using Native American regimens. Spiritually infused, the company has been built by combining expert talent into teams both in the United States and abroad.

From all his experience, Dwight distills the following formula for success: "This whole business has to do with relationships. Solid craftsmanship along with your personality and ability to communicate are the skills that will make you great. Just a small amount of effort can make a good haircut a great haircut." He added, "The most important thing to know is what you want to do. If you know what you want, then doing it is always a focal point for your future."

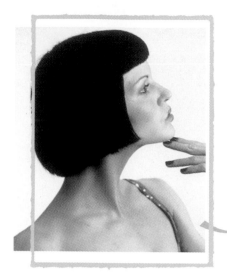

Horizontal blunt cut

Blunt Haircutting

Blunt haircuts that are executed properly are beautiful to behold! These cuts go by a variety of names—one-length or one-level, the solid form, and, of course, the now-famous bob first popularized by women in the Roaring Twentys and later revolutionized by Vidal Sassoon in his geometric cuts of the early and mid-60s. The blunt cut is also referred to as a naturally falling shape. The freedom and the wash-and-wear nature of this shape make it very manageable and versatile.

The classic blunt cut is worn by multitudes of women, and in the salon many of your clients will request some variation of this timeless silhouette, which suits just about everyone. The client who wears the smooth or textured version of the precise all-one-length blunt cut will be a very loyal client, returning to you regularly for a maintenance trim to keep the shape fresh and exact.

The blunt silhouette has a solidity to it that swings and bounces with the movement of the wearer. Mastery of the blunt cut—technically and creatively—will provide you with a very strong foundation upon which to progress and evolve in the salon. A grown-out line or minor errors in the cutting procedure can be very obvious. Cutting a precise horizontal bob is one of the most challenging haircutting tasks—a challenge that you as a professional will undertake and revisit with many clients throughout your career.

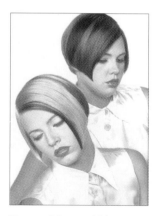

Diagonal forward blunt cut

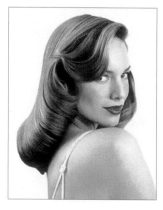

Diagonal back blunt cut

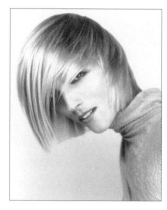

Horizontal blunt cut

*C*onnect
The Blunt Shape and Length

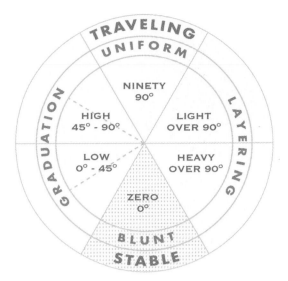

Haircutting angle guidelines

This shape, no matter what the length, falls to one level on the anatomy—i.e., the shoulder, jawline, lip-line, or earlobe. You can choose your length based on your client's body type, head shape, and personal needs. (Describing the length in terms of the anatomy makes it easier for the client to visualize the effect.) The surface appearance of the blunt shape is smooth, with unbroken lines. Naturally, a different appearance is created when texture is introduced.

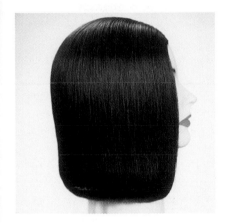

Blunt shape with weight line at shoulder

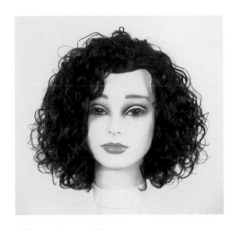

Blunt shape with texture

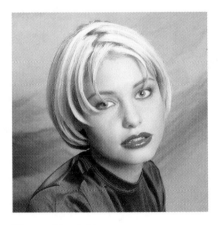

Diagonal back blunt cut

Weight Line

The level at which a blunt cut falls creates a weight line. This is where all the ends of the hair "hang out" together. The weight line can create an illusion of thickness for fine, less dense hair. Also, the introduction of texture can create more of a triangular-looking shape in the finished blunt cut. Whether this cut's expression is high-fashion and dramatic or classic, the weight line is its hallmark.

Creating Line

Just as a client chooses different lengths and personal statements in the hemline of her dress or skirt, so her haircut is a means of self-expression. You create the "line" of its shape according to her head shape, bone structure, facial features, and desired results. In cutting blunt shapes, you may work with a horizontal or a diagonal line. The horizontal line is calm; it is the most stable in nature. It will hold its shape the best. Diagonal lines impart a sense of dynamic movement as the eyes travel along them in a given direction. In blunt cutting, this may be achieved with either a diagonal forward or a diagonal backward line.

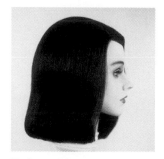
Horizontal line

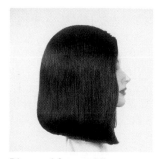
Diagonal forward line

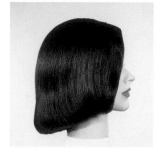
Diagonal backward line

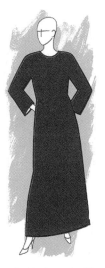
Ankle-length skirt

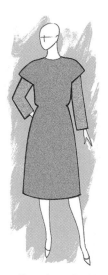
Knee-length skirt

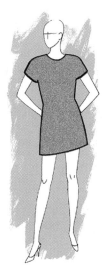
Mini-skirt

Holding Position: Natural Fall

The holding position—the position in which you comb or hold the hair for cutting—is in natural fall, at zero degrees, for blunt cuts.

The hair flows over the curved crest region of the head in a downward direction. It is important to maintain this downward holding position. If you shift the hair out of natural fall, you will create not only an irregularity in the line, but also some unwanted texture along the bottom edge. The front hairline area is the only area where you may bring the hair out of its natural fall, in order to contour it around and into the cutting line.

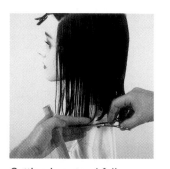
Cutting in natural fall

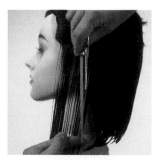
Bringing the hair out of natural fall.

56

Cutting Position

For cutting blunt shapes, the cutting position (the line that the scissors cut at your fingers), may either be horizontal or diagonal, as these are the lines that may be defined in naturally falling hair.

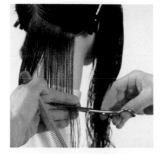

Horizontal cutting position

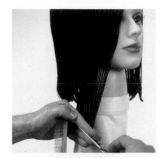

Diagonal cutting position

Scissor Position

The scissor positions most commonly used in blunt cutting are illustrated here. Whether you're holding the hair between your fingers or pressing your hand against the hair and onto the skin, adapt the cutting position as needed. The palm-down position involves cutting to the left of your body; the palm-up position, to the right.

    The palm-away position may be preferred in certain areas, such as behind the ears.

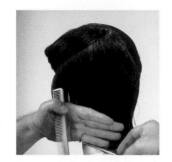

Palm down scissor position

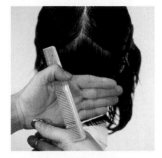

Palm up scissor position

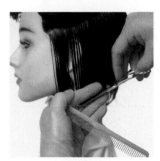

Palm away scissor position

Stable Guide

When you're cutting a blunt shape—whether horizontal or diagonal—the guideline that you follow throughout a given area from the perimeter hairline to the top of the head must be stable. A stable guide stays in a fixed position; it does not move. Thus, you should bring all lengths, section by section, to the initial, or original, guide—which must not change or move. If it does, this will create unwanted graduation (texture and irregularities) in the line. Make sure that your guide is visible.

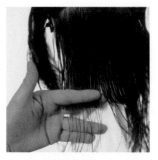

Blunt stable guide

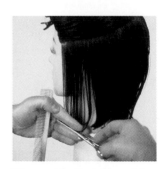

Diagonal back stable guide

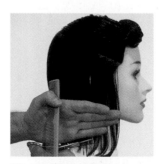

Diagonal forward stable guide

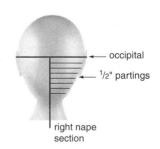

occipital

¹/₂" partings

right nape section

Stable guide diagram

Partings and Sections

Partings are the lines that you create with a comb to divide one group of hair or section from another. As you work from one area of the head to the next, take partings through the hair to release sections for cutting. Consistently clean, neat partings will allow you great control as you work through the haircut from beginning to end. Select the distance between partings according to the density of the hair and the size of the comb you're using. It is very important to see the guideline through the hair—if you can't, your partings are too widely spaced. This will result in an imperfect haircut.

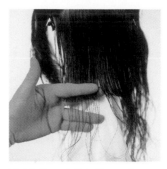

Guideline visible through the hair

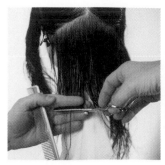

Cutting released section

Are You Right-or Left-Handed?

Many studies have concluded that among creative people, a higher percentage are left-handed, and parts of the brain are more highly developed than with righties. Even so, most of you using this program are right-handed. For the sake of simplicity, we've written the instructions for the following technicals with a right-handed person in mind. If you're a lefty, all you need to do is switch hands and with all that extra brain matter, that shouldn't be a problem for you!

Let the Dance Begin

Pride in your technical ability is of paramount importance. The way in which you work through a haircut—from the parting and sectioning to the position of your body, the cutting position, and the tool positions, to your body language—all will make for a presentation that shows your ability and confidence to your client. Cutting hair is indeed beauty in motion—a dance, if you will. There is a rhythm to it that will show your client a high level of professionalism as well as your joy in what you do.

This is only the beginning of that dance. Enjoy the first steps that follow!

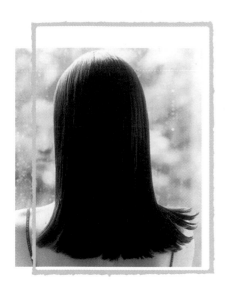

Horizontal Blunt Cut

Overview

This is a smooth, sleek, and shiny shape that, when straight, contours to the curve of the head and has minimal volume, yet offers freedom of movement. When texture is added, the silhouette takes on a completely different look—it has enhanced volume and an expanded shape; the surface of the shape is of sculpted wave formations that create visual interest and a different type of energy. The result is a style quite different from sleek, smooth hair.

In this design, all hair lengths come to one hanging level, and the perimeter is horizontal.

Connect

Natural Part or Artificial Part

In this haircut, you'll learn the difference between a natural part and an artificial or a design part. An artificial part is any part that is not a natural part. One example would be one that you create by parting from the front hairline (upward from the center of the eye) and curving gently back to the center crown area. A natural part is created by combing the hair from the front hairline to the back, then pushing the hair toward the front hairline, which allows the natural part to fall into place.

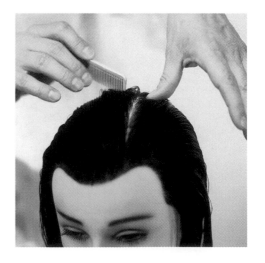

Head Position—Maintain the head in an upright position throughout this cut. This will give you the proper perspective to create a precise horizontal line.

Parting—Part the hair on the back of the head down the center, from the crown to the nape; this will help you control the hair when cutting. Within each of these two areas, create subtle diagonal forward partings to help you distribute and cut the hair section by section.

Holding Position—The natural fall of the hair around the curve of the head—zero-degree (0 rad) elevation—is the position for cutting. This is key in creating a one-hanging-length haircut. The hair at the front hairline, however, must be dealt with differently to create a line that will remain straight as the hair will be worn. Comb it to the side area; shift, or overdirect it beyond its natural fall; and comb it from the side part to the cutting line. Continue to use the zero-degree (0 rad) elevation.

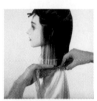

Length Guides—The horizontal blunt can be adapted to any length past the shoulder. Here it falls approximately two inches (5 cm) past the shoulder blades. On your mannequin, this is probably several inches below the bottom of the neck band.

Cutting Position—Keep your fingers in a horizontal cutting position throughout this haircut.

Scissor Position—Face your palm to the floor so that the blades of your scissor are horizontal and parallel to the floor. You'll move the scissors to the left side of your body.

Stable Guide—The first section that you cut horizontally will serve as your guideline for all following sections. This guideline must remain stable; your holding position and cutting position must stay the same. Cut horizontally throughout using zero elevation.

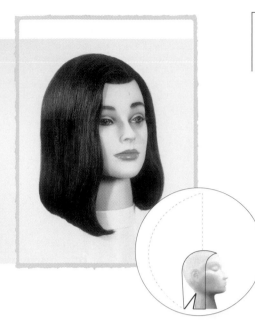

A pply

Blunt Haircutting

With your clients, these technical steps will follow the consultation and shampoo.

Shown here is the sleek, all one length horizontal blunt cut. Whether styled for symmetry or asymmetry, all lengths fall to one line

1. Gently comb the wet hair. (See chapter 6 in your Standard Textbook of Cosmetology.) Create a natural part or an artificial part. To find the natural part, comb the hair back from the hairline at the forehead.

2. Push the hair forward until the natural part breaks. Comb the hair down from around natural part.

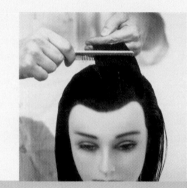
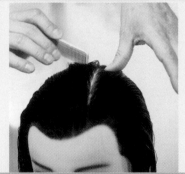

3. To create an artificial part, position the thumb at the natural crown area and the tip of the comb at the front hairline, then trace through from the front hairline to the crown.

4. Separate the hair so that the part is clearly visible.

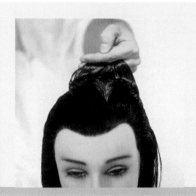
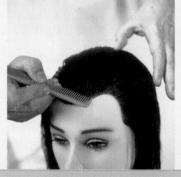

5. Now move to the back and comb the hair into natural fall. Comb all around the crown, making certain all the hair is evenly distributed.

6. Part the back from the crown straight down to the nape, dividing the back into two equal sections.

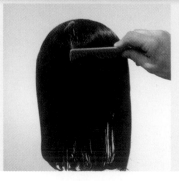
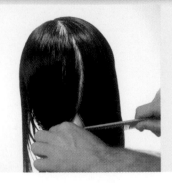

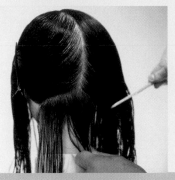 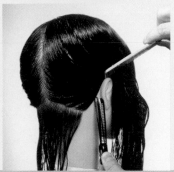

7. Starting on the left side of the nape, part off a 1/2" (1.25 cm) diagonal section from the center moving to below the ear.

8. Comb the remaining hair up and over the ear and clip in place. Repeat on the right side. Comb the remaining hair straight down. Notice how the diagonal lines for the part create an inverted V.

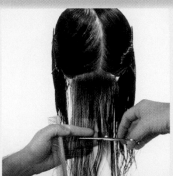 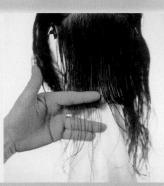

9. Hold the hair horizontally between the fingers of your left hand while holding the scissors horizontally in your right. With moderate tension, cut the left side, starting at the center and moving to the edge. Repeat on the right, cutting from the exterior to the center.

10. Release the next 1/2" (1.25 cm) section on both sides. You should be able to see the previously cut line—which is your cutting guide. Cut the section exactly on this guide.

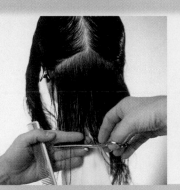 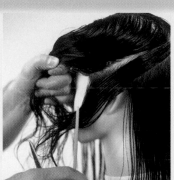

11. Continue releasing 1/2" (1.25 cm) sections, cutting one side and then the other until you reach the crest. Maintain the diagonal partings and horizontal cutting position.

12. When you reach the point that's about 1/2" (1.25 cm) above the ear, take a diagonal part from the center back and bring it all the way through the entire side section to the front hairline on both sides.

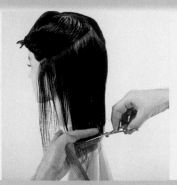 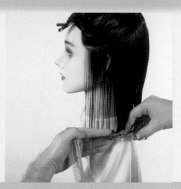

13. Comb the section into natural fall. Begin cutting it from the back, moving toward the ear.

14. Continue cutting toward the front. Comb the hair into natural fall and cut horizontally.

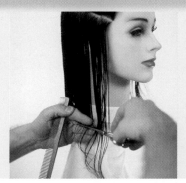 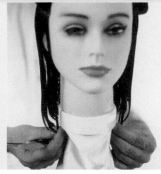

15. Move to the opposite side and repeat the procedure.

16. Before proceeding, cross-check for balance by holding the two front side sections down and ensuring that they are the same length.

17. With the side length established, continue working up the side, bringing down 1/2" (1.25 cm) diagonally parted sections.

18. Cut the section to the established horizontal guideline. Complete the entire side up to the previously established part.

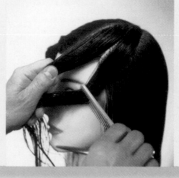
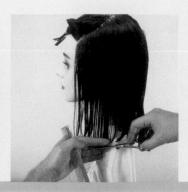

19. Once you have established the length, you can cut from front to back, using the previously cut sections as a guide. Continue bringing down 1/2" (1.25 cm) diagonal sections and cutting them.

20. When you reach the recession area at the corner of the eye, part out the front section.

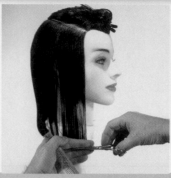
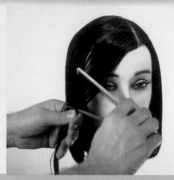

21. Clip the front section out of the way and continue cutting the side until it's complete.

22. Unclip the front section and comb it down neatly toward the side. Hold it to the side so that all the hair passes the eyebrow at the same point.

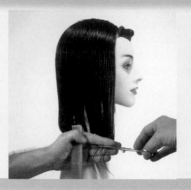
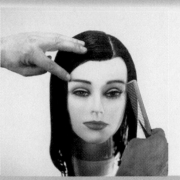

23. Hold the hair at the eyebrow with your forefinger and comb the rest of the hair into natural fall.

24. Cut the hair in this position, using the side section as your guide. Check the nape length by directing the head forward and, if needed, cleaning up the line.

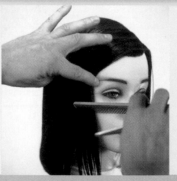
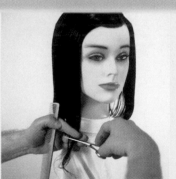

25. Apply the appropriate liquid styling formula before blow-drying into the sleek, blunt finish seen here.

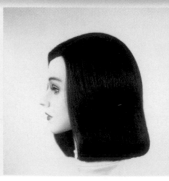

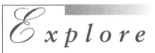

Reflect

Explore

Apply this technique to different lengths, colors, and textures for almost endless possibilities.

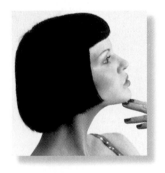

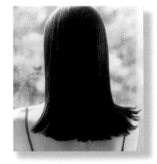

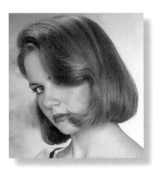

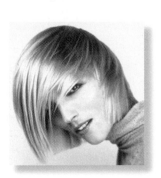

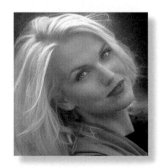

Setting Goals
for your
Success

Before anything else, getting ready is the secret of success.

Henry Ford

Although sometimes it may seem so, very few people become successful "by accident." Yes, there are those who do seem to stumble upon their success, but most successful people had at least one goal—to be successful! To achieve that big goal, they had to set a number of smaller, step-by-step goals and then work to achieve them, so that, when opportunity knocked, they knew how to open the door.

You have proved that you can set goals. By enrolling in a cosmetology program, you set a goal for yourself: to become trained and licensed in the art and science of hairstyling and design. Now come smaller, step-by-step goals for you to set and achieve. They include:

- ◆ **Attending classes and workshops**
- ◆ **Practicing newly acquired skills**
- ◆ **Completing "clock hours" for graduation**
- ◆ **Taking and passing state board examinations**

After you achieve one goal, you go on to the next, and it helps to know in advance what that next goal is. Once you become licensed, you're going to want to get a job. Do you know where you'd like to work? Do you want to work in a salon, a photo studio, a hair product manufacturing company? Maybe you want to start out in a job where the demands aren't too great, so that you can slowly build your confidence. Or perhaps you're in a hurry to get to the top. Now is the time to set your goals for your first job and figure out what steps are necessary to achieve it.

Is a job in a high-fashion, upscale salon for you? Then set that goal, and every day do something, take one step—no matter how small—toward achieving it. Set your next goal today—and write down the steps necessary to achieve it!

Luck is when preparation meets opportunity.

—unknown;

attributed to Oprah Winfrey

MY GOAL #1:

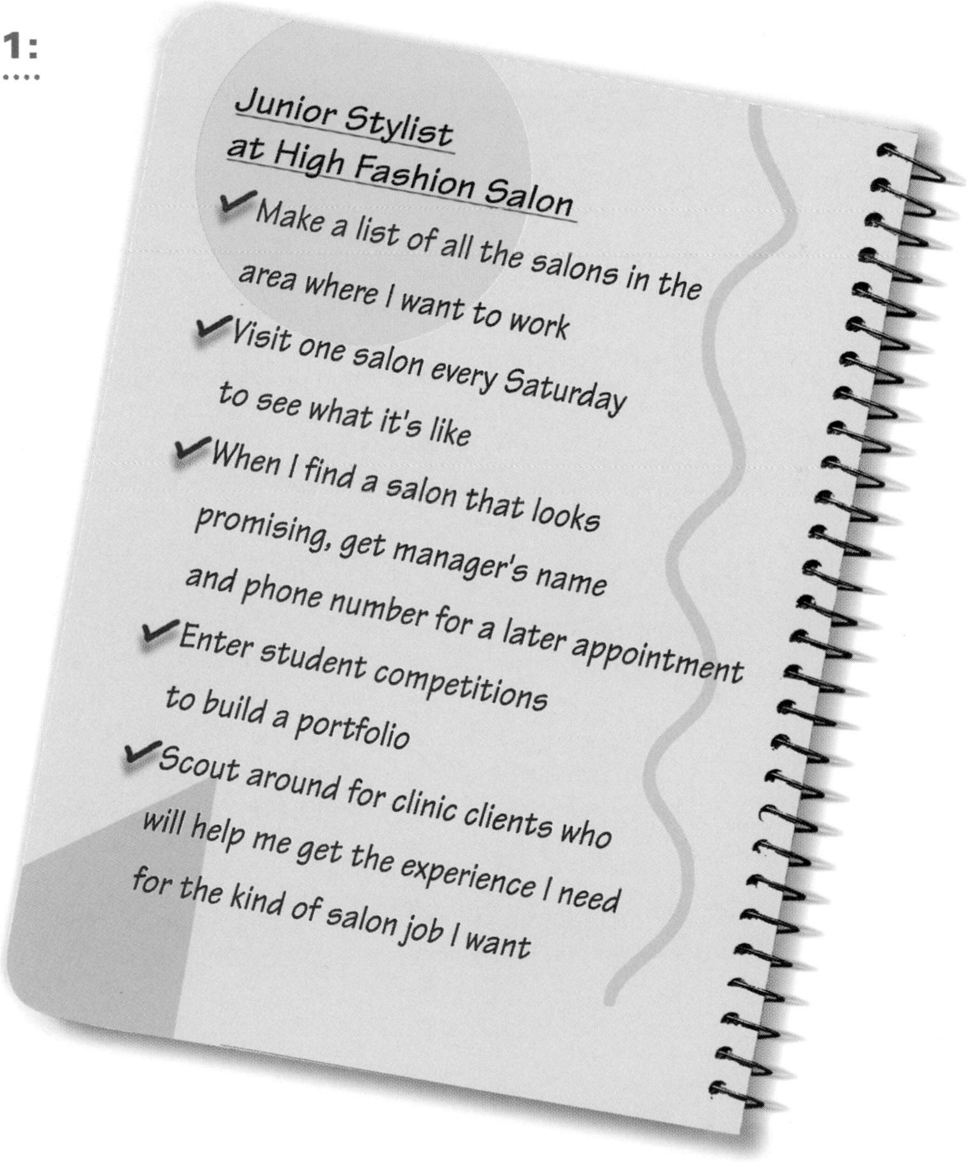

<u>Junior Stylist at High Fashion Salon</u>

✔ Make a list of all the salons in the area where I want to work

✔ Visit one salon every Saturday to see what it's like

✔ When I find a salon that looks promising, get manager's name and phone number for a later appointment

✔ Enter student competitions to build a portfolio

✔ Scout around for clinic clients who will help me get the experience I need for the kind of salon job I want

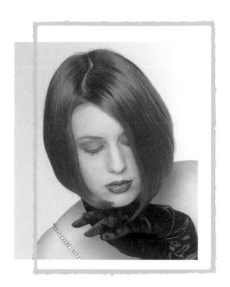

Diagonal Forward Blunt

Overview

A true classic, this cut was first introduced in the Sassoon Salon and later referred to as the A-line or bias-line. The dynamic diagonal line gives it a swingy, free-moving quality. It's cut shorter at the center back area, then lengthens as it travels to the front. The shorter hair will push and direct the longer hair, making the A-line cut move forward. The side parting makes for an evocative and dramatic sweep of hair as it frames the face.

Focus

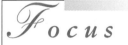

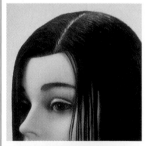

Artificial Part—Create a side part from the front hairline toward the center crown area.

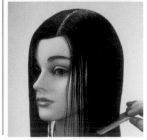

Natural Fall—Comb the hair down around the curve of the head off the side parting you just created.

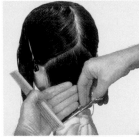

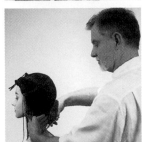

Head Position—To cut the nape area, position the head slightly forward. Move the head to an upright position for the remainder of the cut.

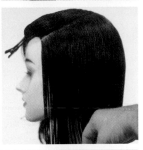

Body Position—Remember to stand in relation to the area of the head that you're working on. This will help ensure accuracy.

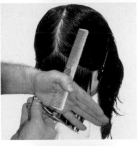

Cutting Position—Use the diagonal cutting position on both sides of this cut. The diagonal lines begin at the center back and travel toward the front on either side. Through the nape area, use the back of your hand to exert pressure or tension against the hair while you cut on the skin. Move the scissors along the bottom of your pinkie, which you should align diagonally. Above the nape area, this position should still be diagonal; hold the hair between your fingers, however.

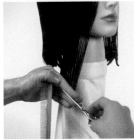

Scissor Position—Use the palm-down position on the left side of the head. On the right side of the head, however, you'll use a new position. Notice how the palm turns upward? This puts the scissors in the ideal position for cutting a diagonal line, and is suited to cutting on the skin as well. Notice how the scissors follow the angle of the hand. Visualize an imaginary line that runs straight down the center of your body; your hands should move to the right or left of this line as you cut from side to side.

Stable Guide—Do not lift the hair away from the head while cutting. Use the section previously cut as your guide. Maintaining it in a stable position, bring all the remaining sections down to it. This ensures the creation of the blunt effect. Remember that you should always be able to see the previous section through your new parting.

> *Reach high, for stars lie hidden in your soul. Dream deep, for every dream precedes the goal.*
>
> *Pamela Starr*

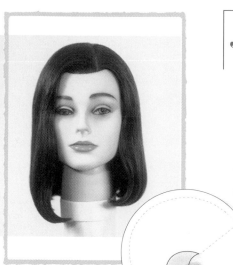

Apply
Diagonal Forward Blunt

With your clients, these technical steps will follow the consultation and shampoo.

In the diagonal forward blunt cut, lengths progress from the exterior area to the interior. All lengths fall to one level along the forward diagonal perimeter frame.

1. Establish a side part and gently comb the hair into place with the head held upright. Comb all the hair in natural fall. Make certain the ends are combed neatly in place.

2. Part the back from the crown straight down to the nape, dividing it into two equal sections.

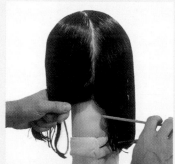
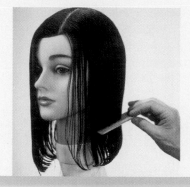

3. Take a 1/2" (1.25 cm) diagonal parting from the center to the ear and comb it down.
4. Clip the remaining hair out of the way and repeat on the opposite side. Begin cutting on the left side. Comb the section down. Holding the hair straight down with the back of your hand, angle your fingers from the center of the back to create a diagonal forward line. Maintain moderate tension as you cut against the neck, along the bottom of your little finger.

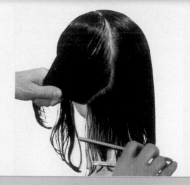
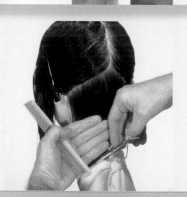

5. Move to the right side. Comb the hair down and place your hand so that it forms a diagonal forward line. Standing just to the left of this section to allow for comfort, hold the hair with your left hand and cut with your right. Using consistent tension, cut against the neck, from the center to the side. Notice that the scissors are held palm up.
6. Return to the left side. Continue to bring down 1/2" (1.25 cm) diagonal sections from both sides and cut to match the length and angle of the previously cut section.

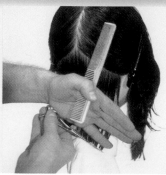
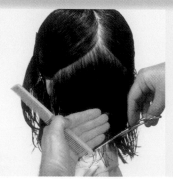

70

STUDENT COURSE BOOK

7. Repeat the procedure on the right side, again cutting the new 1/2" (1.25 cm) section to your established guide. When you move from the left to the right side, switch from holding your scissors palm down to palm up.

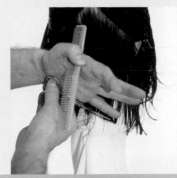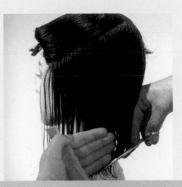

8. Continue in this manner until you reach the crest. Standing in front of your mannequin, take a diagonal parting that moves all the way from the center back, through the side, to the front. With the head straight up, comb the sides and back in natural fall and continue diagonal cutting from the center back toward the front.

9. When you reach the ear, move toward the side. Holding the hair between your index and middle fingers, complete the diagonal forward line by bringing down subsequent 1/2" (1.25 cm) sections until the entire side is cut.

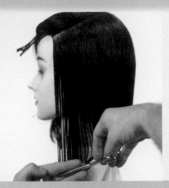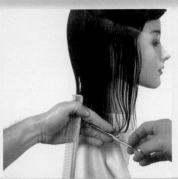

10. Move to the opposite side and repeat the procedure, bringing down 1/2" (1.25 cm) sections and cutting to establish the diagonal forward side lengths. Move the head forward as you cut the back area against the skin. Position the head upright as you cut the side area between the fingers along the diagonal forward line.

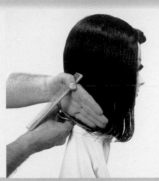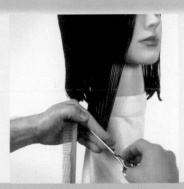

11. Continue bringing down sections until you reach the recession area up from the outside corner of the eye. At this point, section out the top front area, clip it out of the way, and complete the right side, bringing down 1/2" (1.25 cm) sections and cutting them along the established diagonal forward line.

12. With both sides complete, bring down the front section, comb it in natural fall, and cut it diagonally to blend with the already established line.

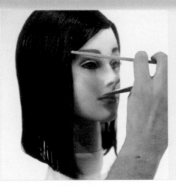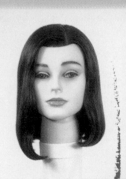

13. To check the line of the cut, push the heavy right side back at the eyebrow to match the hair combed into this position on the opposite side. Check the lengths for balance. Refine the line, if necessary.

14. The finished cut exhibits a gentle diagonal perimeter line around the face. The weight line provides for great freedom of movement.

The journey of a thousand miles begins with a single step.

Chinese Proverb

Reflect

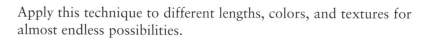

Explore

Apply this technique to different lengths, colors, and textures for almost endless possibilities.

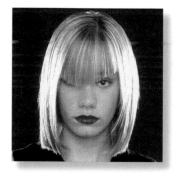

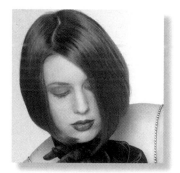

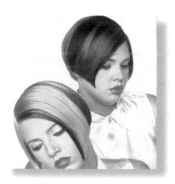

Planning Your Work
and
Working Your Plan

"If you don't know where you're going, any road will take you there."

If you've grown up in, say, coastal Georgia, and one day you decide to drive to visit a friend in Washington State, how would you go about it?

If you're like most people, you'd probably start by getting a map of the country and looking at the major highway routes. You'd check the mileage between cities and, based on how many miles you wanted to drive each day, plan what cities you'd stop in each night. You might get some information about lodgings at each stopover, and figure out roughly how much money you'd need for fuel, food, lodging, and entertainment. You'd arrange for someone to take care of your mail, pets, and plants at home, and tell a friend about your plans.

Life is a lot like that. You start in one place, end up in another. There are many possible routes to take. You can wander aimlessly, stopping here and there, whenever something looks interesting. Or you can make a plan for where you want to be next year . . . in five years . . . in ten years, and work to make that plan happen.

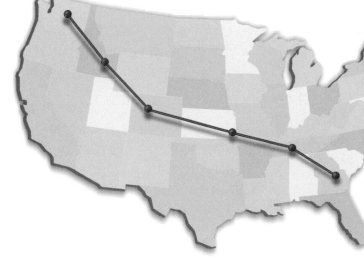

Do you want new furniture next year, a new car in three years, maybe a trip to London in five years? You can have all those things—anyone can—as long as you make a plan. Suppose in three years you'll need $5,000 for a down payment on a $25,000 car. If you receive a weekly paycheck, you'll need to save about $30 every week for three years to get that down payment, and then you'll need to be able to make a car payment of around $450 each month for the following four years.

In order for your earnings toprovide what you desire, you must plan your work and work your plan.

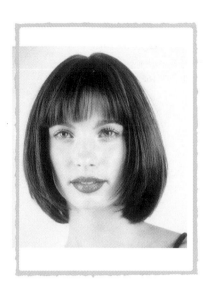

Diagonal Back Blunt

Overview

The Diagonal Back Blunt has a curvy, continuous perimeter line, creating a fluid look. Shorter at the front, then lengthening at the center back, this style—also called a pageboy—provides much versatility in its styling options. The line allows for great freedom of movement, perhaps one reason why Sassoon chose this cut—originally created for the famous dancer Isadora Duncan—to reinterpret. This shorter version of the "Isadora" cut is indeed poetry in motion.

Focus

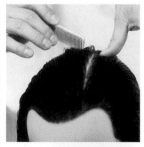

Artificial Part—In this look you will create an artifical or design part from the front hairline to the center crown area. (Refer to page 60 for information on making a natural versus a design part.)

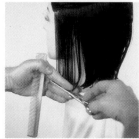

Holding Position—You'll comb and hold the hair in a natural fall or zero-elevation throughout most of this haircut. Around the front hairline, bring the hair on the heavier side of the part over and around the curve of the head into the line you're cutting; continue to hold it in elevation to ensure the blunt effect. Cut the hair in the nape area by holding it against the neck with the back of your free hand.

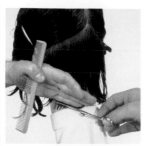

Head Position—Position the head forward as you cut from the nape hairline area up to the crest—where the partings extend through to the front hairline from the back. At this point, bring the head to an upright position. This will give you the proper perspective to create the diagonal back line.

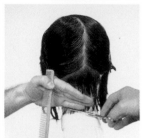

Cutting Position—On either side of the nape area, align your hand along the diagonal back line and cut along the bottom edge of your pinkie. Above the nape area, hold the hair between your fingers along a diagonal line.

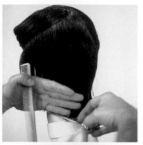

Scissor Position—Use the palm-down scissor position on the entire left side of the head. Use the palm-up position on the right side of the nape; then switch back to the palm-down position for the remainder of the right side.

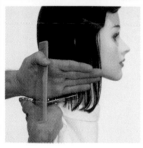

Stable Guide—Use a stable guide throughout this cut to ensure a blunt result. Make sure that this stable guide is always visible as you release new sections to be cut.

Life is like a garden.
The thoughts you plant
are like seeds that
develop into experiences
later on.

Louise Hay

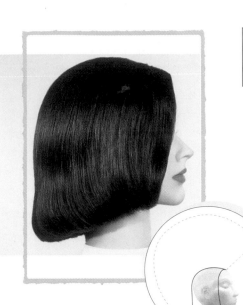

Diagonal Back Blunt

With your clients, these technical steps will follow the consultation and shampoo.

The diagonal back frame moves from just below the jaw to the collar area at the back of the head.

1. Prepare for this cut by parting as in the previous blunt cut. On the left side, position the back of your hand against the head so your fingers point down toward the nape and your wrist is slightly elevated. Hold both hands left of the center of your body. Using a palm-down cutting position, cut diagonally from the center back to the side.

2. For the right side, use the palm-up cutting position. Angle your hand by dropping your wrist, with fingers pointing toward the ear. Both hands are to the right of the center of your body. Cut from the center back toward the side.

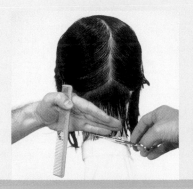
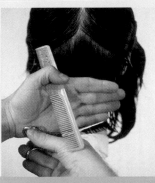

3. Return to the left side, part off another 1/2" (1.25 cm) diagonal section of hair, and cut, moving your hands to the left of the center of your body and using the palm-down cutting position. The fingertips of the hand holding the hair should angle downward, elevating the wrist slightly.

4. Continue moving side to side and cutting 1/2" (1.25 cm) diagonal sections up to the crest. Maintain 0 {deg} elevation, even tension, and the diagonal back cutting line.

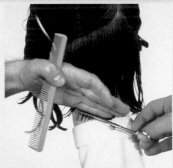
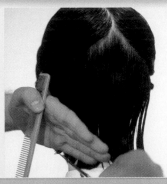

5. When you reach the crest, take a 1/2" (1.25 cm) diagonal parting that moves all the way from the center back, through the side, to the front. With the head straight up, comb the sides and back in natural fall. Cut the side section, using your hand to continue the diagonal back line from the back section you just cut to the front.

6. As you reach the front, move your body into position at the side. Bring down subsequent sections and complete the left side.

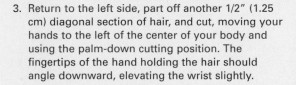
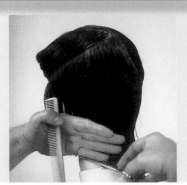
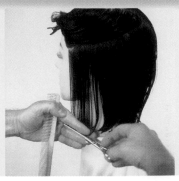

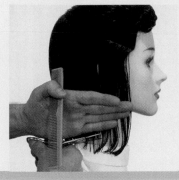
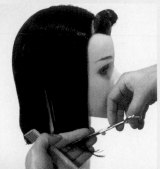

7. Move to the right side. Take a parting from the back through the side, and cut. Use 0{deg} (0 rad) elevation and position your hand to continue the diagonal back line.

8. When you reach the recession area at the corner of the eye, clip the front fringe out of the way and complete cutting the right side.

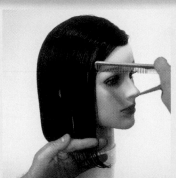
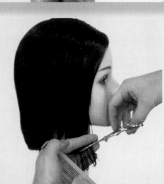

9. Check the cut for balance, making certain both sides are cut to the same length, at the same angle. Release the front fringe and comb it down. Push the heavy right side back at the eyebrow to match the position of the hair on the opposite side.

10. Holding the front section and the side guide together, cut the front section.

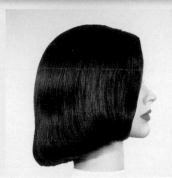

11. In the finished cut, the strong diagonal back line is evident.

Success is the sum of small efforts, repeated day in and day out.

Robert Collier

$\mathcal{R}$ eflect

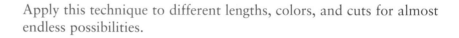

$\mathcal{E}$ xplore

Apply this technique to different lengths, colors, and cuts for almost endless possibilities.

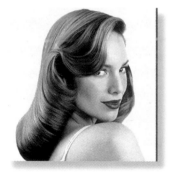

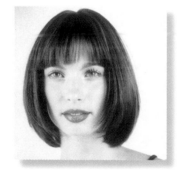

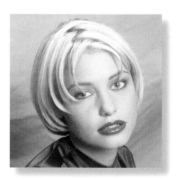

Attitude

Ability is what you're capable of doing. Motivation determines what you do. Attitude determines how well you do it.

Lou Holtz

Attitude is everything.

Francie Baltazar-Schwartz

Jerry was the kind of guy you love to hate. He was always in a good mood and always had something positive to say. When someone would ask him how he was doing, he would reply, "If I were any better, I would be twins!"

He was a unique manager because he had several waiters who followed him around from restaurant to restaurant . . . because of his attitude. He was a natural motivator. If an employee was having a bad day, Jerry was there telling the employee how to look on the positive side of the situation.

Then one day Jerry did something you are never supposed to do in a restaurant business: He left the back door open one morning and was held up at gunpoint by three armed robbers. While trying to open the safe, his hand, shaking from nervousness, slipped off the combination. The robbers panicked and shot him. Luckily, Jerry was found quickly and rushed to the local trauma center. After 18 hours of surgery and weeks of intensive care, Jerry was released from the hospital with fragments of the bullets still in his body. I saw Jerry about six months after the accident. When I asked him how he was, he replied, "If I were any better, I'd be twins. Wanna see my scars?"

I declined to see his wounds, but did ask him what had gone through his mind as the robbery took place. "The first thing that went through my mind was that I should have locked the back door," Jerry replied. "Then, as I lay on the floor, I remembered that I had two choices: I could choose to live, or I could choose to die. I chose to live. . ."

Jerry lived, thanks to the skill of his doctors, but also because of his amazing attitude. I learned from him that every day we have the choice to live fully. Attitude, after all, is everything.

Now you have two choices. You can choose to remember Jerry's story and the lesson it teaches, and approach the rest of your life with a positive attitude. Or you can forget it.

The choice is yours. The life you lead—be it happy and fulfilling, or otherwise—is yours for the making.

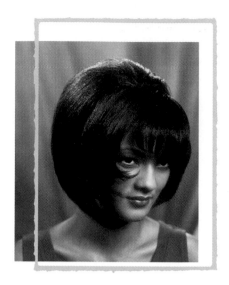

Blunt Cut

on dry hair

Overview

Time management is a top priority for today's hectic pace of living. A good time management technique for your clients with very curly or kinky hair is to invest more time in chemical relaxer services, conditioning treatments, and preparation of the hair by blow drying smooth (pre-prep) before you begin cutting and finishing.

Hair that is highly textured (curly or kinky, for instance) appears completely different when wet. When this kind of hair dries, it contracts in length as the kink or curl pulls it up. Cutting hair of this type dry gives you more control over the creation of the shape. Once the hair is relaxed to be straight and smooth, an unlimited variety of sculpted styles can be created from this foundation.

The dry cutting technique is a classic, condensed cutting and finishing concept.

Focus

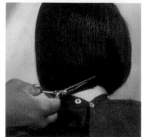

Notching Technique—Notching is a form of cutting that creates serrated points along the edges of the hair. To notch the hair around the face, comb it either between the fingers or against the skin and cut V-shaped notches into it. This is where your true artistry may come into play! Adjust the depth and amount of notching according to the desired results, from subtle to dramatic.

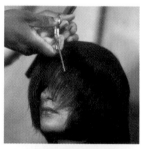

Blunt Weight Line—The blunt weight line falls to one level on the anatomy. The surface appearance of the blunt shape is smooth, with unbroken lines.

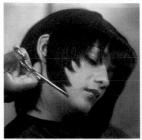

Head Position—Tilt the head back while you comb the hair onto the face and cut notches in the fringe area. Move it to one side to allow you to notch the perimeter of the opposite side. For the blunt back line, position the head upright for natural fall.

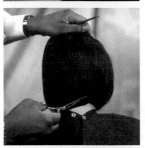

Cutting Position
Cut the hair to be notched flat against the skin. Cut the blunt back perimeter against the nape in natural fall.

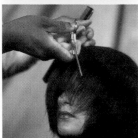

Scissor Position—Use the palm-down scissor position on the left side of the head. Use the palm-up position on the right side. For notching, use the palm-up position.

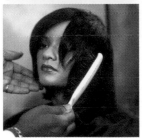

Length Guide
Use the eyes and the nose as guidelines in the fringe area, and frame the hair diagonally along the cheek to under the ear. In the back, create a blunt line at mid neck.

The first and most important step toward success is the feeling that we can succeed.

Nelson Boswell

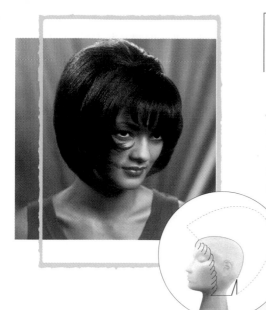

Apply *Blunt Cut*
on dry hair

With your clients, these technical steps will follow the consultation. The relaxer is performed first followed by the conditioning and color treatments. Refer to the Texture and Color sections for these techniques.

To prepare for the cut, blow dry the hair smoothly. Refer to this technique in the Hairstyling section (see page 192).

Pre-existing internal layers flow over the perimeter blunt weight line. The notched areas around the front hair line are cut bluntly.

1. After blow drying, use a dry wrapping technique to straighten, control, and smooth the hair for dry cutting. Brush or comb all the dry hair around the head, then blow dry for a few minutes or put under a warm dryer to "set" the wrapped hair direction.

2. This will create natural-looking curved movement, with the hair contouring close to the head shape, a result that is not generally achieved by chemically relaxing, blow drying, or ironing hair.

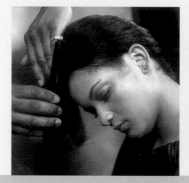
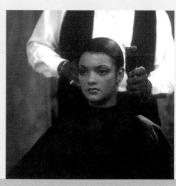

3. Now the hair is ready for a dry designer cut.

4. Brush the hair in the direction of the desired cut.

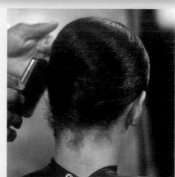
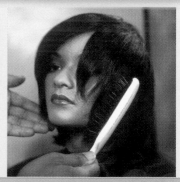

5. Diagonally blunt cut a line over the left eye. You will do notching on either side of this line. This technique is freeform in nature—you are notching into the lengths around the front hairline at measured, slightly irregular intervals.

6. After completing the fringe area, move to the right side. Continue to create your design around the face using the notching technique. Repeat on the left side.

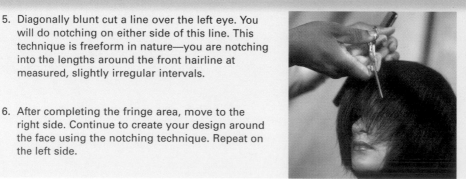
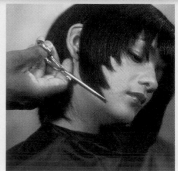

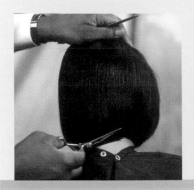

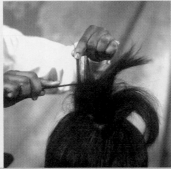

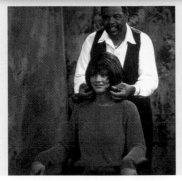

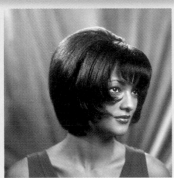

7. After completing the left and right sides, move to the back section. Create a blunt weight line at the desired length.

8. Backcomb the hair on the top of the head to create a base for volume through the crown area. Smooth and curl the hair. You have an entire head of hair that is consistent in texture, with soft curls for movement.

9. Spray the hair for hold. Spray on fingers and detail around the face. The client's makeover is complete. Her hair has been transformed!

10. The consistent texture and soft movement complement the closely contoured blunt shape, results that are accentuated through the dry wrapping and cutting techniques. The finished style is progressively classic, with hair that is shiny and silky.

*R*eflect

Teamwork

Synergy: When 1 + 1 = 3

Teamwork creates synergy, and the best way to describe synergy is that it's what happens when one plus one equals three. Whether you're just getting the everyday work done or putting your heads together to solve a problem or make great new things happen, salon teamwork benefits everyone: the salon, the clients, and the employees.

Teamwork doesn't exist in all salons. If stylists believe the clients sitting in front of them are "their" clients, and thus pay attention only to "their" clients' needs, you don't have a salon team. You have a lot of independent stylists working under the same roof, but not working together.

When this happens, clients sense the tension. A well-known fashion magazine once interviewed salon clients about their salon experiences. Every woman interviewed said she would go to a new salon before she would change stylists within a salon. Clients sense the possessiveness and jealousy of stylists in salons where teamwork doesn't exist, and both stylist and salon lose business.

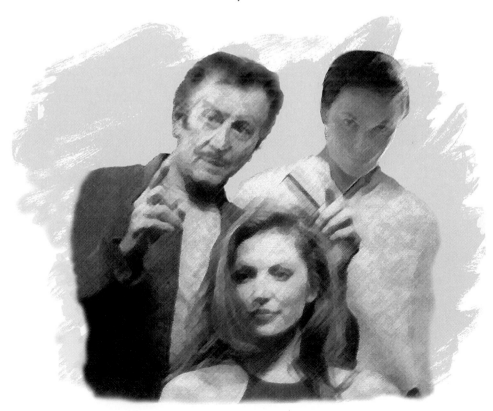

When you're part of a strong salon team . . .

◆ **You get help from co-workers at times when you're swamped and at other times return the favor**

◆ **You can refer your clients to coworkers when you're ill or on vacation, knowing they'll be "handled with care"**

◆ **You teach and learn from each other**

◆ **You work to project a unified, professional salon image**

◆ **You work in an atmosphere of colleagues helping colleagues rather than competitors fighting over clients**

◆ **You enjoy greater success and career opportunities**

Start your career in a salon that encourages teamwork, and your career will soar.

When spiderwebs unite, they can tie up a lion.

Ethiopian Proverb

Graduated Shapes

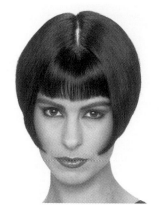

Graduated blunt cut

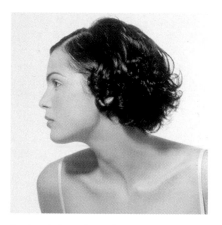

Horizontal graduated cut

Overview

Graduation is one of the most popular haircutting methods. Clients enjoy the versatility that the graduated cut gives them. Graduation takes the edge or weight off the line, which allows great movement and flexibility. The expansion or volume possibilities—both styling and adding texture—make this cut even more desirable. The angled edges of the graduated cut will stack out to create a more triangular shape. The graduated effect may be combined with other shapes, or used alone to create a style.

The graduated cut popularized in modern times by Sassoon's Firefly became a mainstream hit with the American woman after figure skater Dorothy Hamill wore it in her gold-medal-winning performance in 1976. It became known as the Dorothy Hamill wedge or simply as "The Wedge;" the name reflects its angular, stacked-out silhouette.

As with blunt haircuts, graduation is an exterior concept: The graduation takes place at the perimeter, or exterior area, of the

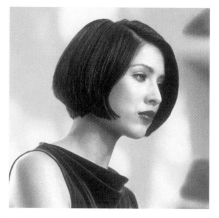

Low graduated cut

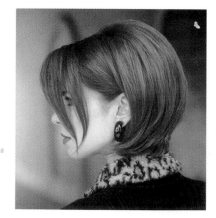

Horizontal graduated cut

haircut. However, in contrast to the single length of the blunt shape, the graduated lengths stack out away from the head at an angle determined by the degree of elevation. This stacking up and out of hair lengths removes weight from the line you're cutting at the perimeter. There will still be a weight area or a ridge line; however this is where the longest length from the interior is brought down and cut to. If you layer over a graduated shape, this weight area or ridge line is diminished—creating a very different result.

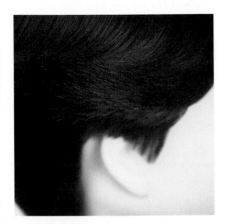

Graduation at the perimeter

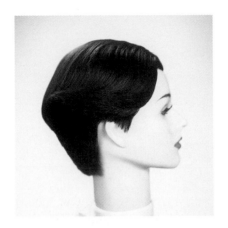

Angular silhouette of the graduated cut

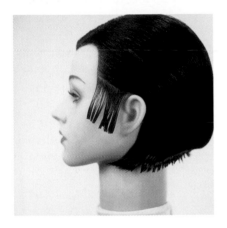

Low graduated cut

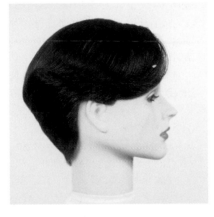

Horizontal graduated cut

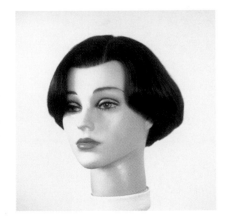

Low graduated cut

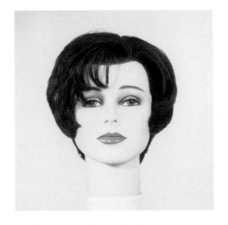

High graduated cut with layers

Low, Medium and High Graduation

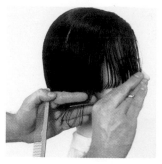

Low graduation

Graduation may be classified as low, medium, or high, depending not only on how the finished style looks but also on the technique used to create the graduation.

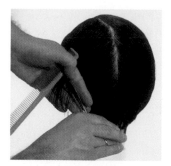

Cutting in, mid to high graduation

Low to mid-graduation uses a stable guide. Remove weight from the line, to allow the line to move along itself.

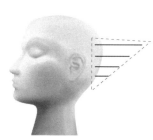

Mid-graduation diagram

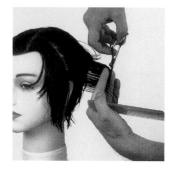

Mid graduation

Mid to high graduation, which is also termed cutting in, uses a traveling guide. This graduation is generally approached from the perimeter. One of the primary methods used in this program for achieving high graduation calls for you to take vertical sections, direct lengths either straight out or downward from the head, and angle your fingers to the desired diagonal guideline. Cross-check the cut lengths horizontally.

Another method is to raise the hair to a given elevation (medium to high) and angle your fingers according to the perimeter line you're creating—horizontal or diagonal.

Connect
Holding Position

This is the position that the hair is combed and held from the head. To create a graduated shape, bring lengths of hair up and out of natural fall. You can hold these lengths at low elevation (higher than the natural fall but lower than medium or 45 degree elevation) or at mid to high elevation (45 degrees up to 90 degrees or straight out). Another method is to bring the hair out of natural fall by shifting off the base parting; if you're working off of vertical sections, you can either shift your holding position diagonally downward (for lower graduated effects), or straight out from the curve of the head. Then angle your fingers to the cutting position desired.

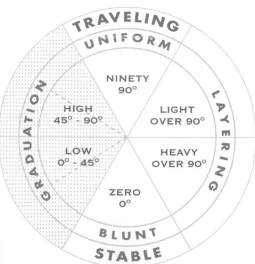

Haircutting angle guidelines

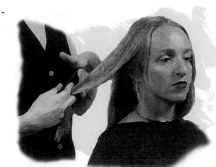

Low elevation holding position

Cutting Position

If you're creating a low to mid-graduation cut along the perimeter line, your cutting position is defined by the line you're creating—horizontal, or diagonal forward or back.

If you're creating a mid to high graduation—directing the hair out from vertically parted sections—then the cutting position is referred to as cutting in. This is generally a diagonal line, and its angle is determined by your finger position—from subtle to extreme.

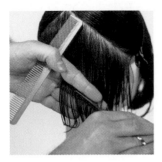
Diagonal forward

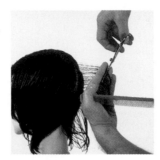
Cutting in

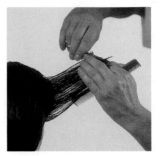
Cutting out

Scissor Position

The classic technique for cutting a graduated style is to position the hand holding the scissors with its palm facing the other hand, which is holding the hair in the cutting position. For a high graduation cut—in which you move the scissors along your fingers, which are holding the hair out from the vertically parted sections—you also position your palm away from you.

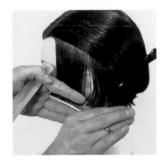
Palm to palm

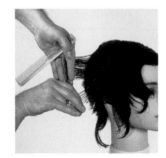
Palm away

Stable or Traveling Guide

To cut low graduation, use a stable guide. Cut an initial guide and hold it at a low elevation; bring all subsequent sections to this stable guide.

To cut a mid to high graduation, use a traveling guide. Hold the hair out from vertical base partings and cut to the desired angle of graduation. With each new section you cut, use the previously cut section as your guide. Each new section then becomes a traveling guide that is brought to the next section.

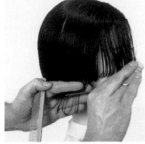
Stable guide

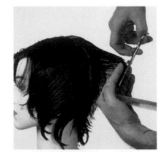
Traveling guide

Tapering—Special Effects Cutting

Within the haircutting part of this program, you will be introduced to a variety of tapering techniques. These may be done with many different tools, including regular and tapering scissors and the razor. This part of the cutting procedure is indeed integral in personalizing the shape. Tapering will render the hair supple, imparting movement and dimension, and breaking up a given area or surface, be it along the ends, the entire strand, or the top surface of the cut.

Remember that this is only a brief introduction to tapering techniques. When done well, tapered effects should be able to "melt" (or blend) into the surrounding hair if desired. Whatever the cut structure, the construction of the shape should include some form of texturizing to create movement and dimension as well as direct lengths and weight, creating a built in support system.

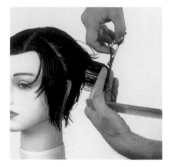

End Tapering

End tapering, using a pointing technique, is effective in creating mobility or softness at the ends of the hair. It may be done around the perimeter frame area of the cut for ornamental effect. Whether on longer lengths or use in short perimeter areas, such as the neckline or sideburns, point into the lengths as held over a comb. This works well to personalize short area influenced by growth patterns.

Point into the hair through the internal lengths of a cut to activate movement through this area. Place the fingers at the depth from the ends related to how far in you would like to taper.

This technique actually channels out alternating short with long lengths for dramatic variegation along the edges. The tips of the scissors snip in at intervals along the fingers.

Notching creates a chunky effect along the edges on internal as well as perimeter frame lengths. Cut in along the fingers at an angle. Adjust the amount and depth of notching for the results desired.

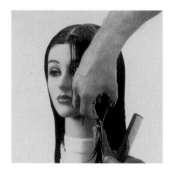

Slide cutting (slicing)

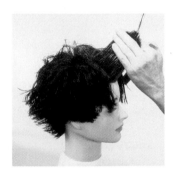

Pointing at the weight corner

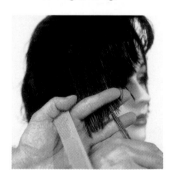

Finger placement determines depth of pointing

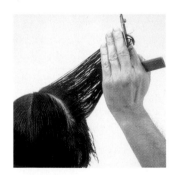

Softening the weight line by pointing

Slide Cutting

Slide cutting, which is sometimes called "slicing" and "slithering," may be done along the top surface as well as individual sections of hair. Glide the scissors through the hair in one fluid motion or slightly open and close as sliding through the hair. Move in the directions that you want the hair to flow. This will create a network of shorter internal lengths that provides expansion, dimension, and directional support. It can be done on damp hair as well as a final step on personalizing dry hair.

A very precise and meticulous tapered effect using slide cutting may be created by picking up small individual strands of hair and slicing in along the strand to carve out fringy, tapered lengths. Place the scissors at that point along the strand where you want the tapered effect to begin. This is an ideal technique to personalize shorter perimeter frames. This slicing of small strands may also be used along the ends of the hair as well. Place the fingers at the area from which you'll slice outward toward the ends.

You may glide out all at once or gently glide out as opening and closing the inside of the blades along the hair.

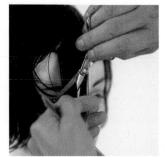
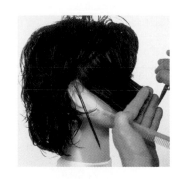

Slide cutting to soften the perimeter

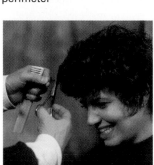

Slide cutting to reduce weight

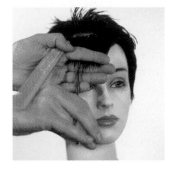

Pointing to create a soft fringe

Razor Tapering

Use the razor to create a wide variety of tapered effects. Pick up small, individual pieces and run the edge of the razor along the top surface to create effects that range from delicate to highly diverse and irregular.

Place the razor along the top of the strand at the point where you want the tapering to begin, then move it out toward the ends to remove the desired length. As in pointing with the scissors, you may taper and cut to the desired length simultaneously.

Contour tapering or what is also call razor rotation is used in areas where a close fitting contoured effect is desired. The razor is rotated with the comb along the surface to be tapered.

Tapering Scissors

The tapering scissors are used for end tapering and creating accentuated movement when desired, and ends that blend for smoother effects. Work through longer internal lengths over the fingers or the comb to insert and cut with the tapering blades.

End tapering is also an excellent final step used over the comb, to work through very short shapes for precision. The ends will blend and harmonize meticulously.

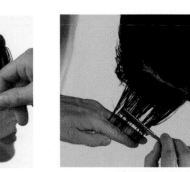

Razor tapering

Razor tapering in 1/2-inch sections

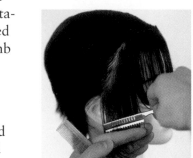
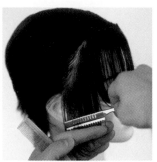

Razor tapering the side

Razor tapering the nape area

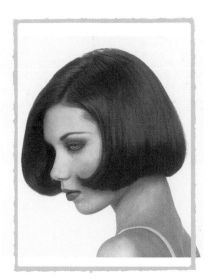

Graduated Blunt

Overview

In this cut you will combine two distinctively different shapes in a harmonious fashion. The graduated nape area flows into a blunt diagonal forward shape toward the front and sides of the design. To create the cut, you will learn several new techniques: the use of graduation through the nape area, and the use of pointing to refine the graduation as well as the perimeter line. This graduated blunt cut—some call it the graduated bob—is modern in its silhouette, and its diagonal forward line gives great freedom of movement. The close-fitting nape area is very sculptural in nature, while the rest of the cut features great structure and shape.

Connect

The Graduated Nape

You'll cut the nape area to create a low graduated effect. Working off diagonal forward partings, bring the first section out at a low (one-finger) elevation and cut it, creating the guide for the following sections up to the occipital. Bring these following sections to the initial stable guide, which you're holding at a low elevation; this creates the graduated effect. At the occipital, working all lengths to the graduated stable guide will start to create a weight buildup. Hold the hair in a downward direction when cutting—do not shift it out of the natural fall direction, as this will distort the shape you're creating.

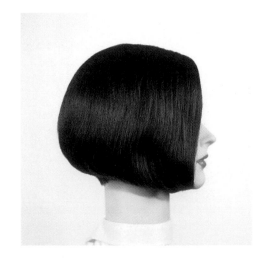

Pointing Technique

You'll use the pointing technique in this cut to refine the graduated area and perimeter line. You can do this over the comb or freehand pointing. Lift up the nape area with your comb, point the tips of the scissors in, and cut; this allows you to check the shape, soften the edges, and render the line very natural looking. Pointing has a wide range of applications. This is only your first exposure to it; you'll also be using this technique in layered cuts.

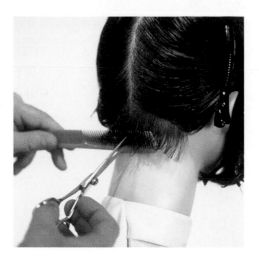

Focus

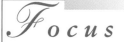

Parting or Sectioning—You'll create an artificial side part from the front hairline area to the crown and extend it down the center back, dividing the back in preparation for cutting. Throughout the cut, you'll use diagonal partings that start at the center part in the nape area, extending forward and down to section the hair.

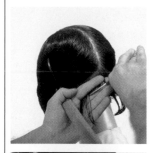

Length—The length at the nape area, where the graduation begins, is approximately one inch (2.5 cm); the hair progresses rapidly toward longer interior lengths. An important factor that you can adapt for your clients is the length of the front of the sides, which is 1 1/2 inches (3.75 cm) below the jaw line. Use facial features or levels on the anatomy to gauge length as you work around the head.

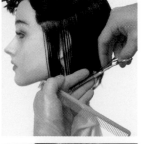

Head Position—While cutting through the nape area, position the head slightly forward; return the head to an upright position to cut the remainder of the shape.

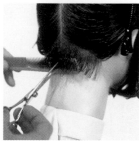

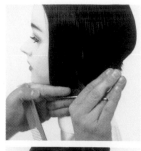

Holding Position—At the nape hairline use a low-elevation holding angle (also called a one-finger elevation), bringing the hair out of natural fall. Bring all subsequent sections to this stable guide. Bring the hair above the occipital down to the last elevated section at the occipital; maintain this throughout the remainder of the back. As you work into the sides, your holding position is at natural fall, other than the top front area that is worked over into the line to be cut on the heavy side of the part.

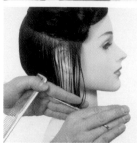

Cutting Position—Use the diagonal cutting position throughout the entire back area and horizontal through the side.

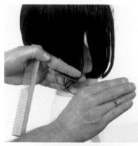

Scissor Position—Use a palm-to-palm scissor position throughout the graduated area of this haircut.

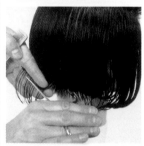

Stable Guide—Use a stable guide throughout the cut.

Hearty laughter is a good way to jog internally without having to go outdoors.

Norman Cousins

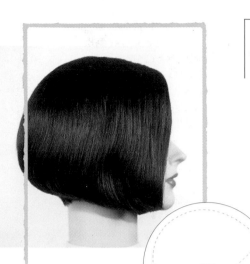

Apply

Graduated Blunt

With your clients, these technical steps will follow the consultation and shampoo.

The graduated blunt cut is a modern classic. The sculpted graduation in the nape falls into a beautifully defined weight area at the sides.

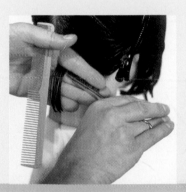
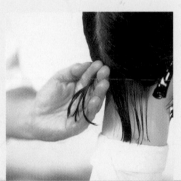

1. In this cut we'll use the palm-to-palm scissor position for the first time.

2. Preparing the hair as in blunt haircutting, begin cutting in the back on the left side. Comb and elevate the hair, holding it one finger's distance from the base area. This is a one-finger elevation or holding position for creating graduation.

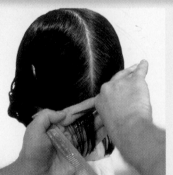
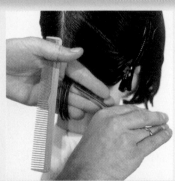

3. Cut the section diagonally along the inside of the middle finger of your left hand, which is holding the hair. Notice how the entire left hand is angled downward to the left.

4. Repeat the procedure on the right side, cutting the hair in the opposite direction.

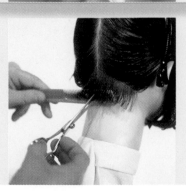
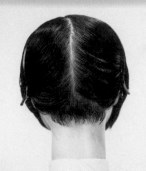

5. To refine the perimeter shape at the nape, hold the section out with your comb and use a pointing technique.

6. When complete, the first section already shows graduation: Rather than lying flat, the hair stacks along the graduated angle you have cut.

7. Release the next 1/2" (1.25 cm) section. You should be able to see the previously cut guide through it.

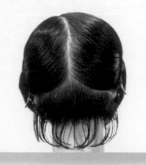
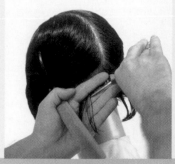

8. Comb the hair down and out at a medium elevation and cut, following the established guideline.

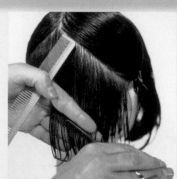

9. Repeat this procedure on the opposite side.

10. Continue to bring down 1/2" (1.25 cm) sections and cut to your guide. This will be the procedure as you work up the back area. Do not shift the hair away from the natural fall direction.

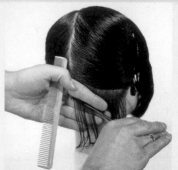
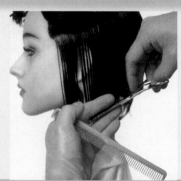

11. When you reach the crest, you will begin to work on the sides.

12. Part all the way through the sides, taking a diagonal forward section that's no more than 1/2" (1.25 cm) over the ear. Bring the head upright. Cut diagonally with a low holding position. Position your fingers to establish the length and create the diagonal line; cut the entire side section, holding the hair as close to the skin as possible.

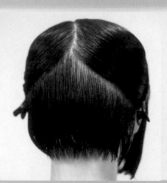
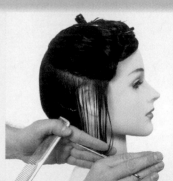

13. Comb the hair against the skin and check the line for accuracy. This will accentuate a blunt line.

14. Move to the opposite side. Bring down a 1/2" (1.25 cm) diagonal parting over the ear. Bring the head upright. Holding the hair low, begin cutting at the graduated back. Cut diagonally forward with the hair in natural fall. Position your fingers to establish the length and create the diagonal line; cut the entire side section, working as close to the skin as possible.

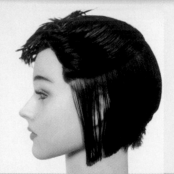
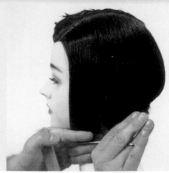

15. Before cutting subsequent partings at the sides, check the lengths on both sides to make certain they are even.

16. Return to the left side. Part out diagonally, releasing 1/2" (1.25 cm) sections. Cut, following the established guideline. Maintain the natural fall direction as working toward the sides, holding the hair as low as possible. Continue to use this technique to the top side parting.

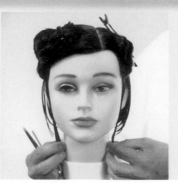

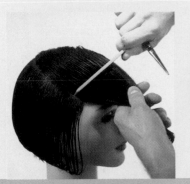
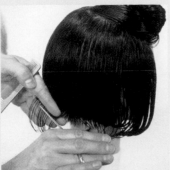

17. Continue on the right side, parting out diagonally to release sections.

18. Maintain natural fall while cutting through the sides, following the established guide. Continue to follow the established guideline to cut diagonally toward the front and sides.

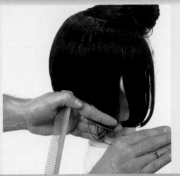
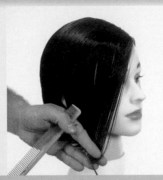

19. Move to the side and cut in natural fall.

20. Section out the top front fringe area, comb it to the heavy right side, and cut it at an angle through the front that blends with the sides. Cutting of the top is performed on the heavy side of the part—the right side—only.

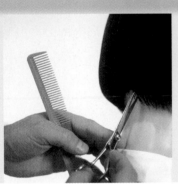
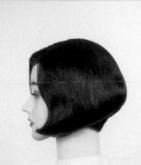

21. Check the entire perimeter using the pointing technique described on page 93.

22. The sculptural silhouette seen here is a magnificent shape to be adapted in a variety of ways. The precision of the shape gives the style a modern appeal.

Tough times never last but tough people do.

Robert Schuller

Reflect

Explore

Apply this technique to different lengths, colors, and textures for almost endless possibilities.

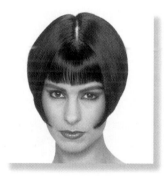

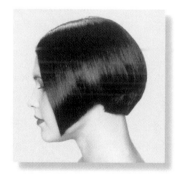

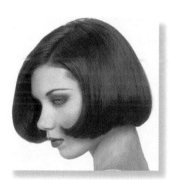

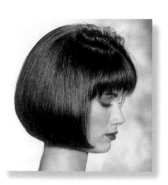

graduated blunt

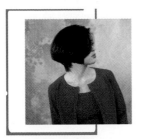

*T*he client wants to update her image for professional reasons. Her hair is in a growing-out phase. The stylist asks all the right leading questions, listening carefully, before making recommendations for the client's approval.

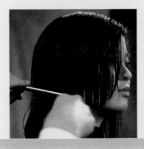 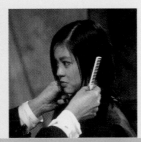

1. Create a side part and establish the desired length at the sides. Angle the comb back to establish the desired diagonal forward line of the cut. Comb the hair in natural fall and cut. Continue cutting the entire side. Work from front to back, maintaining natural fall and the angle of the comb. Repeat this procedure on the other side, adjusting the angle as desired.
2. Check for a harmonious balance on both sides.

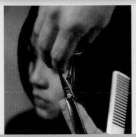 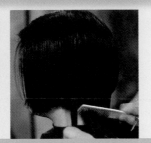

3. Cut the area framing the face on a diagonal back. This will soften the weight corner at the front. Using a reference point on the face, such as the nose, for where you'll begin, hold a 1/2" (1.25 cm) section at the front hairline shifted forward and cut on an angle, as shown.
4. Next you will cut the back area. On the sectioned-out top you will be cutting in for a graduated effect, while at the nape you will be cutting out for a layered effect. Move to the back area and vertically part off a section, directly behind the ear and the newly cut side length. Comb this section down diagonally.

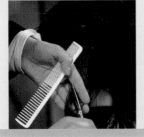 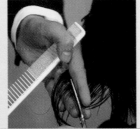

5. Begin cutting out from the length established at the back of the side. This will serve as a guide through the lower nape.

6. Having clipped the top area out of the way, continue to part out vertical sections. Direct the nape lengths down diagonally and cut for a length increase. You will cut all nape sections using this technique to the center back.

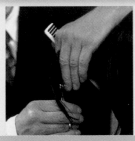 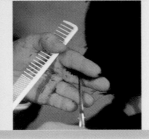

7. Release the top sections, comb, and hold the hair out from the base. Begin cutting in to create a graduated effect. Repeat this procedure as outlined on the opposite back side.

8. Take sections through the back and point into the ends to detail and soften the edges. Work toward each side, pointing in as you cross-check the line.

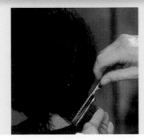

9. When you are satisfied with the back line, comb down the nape, and cut it to the desired length, using a razor. Taper the top surface for a feathery effect as you create the line. In the finished cut, the geometry of the heavy right side is evident. The soft, wispy nape moves into the graduation over it.

It's About Time

Time is the scarcest resource of the manager; If it is not managed, nothing else can be managed.

Peter Drucker

"Time marches on."

"Time flies."

"Take some time."

"Time heals all wounds."

"Time wounds all heels."

"Time and time again."

"What time is it?"

"Do you have the time?"

"Is it time yet?"

"I have no time for this!"

"Where did the time go?"

Bet you've heard all of these before! And here's another one that's key to your career as a stylist:

"Time is money."

What does this mean to you as a stylist? Certainly, the faster you work, the more money you make. Or do you? If you aren't careful to balance quantity of work with quality of work, your clients won't be satisfied with the results and won't return. Then you won't make much money at all.

As a stylist, you can make time your enemy or your friend. You can have too much or too little, or you can learn to manage it wisely for:

◆ **Income and career advancement**

◆ **Client satisfaction and retention**

For some new stylists, it can seem that all they have is time. The hours tick by slowly while they wait for a new walk-in client to be assigned to them, or to be asked by a busy senior stylist for help. Many of today's most successful working stylists remember the agony of standing around on that first salon job and waiting for their career to begin.

Time is important to clients, too. Keeping a busy client waiting, or taking too much time to perform a service, can send her in search of a more time-oriented stylist. On the other hand, making a client feel rushed through a service can cause problems, too. That's why salons have time standards for
each service.

To make time your friend, learn to manage it wisely. We've already mentioned the importance of setting goals and planning your work. It helps to have a plan for downtime, too. Whether it's creating and mailing flyers that offer new clients 20 percent off your services, sending thank-you notes and appointment reminders to clients, studying a new design technique, or helping out in the nonservice areas of the salon (such as the retail area or the dispensary), if you use your time wisely, you will enjoy a more successful future.

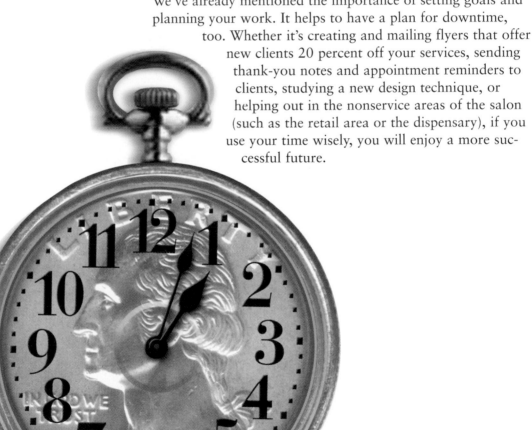

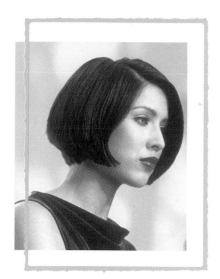

Low Graduation

Overview

In this classic graduated shape, lengths flow diagonally back away from the face. This mid-length style is perfect for the client who likes the look of long hair but appreciates the control and manageability of a short cut.

After you create the graduated shape, you will soften the edges of the graduated weight line by removing the weight corner. This will modernize the shape and create softly rounded edges.

Focus

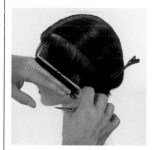

Head Position—Maintain the head in an upright position throughout this entire haircut.

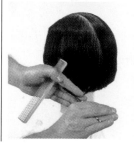

Holding Position—Use one-finger low holding positions to create this graduated effect.

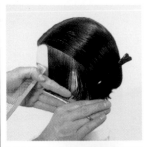

Cutting Position—The cutting position used throughout is a diagonal back line. An exception is the long fringe, which you comb into natural fall and cut to create a slight length increase toward the lip line (see page 105). When you then comb the fringe back into the diagonal back line, the heaviness of the line will be maintained.

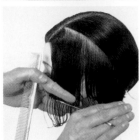

Scissor Position—Use the palm-to-palm scissor position with a straight wrist for comfort and ease while cutting the sides. In the back perimeter, fringe area, and interior, the scissor hand is palm down.

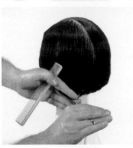

Blending—In this cut, the diagonal back line will blend into the shape you already created at the center back.

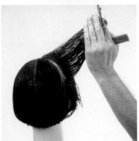

Weight Corner Removal—Softening the weight corner all the way around the haircut is optional; doing so will soften the shape, making it curved instead of angular. Take sections straight out from radial partings. The corner may be cut off bluntly or pointed or notched in, to soften the effect even more.

I can't change the direction of the wind, but I can adjust my sails to always reach my destination.

Jimmy Dean

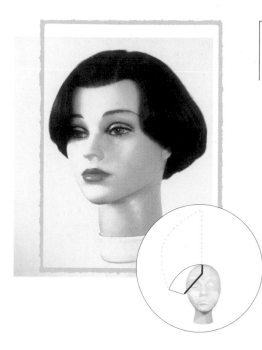

Apply
Low Graduation

With your clients, these technical steps will follow the consultation and shampoo.

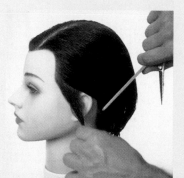

This very popular, commercial style features a graduated frame that flows back off the face. The mid-length shape features a line that travels from the tip of the nose to approximately one inch below the nape area in the back.

1. Establish a side part, combing the hair into natural fall with the head upright. Make sure the ends are neatly combed. Working off a side part, comb the hair back over the ear. Diagonally part a 1/2" (1.25 cm) section just in front of the ear, moving from the front hairline back over the ear.

2. Use a low (one-finger) elevation. Angle the fingers holding the hair from the tip of the nose to the ear lobe. Use the palm-to-palm scissor position as you cut.

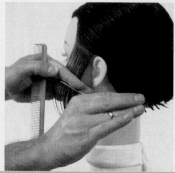

3. This diagonally angled line will be your cutting guide. Notice that it angles from the nose to the ear lobe.

4. Part off the next section, angling down from the hairline to the back, so the part line falls 1/2" (1.25 cm) above the top of the ear. Comb the hair into the natural fall direction and cut on the diagonal, following the established guide.

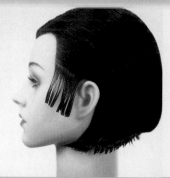

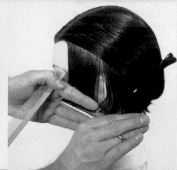

5. Hold your scissors low in a palm-to-palm position. Taking care not to cut past your second knuckle, extend the guide through to back.

6. Continue bringing down 1/2" (1.25 cm) sections and cutting to the previous guide. (Make certain you can see the guide through each new section.) Cut exactly on your guide.

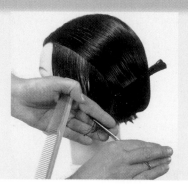

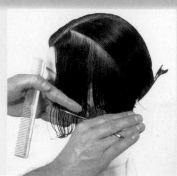

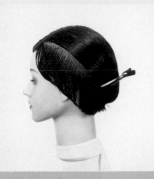
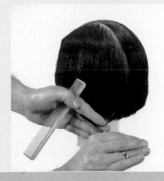

7. The completed sections should form a perfect diagonal line from front to back.

8. Complete the entire side, diagonally parting out 1/2" (1.25 cm) sections and following the guide. Maintain the low one-finger elevation. Comb the lengths against the skin and refine the perimeter line. Comb the line between the fingers and point into to blend and refine the back area.

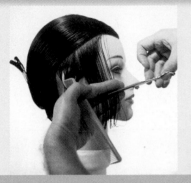
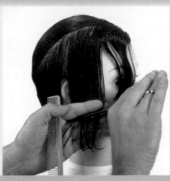

9. ,10. Move to the opposite side. Establish a guide as described in step 3. Cut subsequent sections as in steps 5 through 9 until you reach the recession area.

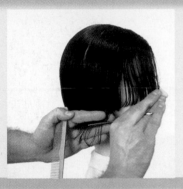
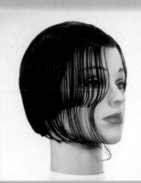

11. Part through from the center front hairline. Notice that the front hairline is left out. Cut through from the side to the nape. Blend and cut the fringe in natural fall. The horizontal finger position is aligned with the tip of the nose. Continue working upward using this procedure. Cut the sides to the guide then cut the fringe to the guide. Remember to use the natural fall direction and low elevation.

12. Comb all the top hair and front fringe down in the natural fall direction. Here you can see the guide through the final, front section.

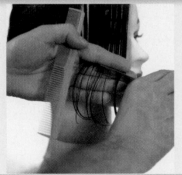
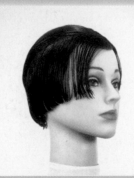

13. Cut the fringe line to adapt to the needs and desires of your client.

14. The completed side shows that the front piece extends toward the tip of the nose.

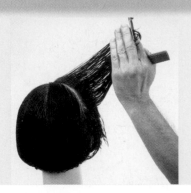
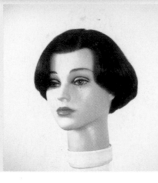

15. If you wish to soften the weight line by removing the corner, work radially through the interior, bringing sections up and out and taking the weight corner off. You can do this blunt, or pointed or notched in.

16. The graduated diagonal back silhouette flows into a softly rounded back area. The weight area, having been rounded, creates a soft shape.

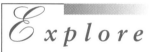

Reflect

Explore

Apply this technique to different lengths, colors, and textures for almost endless possibilities.

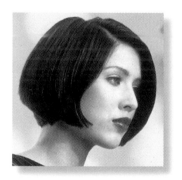

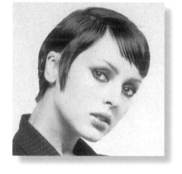

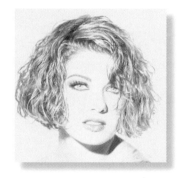

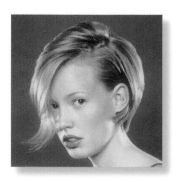

Dressing for
Success

You must begin to think of yourself as becoming the person you want to be.

David Viscott

Dress for the job you want, not the one you have.

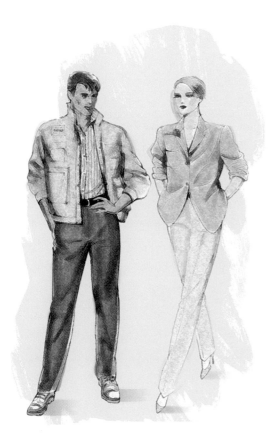

*S*uccessful people in all professions follow this advice. They carefully observe others who occupy higher positions, noting how they dress, talk, and conduct themselves.

Dressing for success is different for different jobs, different industries, and different situations. From dark, two-piece suits in a Wall Street investment firm to jeans and T-shirts at a California computer software company, each individual workplace has its own dress code. Observation is the best way to learn the code.

Dressing for success in the salon could mean anything from the most conservative, traditional looks to totally progressive fashion and hair design. It all depends on the clientele and what makes them comfortable. When you're interviewing for a salon job, visit the salon first and see what the stylists–and the owner or manager–wear. Then plan your interview wardrobe, hair, and (if applicable) makeup accordingly.

Even if you don't yet have a lot of money to spend on clothing and accessories, you can still dress for success by making sure what you wear is clean and pressed, free from stains and damage, and complemented by appropriate accessories, hair, and makeup. In all but the most fashion-forward salons, less is usually more. If you cannot afford a lot of clothes, purchase a few good items that can be mixed and matched, and keep them clean and in good repair. Similarly, your shoes should always be clean and polished.

Many things about you work together to determine what impression you make. Even the most appropriate, well-tailored suit won't win you points if your fragrance is too strong or your breath unpleasant. Make sure everything about your appearance–from clothing to grooming, scent, and smile–combines to make a memorable and pleasing impression on others.

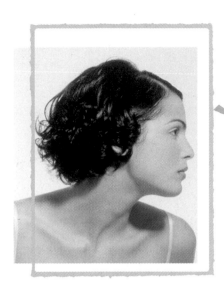

Horizontal Graduation

Overview

In this silhouette, a uniquely geometric front and sides contrast to the highly graduated nape area. This short, contoured nape harmonizes beautifully with the low graduation cut horizontally at the front of the design.

Connect
Length Lines

You'll cut the short lengths within this shape along two distinctly different lines. Cut the front and side lengths to a horizontal line adjacent to the tip of the nose; cut the lengths throughout the back area along a diagonal line that follows the hairline behind the ear on either side.

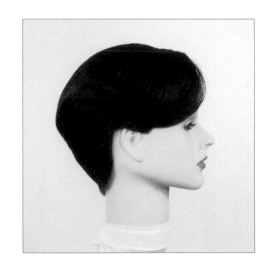

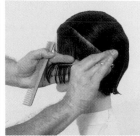

Holding Position—On the sides, use a low (one-finger) elevation holding position. At the back, cut the first line behind the ear with a low elevation holding position, then change to a medium elevation as you work toward the center back.

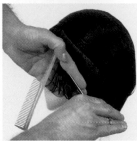

Stable and Traveling Guides—Use a stable guide to establish the low graduation through the sides. Use this as a guide to work into the back area. This guide is then used as a traveling guide with subsequent sections you cut through the back. Bring them to a medium-elevation holding position that moves from section to section.

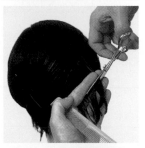

Cutting Position—On the sides, use a horizontal cutting position. At the back, use a diagonal cutting position, traveling from the edge of the horizontal line over the ear into a diagonal back line along the nape hairline.

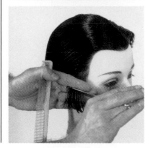

Scissor Position—The scissor position throughout this cut is palm-to-palm.

Dream what you dare to dream.
Be where you want to go.
Be what you want to be.

Richard Bach

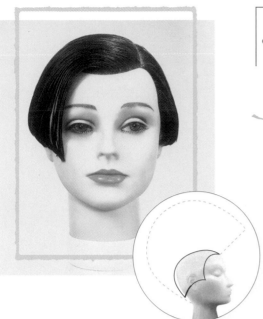

Apply

Horizontal Graduation

With your clients, these technical steps will follow the consultation and shampoo.

This short, exacting cut may be styled back off the face as seen here to accentuate the flow of graduation. This is an easy care, easy wear shape given the precise lines of the graduated shape. Horizontal lines at the sides move into the diagonally graduated back.

1. Establish a side part, combing the hair into natural fall with the head upright. Make sure the ends are neatly combed. Part the back from the crown straight down to the nape, dividing it into two equal sections. After establishing a side part, comb the hair on the left side over the ear. Diagonally part out a 1/2″ (1.25 cm) section in front of the ear, comb it in natural fall, and establish the length, using a horizontal cutting position and low elevation holding position.
2. Release the next diagonal back section and cut to the horizontal guide, holding in low elevation.

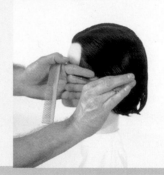
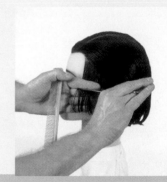

3. Diagonally part another 1/2" (1.25 cm) section from the front hairline to the nape, following the perimeter hairline. Cut the side horizontally to the established guideline using low elevation. Continue the line behind the ear diagonally, using a low elevation. The hair through the back is shifted out of natural fall toward the diagonal guideline created behind the ear.

4. Cut the entire section behind the ear to the nape in this manner.

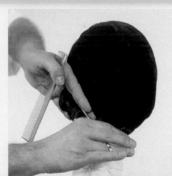
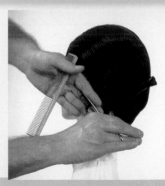

5. Bring down the next 1/2" (1.25 cm) diagonal section from the front hairline to the nape. Comb the hair neatly into the natural fall. Cut the side horizontally, using a low elevation. You're beginning to build graduation.

6. Angle your fingers down toward the nape to blend the back of this section into the diagonal back guide and continue cutting, using a medium elevation with the traveling guide.

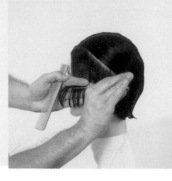
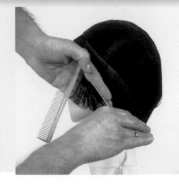

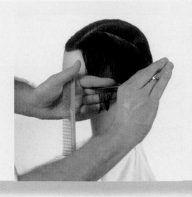
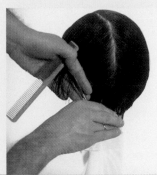

7. Complete the entire side, cutting the section in front of the ear horizontally.

8. Use the traveling guide with medium elevation to continue cutting the back section on a diagonal.

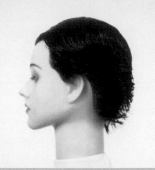
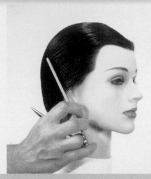

9. The completed left side shows activated graduation.

10. Move to the right side and comb the hair diagonally, toward the back.

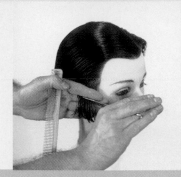
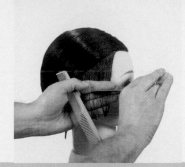

11. Diagonally part a 1/2" (1.25 cm) section, comb it down, and cut it horizontally, as you did before, using low elevation.

12. Bring down a second diagonal parting and cut it in the same manner.

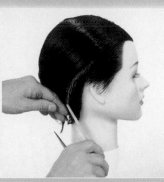
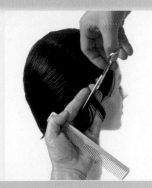

13. Take a diagonal parting from just above the horizontally cut sections all the way to the nape, following the hairline.

14. Cut the side, then starting at the back end of the horizontal guide, cut the back section along a diagonal, using the low elevation holding position.

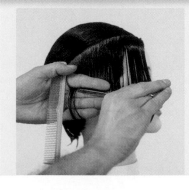
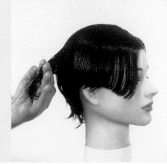

15. Return to the front. Bring down another 1/2" (1.25 cm) diagonal section. Cut the side area horizontally, leaving out the front fringe section.

16. Follow this section into the area behind the ear, using a traveling guide with medium elevation.

17. Continue to graduate the lengths along a diagonal line until you reach the center back.

18. Direct the front piece that you left out toward the side. Cut the front piece at an extreme angle toward the lip line.

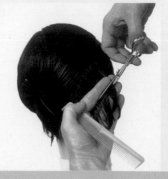 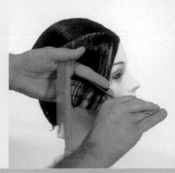

19. Continue working to the top using the techniques as outlined. Continue into the back area using consistent holding, cutting, and scissor positions as established. Check both sides at the center back by combing the hair straight out.

20. As a final step, check upward horizontally through the center back.

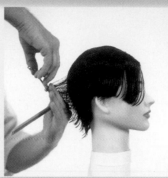 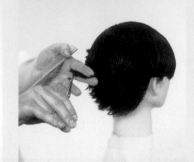

21. Here the finish is styled in its natural flow and direction to highlight the horizontally cut front. There is a subtle asymmetry at the frame area. The hair styled back off the face accentuates the graduated effect. A slight graduation around the sides flows into a more highly graduated back area that contours to the curve of the head.

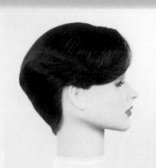

Follow your bliss.

Joseph Campbell

Reflect

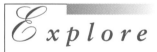

Explore

Apply this technique to different lengths, colors, and textures for almost endless possibilities.

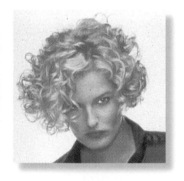

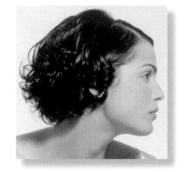

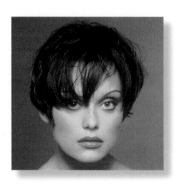

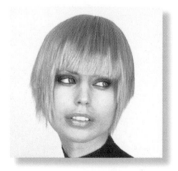

*Do your work with
your whole heart,
and you will
succeed–there's
so little competition.*

Elbert Hubbard

In surveys conducted with salon owners all over the country, one complaint is heard over and over. "My younger employees don't have a strong work ethic," goes the refrain. "They don't work as hard to get ahead as my generation did when we were starting out."

What are salon owners talking about? What exactly is "work ethic"?

Webster's Dictionary defines work as "purposeful activity" and work ethic as "a belief that work is of central importance to life, and that hard work builds good character qualities."

Some people believe that those born in the last half of this century, after the Great Depression and World Wars and during a time when the rapid growth of technology changed the way work gets done, do not display a strong work ethic because "they never had it as hard" or "they've been given too much without having to work for it."

The truth is, every generation faces its own hardships. Our ancestors may have made many sacrifices through the Great Depression and World War II; but the current generation, while they may have plenty to eat and wear, faces a stress-filled, hurry-up world in which families are far flung and people often must face their problems without the support of family. It is no one's place to say who suffers more.

The truth is, work ethic is alive and well, and every person can have one–simply by choosing to. Here's our Top Ten List of the behaviors and practices that will lead employers to think of you as a hard worker with a good work ethic.

*Work to do and
someone to love
are the only two
reasons to get up
every morning.*

Sigmund Freud

Top Ten Ingredients
of Good Work Ethic

1 Arrive at work promptly, well rested, and appropriately dressed and groomed.

2 Perform your duties with a positive attitude and to the best of your skills and abilities.

3 Maintain your station and tools in a clean, sanitary, attractive matter.

4 Do not take or make unnecessary personal calls during work hours.

5 Communicate properly and politely with clients and coworkers. Refrain from personal conversations with coworkers when performing client services. The clients are your main focus.

6 Do not take more than the allowed number of personal and sick days, and do not keep rearranging your work schedule to fit your social life.

7 Understand and support the rules, policies, and goals of the salon business. Contribute your ideas and creativity to help make the salon more successful.

8 Volunteer for additional work that will help the salon and teach you new skills.

9 Continue your education and develop your skills.

10 Go the extra mile. Stay a little late. Take the extra client. Help out a coworker who is struggling.

Remember, you get from work and life what you put into them. The character qualities that come from being a dedicated worker will serve you well.

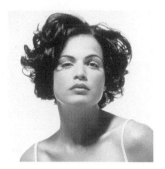

Layered square cut

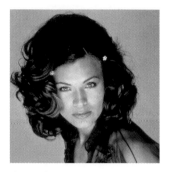

Heavy layer cut

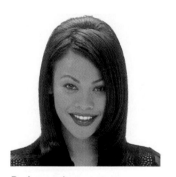

Perimeter layer cut

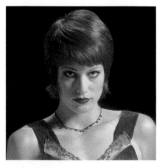

Full layer cut

Layered Shapes

Overview

In creating layered shapes, you are heading into new territory. The technique of layering results in a very textured appearance on the surface of the hair, in contrast with a smooth unbroken surface, and offers about as much variety as you can get. Any length of hair can be layered, from very short to very long. It is important to know toward what point you want to distribute weight and length in the haircut.

Whether full and voluminous or close and cropped, layered shapes will be a mainstay in your repertoire of skills. You'll use them again and again with your clients. This program will expose you to the fundamental layered shapes; as you work, you will expand your knowledge of this useful technique.

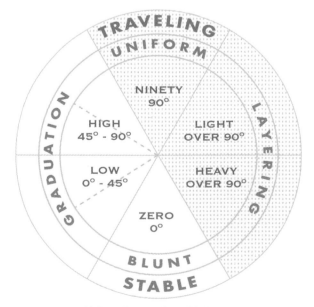

Haircutting angle guidelines

Compare the layered silhouette (first photo) seen here to the graduated or blunt shape (2nd photo). Do you see how the ends of the hair are spread out around the curve of the head? In this traditional, or classic, layered shape, the lengths actually increase (go from shorter to longer) from the interior area of the head toward the exterior. This was achieved by bringing all lengths up to a guide in the interior area of the head and cutting. When those lengths are released, they fall toward longer lengths at the perimeter area. This is only one of the many possible ways to layer the hair. Layering is also very often used through the interior over a perimeter shape that is blunt or graduated. Generally, however, layered cuts have hair lengths that move from shorter in the interior to longer at the exterior, or lengths that are the same throughout the entire head.

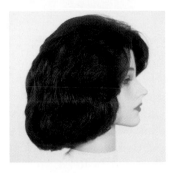

Heavy layers

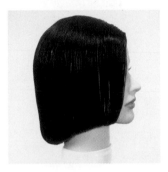

Diagonal back blunt

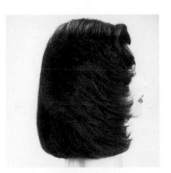

Shorter layers in the interior moving to longer layers at the exterior

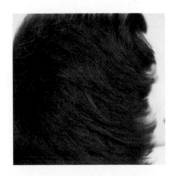

Closeup shot of above picture

Square Layers

In this cut, the technique is to build weight and length toward the front hairline area as well as behind the ears on each side. The resulting weight corners in the layers give this shape dimensional interest, so it's particularly useful if adding some definition will accentuate your client's head shape. To do this, use a section that extends from ear to ear to bring lengths to the side, holding them horizontally out from the head and cutting them vertically. You'll bring all lengths on each side to this guide. Then cut a center back parting using this same approach—again, bring all surrounding hair lengths to this guide. Finally, work through the top with the same concept, bringing all lengths to a central guide, in order to distribute the weight in the desired direction.

Holding Position

Through the sides and back, the holding position is horizontal. Through the top, the holding position is vertical or straight up from the top of the head.

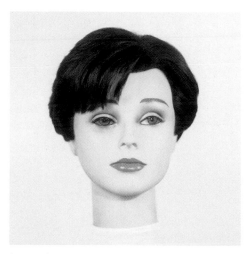

Layered square cut

Cutting Position

The cutting position is vertical through the sides and back. Through the top, the cutting position is horizontal.

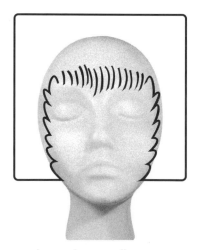

Layered square diagram

Guides

You will use stable guides throughout the cut. Create three separate guides (over each ear and in the center back) and bring all lengths to them.

Light and Heavy Layers

To create light layers, you will use a stable guide, which produces longer lengths in the opposite direction from where you're holding the hair. This type of layering is generally approached from the top of the head. You can also create face-framing layers by establishing a stable guide around the front hairline; bring all lengths forward to it.

To cut heavy layers, you will use a traveling guide, which develops a lesser amount of weight emphasis or length than light layers do. Heavy layers are also approached from the interior area of the head.

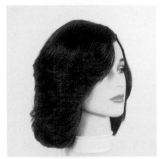

Light layer cut

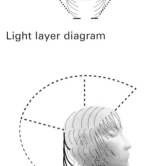

Light layer diagram

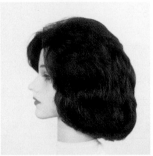

Heavy layer cut

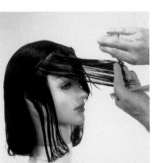

Heavy layer diagram

Holding Position

In creating either light or heavy layered effects, the holding position you use will depend on the elevation at which you're holding the stable or traveling guide from the head—either low, medium, or high. For a total progressively layered shape, use the straight-out holding position: Hold sections straight out from base partings. Cut out or diagonally from the interior outward to the exterior.

Cutting Position

The cutting position for light or heavy layers may be horizontal, vertical, diagonal (cutting out), or parallel to the curve of the head.

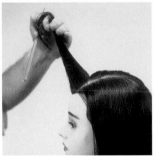

Straight up holding position

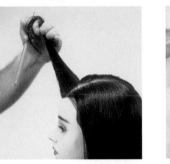

Straight out holding position

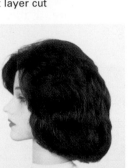

Horizontal cutting position

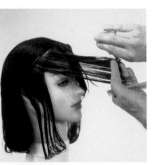

Vertical cutting position

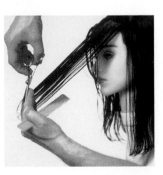

Diagonal cutting out position

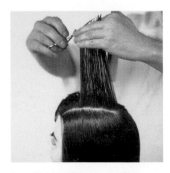

Parallel to the curve of the head position

Uniform Layers

Uniform shapes are heavily layered. All lengths within a given area—
or throughout the head—are evenly cut to echo the curve of the head.
Because it's round, a uniform shape is a low-maintenance, short, and
sassy haircut. As you cut the uniform shape, you must be sensitive to
the curves or different planes of the head.

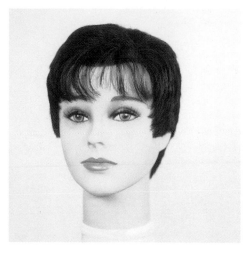

Uniform length cut

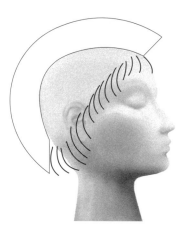

Uniform length diagram

Holding Position

The holding position for the uniform shape is
straight out from the curve of the head.

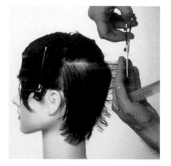

Hold straight out

Cutting Position

Cut parallel to the curve of the head, or even with
the surface of the head.

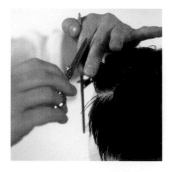

Traveling Guide

Use a traveling guide throughout this cut in order to
evenly encircle and cut around the head.

Cut parallel to the head

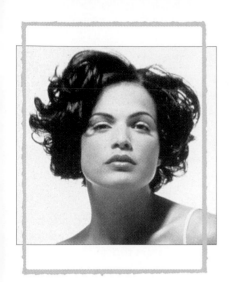

Layered Square Shape

Overview

This dynamic short shape will provide your client with a silhouette that features weight emphasis and length to frame the face and add volume to the back of the head. The shape is more closely contoured or layered above the ears and through the top area of the head. It's a very wearable, distinctive geometric shape that can be styled in a variety of ways—ideal for the client who likes to wear her hair short, as well as for the client who may have a less-than-perfect head shape. You'll revisit this cut again and again.

This cut progresses from the previous one, Horizontal Graduation on page 108, where the lower nape lengths are already established as graduation. When performing this cut on a client in its entirety, you would first cut the perimeter frame along the desired lines either as a blunt or graduated shape.

Focus

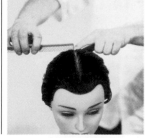
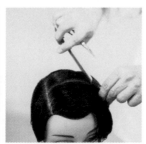

Parting—In this cut you'll create a center design part that you'll cut around symmetrically. Shown here is the parting pattern you'll use throughout the head. As you begin to cut this shape, pivotal partings radiate around the crown of the head. Then, as you layer through the top, you will bring all lengths to a central top guideline.

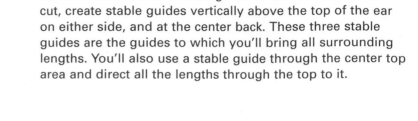

Focus

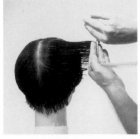

Stable Guide—To work through the external areas of this cut, create stable guides vertically above the top of the ear on either side, and at the center back. These three stable guides are the guides to which you'll bring all surrounding lengths. You'll also use a stable guide through the center top area and direct all the lengths through the top to it.

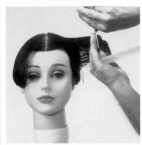
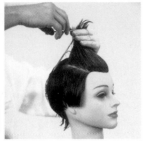

Holding Position—Hold the hair in a horizontal position, parallel to the floor, through the external areas of the cut. You will hold the hair straight up from the top of the head.

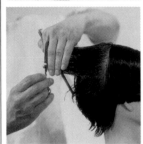

Cutting Position—While creating the shape of this cut, the cutting position will be both horizontal and vertical, always perpendicular to the stable guide.

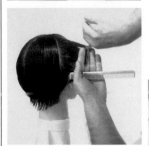

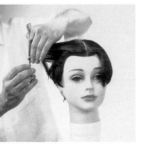

Scissor Position—Your scissor position will change, depending on the area of the head that you're cutting. Through the external area of the cut, use the palm-to-palm scissor postion. Through the top area, your palm is down.

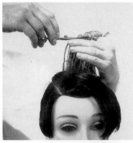

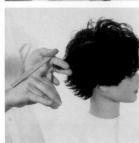

Pointing Technique—Variations on the pointing technique are used throughout this cut. Point into the front fringe, the sideburn area, and the weight corners, to soften the edges and personalize.

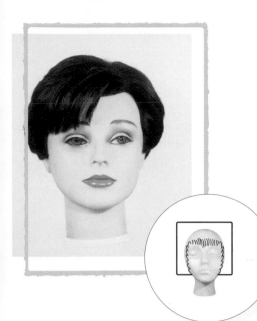

Apply Layered Square Shape

With your clients, these technical steps will follow the consultation and shampoo.

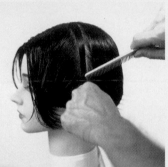

Shown here is the finished layered shape. The weight areas within this haircut emphasize a unique dimension. This haircut is suitable for a wide range of clients, and the geometry of the layers may work well for the client with a less than perfect head shape.

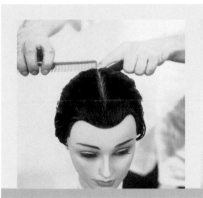

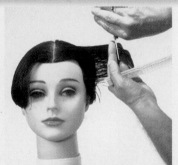

1. First, comb the hair in natural fall. Establish a center part.

2. Part out a 1/2" (1.25 cm) vertical section from behind the ear to establish a guide. Comb this hair straight out from the side of the head into a horizontal holding position. In this cut, the guide will be approximately 3" (75 cm), out from the ear area.

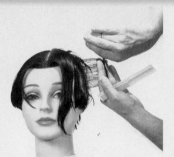

3. Cut this section along a vertical line.

4. Bring the front area, 1/2" (1.25 cm) section by section, back to the guide.

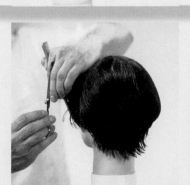

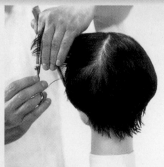

5. Notice that while you're holding the hair straight out from the side, the cutting position is vertical. Notice that the scissor position is also vertical.

6. Bring sections from the back forward to this guide and cut, using 1/2" (1.25 cm) sections. Work all the way to the center back with sections that pivot around the crown.

7. Repeat the procedure outlined for the side area, bringing 1/2" (1.25 cm) sections from the top and sides back to the guide at the ear and then cutting.

8. Take a 1/2" (1.25 cm) vertical section from directly behind the ear and cut to the guide.

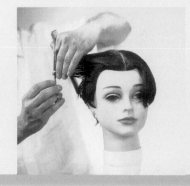 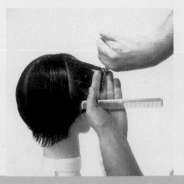

9. Using pivotal partings, bring sections from the back forward, toward the side guide, and cut. Work all the way to the center back.

10. In preparation for cutting the back, take a 1/2" (1.25 cm) vertical section from the center of the back. Hold it straight out from the curve of the head, and cut it vertically.

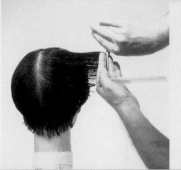 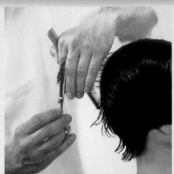

11. Bring the hair from both sides back to this stable guide and cut. Again, use 1/2" (1.25 cm) sections, and direct the hair back to your stable guide until you run out of length toward the ears.

12. Establish a guide for cutting the top front and crown areas. Part a horizontal section across the top of the head, positioned upward from the top of the ears.

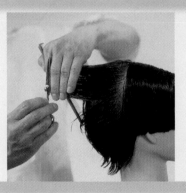 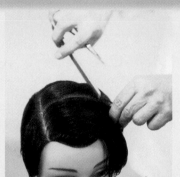

13. Comb and hold this section straight up, then cut it horizontally to establish your length guide.

14. Bring all the hair in front of this section back to the guide and cut.

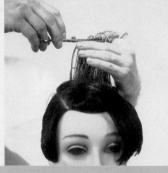 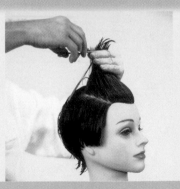

15. Part upward from the top of the ear as a guide to begin sectioning into the crown area of the head. Bring the crown sections forward to the stable guide and cut.

16. Use 1/2" (1.25 cm) sections for control and cut until you no longer have enough length to reach the guide.

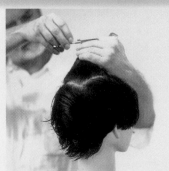 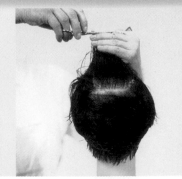

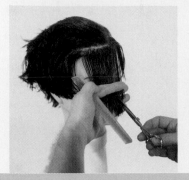
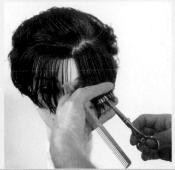

17. Part off the fringe to cut the front perimeter into the desired shape.

18. Use a pointing technique to create a softened edge.

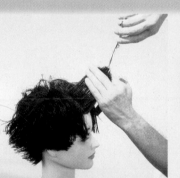
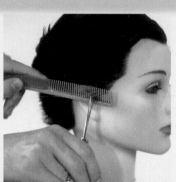

`19. The layering technique used in this haircut has created weight corners.

20. These weight corners may be softened by holding the hair straight out from the curve of the head and pointing into the lengths to diffuse the edge.

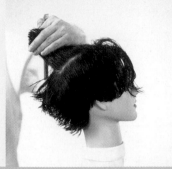
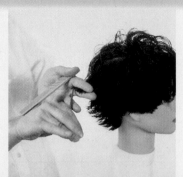

21. Use the pointing technique at the weight corner areas throughout the head.

22. Use the pointing technique in front of and over the ear, holding the hair with the comb.

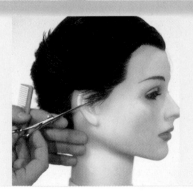
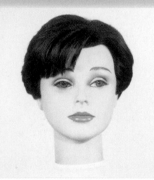

23. To complete the cut, refine the side edges. Strive for a soft, wispy effect, using variations on the pointing technique.

24. The finished style has dynamic movement and texture with a shape that allows for easily created volume and dimension.

Reflect

Explore

Apply this technique to different lengths, colors, and textures for almost endless possibilities.

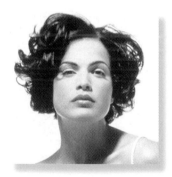

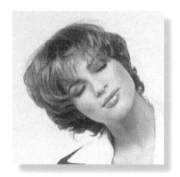

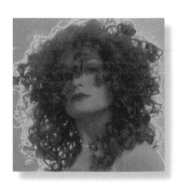

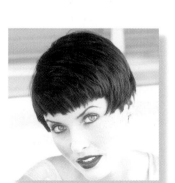

Money
Management

I finally know what distinguishes mankind from the other beasts: financial worries.

Jules Renard

$\mathcal{R}$are is the person who can say she has never worried about money, either how to get more or how to keep what she has. But money is like anything else—life, school, career, relationships—in that, if you do a little planning and some careful managing, it will give you what you want.

To give you a head start on managing your money once you get that first job, study this sample budget:

Monthly take-home pay	$1,200
Savings (15%)	$ 180
Rent and utilities (these should be no more than 25% of the gross)	$ 300
Food (20%)	$ 240
Transportation (20%, including car payments, insurance, gas, and repairs)	$ 240
Clothing, accessories, and personal care (15%)	$ 180
Medical insurance premium (5%)	$ 60
Total	$ 1,200

Notice we put "savings" at the top. That's called "paying yourself first." You may be saving for a vacation, a house, or to start your own business, but you should save, every month, at least 15 percent of your take-home pay.

Once you have developed a budget, you'll know what you can afford. On the budget above, you can't afford to rent a $500-per-month apartment by yourself, for example, but you can afford it if you share rent and utilities with a roommate.

As long as you faithfully budget "by the numbers," then when your income goes up, you'll know how much to increase each of your spending categories. At $2,000 per month take-home pay, you can afford $500 for a roof over your head. Or you can keep your expenses the same and save more. Eventually, you'll have whatever you want. What you won't have are financial worries.

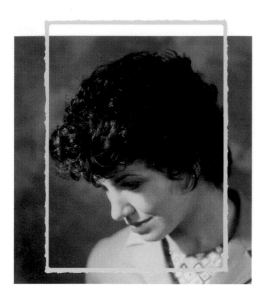

Square Layers

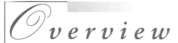
on curly hair

Overview

Hair that has a textural movement, from wave to curl, must be cut with a consideration of final length. Because curl pulls the hair closer to the head, the hair length when wet appears longer than it does dry. Curly hair contracts as it dries, and to keep the length closer to what it will be when dry, work with damp hair rather than wet. As you cut, remist the hair with water only as needed. Adjust the cutting length to allow for this. Work with a minimal tension on the hair to allow for curl and natural growth patterns as you cut.

In this cut you will use both stable and traveling guides to create the desired weight distribution. This cut is a variation of the square geometric layered shape you created on your mannequin. You will use a pointing technique to diffuse any hard edges. The overall effect is one of soft movement over the entire head.

Focus

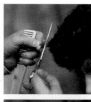

Slide Cutting—In this cut, you will be using a form of slide cutting, called slithering, to reduce weight around the fringe and perimeter hairline. For more on slide cutting, refer to page 134.

Pointing Technique—Use the pointing technique in this cut to reduce weight and soften any edges. You can do this over the comb or freehand pointing. Lift up the nape area with your comb, point the tips of the scissors in, and cut; this allows you to check the shape, soften the edges, and render the line very natural looking.

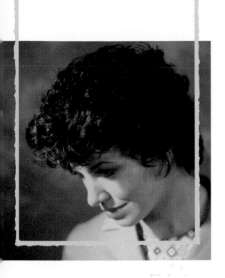

A pply

Square Layers
on curly hair

The shape of this cut places weight corners or edges to frame the face and neckline as well as create fullness through the crown. This definitive shape complements not only the client's natural hair texture, but also her personality and her sense of style.

For this cut, you will begin with damp hair. Remist each section with water as needed prior to cutting and comb through.

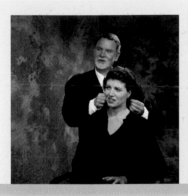

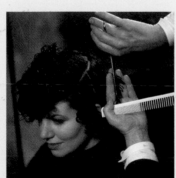

1. The fully layered cut chosen here will feature shorter layered lengths from ear to ear and through the back. Lengths will increase from these areas—toward the front hairline, the crown, and the nape.
2. Dampen the hair and comb it out evenly deciding where you want the final length to fall. To begin, part off the top section, using the hairline recession areas and the crown as your guides. Part a 1/2" (1.25 cm) vertical section above the ear, hold it out horizontally, and cut vertically. This will establish your stable guide for the side.

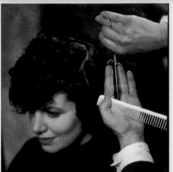

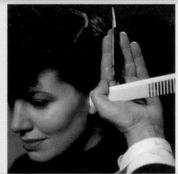

3., 4. Move toward the front, take the next vertical parting, direct lengths to the stable guide, and cut vertically. Work toward the hairline, continuing to direct lengths to the guide above the ear. Hold the hair straight out from the curve of the head and cut vertically. Check the hair's natural movement as you work to ensure that the desired shape is developing.

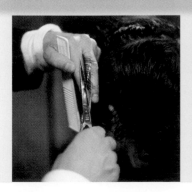

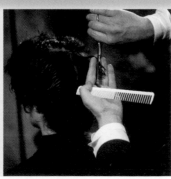

5. Direct the lengths over the ear to the stable guide, which you hold straight out from the side of the head. Cut vertically to this guide. Using the section from behind the ear as the traveling guide, direct lengths through this back side section out from the side of the head and cut to the established guideline. This will create a slight increase toward the back area.
6. Rounding the curve of the head into the back area, bring the lengths straight out from the curve of the head and cut to the traveling guide established through the area behind the ear.

7. Use this traveling guide to cut to the center back. Maintain the vertical cutting position. This will create a slight increase toward the nape area. Repeat the entire cutting process on the opposite side area into the back.

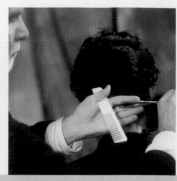
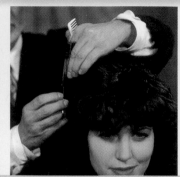

8. Work upward through the center back from the nape area to the crown using horizontal base partings. Comb and hold the hair horizontally from the head and cross-check the line created. Note how the horizontal line meets the weight corner on either side from the lengths cut behind the ear.

9. Next, check the crown lengths in to the back line by directing lengths out from the lower crown area. Cut to extend the line from the back.

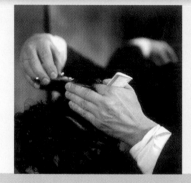
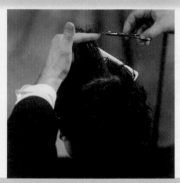

10. Direct lengths from the crest on either side up and out from the crest area above the ear on either side and blend the line.

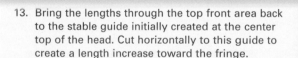

11. At the top area of the head, part out a horizontal section, direct straight up from the top of the head and cut horizontally. This line blends with the crest lengths on either side.

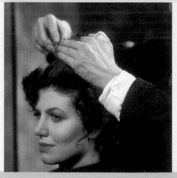
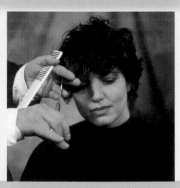

12. Cut the lengths through the top crown area to increase in length slightly by bringing each new section to be cut to the previously cut section. Cut horizontally to the traveling guide, which you hold straight up from the top of the head. Note the scissor position used here, with the palm downward.

13. Bring the lengths through the top front area back to the stable guide initially created at the center top of the head. Cut horizontally to this guide to create a length increase toward the fringe.

14. Part out around the front hairline to direct the front fringe lengths forward. Point into the lengths to refine and soften the fringe.

15. Work upward through the back side areas to refine and soften the weight corners that have been created. Direct the lengths straight out from the curve of the head, then point cut into the weight corner to achieve the desired line and softness.

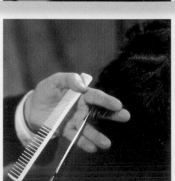
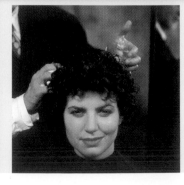

16. For styling, the artist has applied a medium hold conditioning foam for this client to accentuate and control the texture while adding shine. Use the appropriate product for your client's hair type.

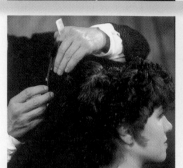

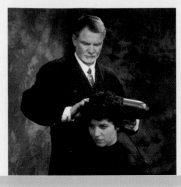
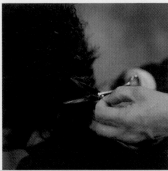

17. Blow dry on a low setting so as not to disturb the curls.

18. After drying, personalize the cut by tapering lengths of hair.

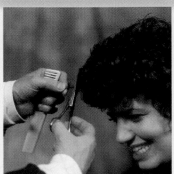
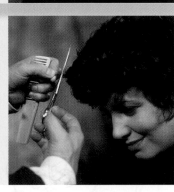

19. Taper the lengths around the perimeter hairline area to further refine and soften the shape. This will accentuate the textural movement while reducing the weight.

20. Taper small sections of hair by slithering the open-bladed scissors back and forth along the strand to create a variegated irregular edge. The blades open and close slightly as gliding the scissors back and forth along the strand. This technique will lighten the hair and enliven the movement.

Reflect

Investing for Your
Success

> *"Never invest your money in anything that eats or needs repainting."*
>
> *Billy Rose*

*T*here's a bit of wisdom from someone who became famous as a producer of Broadway musicals earlier this century. So, it's not exactly expert financial advice. As a "man-about-town," Billy Rose had probably learned the hard way not to bet on horses or spend a lot on houses. At least not with money he was setting aside for a specific goal in the future.

If you save 15 percent of your take-home pay, as we recommended on page 127, you have some choices about what to do with it. You can leave it in your checking account earning interest at a low percentage rate. That will do nothing for you. You can put it in a savings account or certificate of deposit, where it can earn more interest per year. If you leave it there, allowing the interest to "compound," money invested today will double in 12 years at that rate.

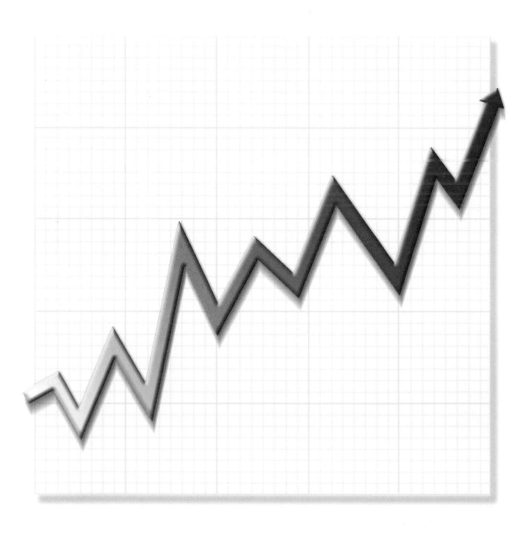

In the past 50 years, the amount of money invested in company stocks has grown even faster than the amount invested in bonds, certificates of deposit, or regular bank savings accounts. Company stocks include both individual stocks or mutual funds, where investors pool their money in a "portfolio" of stocks, and a professional financial manager buys and sells the stock to try to gain the greatest return without losing the investors' money. Through the 1990s, returns of 15 and 20 percent a year were not uncommon. At 18 percent interest per year, it only takes four years to double your money.

Financial advisors will almost always tell you that you should spread out your investments or diversify. That means that you should put some in ready cash savings; some in stocks that you're holding for the longer term for growth; and some in bonds or long-term certificates of deposit, which pay more than savings (though less than stocks), but which are insured and guaranteed. Stocks are not guaranteed, and you can lose everything you invest.

There's not enough space here to give you complete advice on how to invest your money wisely. Our goal is to raise your awareness about investing. Some salon industry people say that, because of the very nature of the hairstyling business and the creative, impulsive people who are drawn to it, money management and investing have not traditionally been high priorities. As a result, very few stylists retire rich, and very few bankers are happy to see a loan application from a salon owner for business expansion.

It doesn't have to be that way. It can change, one smart, savvy stylist at a time. Realize that you do have a future, and it's what you make it. Pick up a book about investing or subscribe to *Money* magazine and start to plan for your own successful investments.

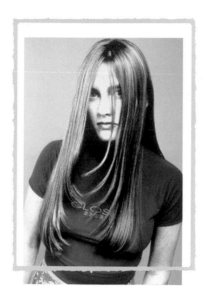

Perimeter Layers

Overview

Long layered shapes are an often-requested design in the salon. They are highly commercial and may be styled for a wide variety of looks. Soft face-framing layers complement the long horizontal bluntness of the remainder of the cut.

To begin, you'll learn a fundamental approach to this cut. As you progress, you will start to introduce some of the many variations on this silhouette into your work.

Connect
Slide Cutting

The primary method used to create this long layered effect is called slide cutting. With this technique, your fingers and scissors glide along the edge of the hair to remove length. It is essential to have sharp scissors so that you can easily slide through the hair with the inner edge of the blades. You'll hold the hair with your fingers so that they serve as a guide to cut along with the blades.

Imagine running the open blades of your scissors through a sheet of wrapping paper or through a lightweight fabric. The blades may glide through smoothly and all at once—or the scissors may glide along the hair as the blades slightly open and close.

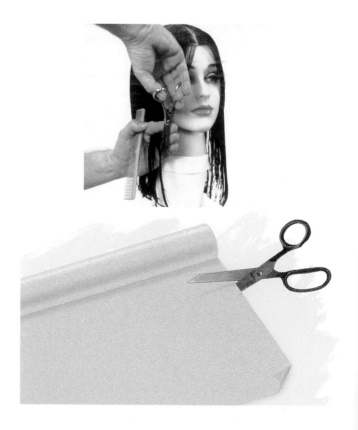

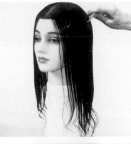

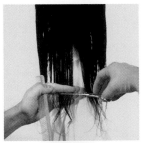

Parting—Use a center parting to cut the perimeter length. At the end of the cut, the blending at the center front will allow for the part to change as you style the hair.

Holding Position—The holding position throughout this haircut is natural fall.

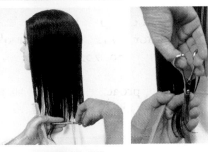

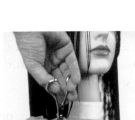

Cutting Position—The cutting position around the lower perimeter area is horizontal. The position for slide cutting around the front hairline is diagonal.

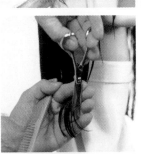

Scissor Position—The scissors in this picture are placed on the front edge of the fingers for sliding along the edge of the hair. A variation would be to place toward the back of the fingers for sliding.

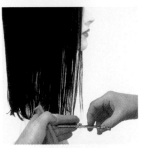

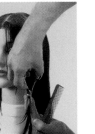

Perimeter Weight Line and Weight Corner—As you cut the perimeter blunt horizontally, you'll create a weight line. The area around the face where this line ends is called a weight corner. Slide cut towards this weight corner from approximately the jaw length downward.

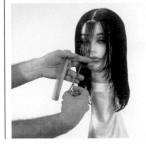

Balance Points—As a final step in this cut, you'll blend and balance the slide cut areas as needed at the front hairline.

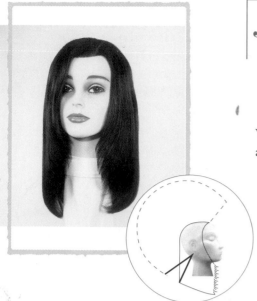

Apply *Perimeter Layers*

With your clients, these technical steps will follow the consultation and shampoo.

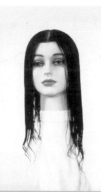

This shape features a horizontal blunt perimeter line combined with long soft layers that flow from the jawline down to the blunt weight line.

1. Comb the hair gently to remove any tangles. Create a center part.

2. Make certain the hair is evenly distributed all around the head in natural fall.

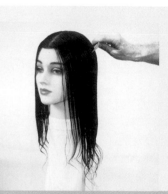

3. Begin removing excess length in the back, starting on the left back side. Use a horizontal cutting position; hold all the hair between your fingers and cut. You can also hold the hair flat with your comb and cut, using comb control alone.

4. Cut toward the side, using the horizontal cutting position with your palm downward. Complete this side.

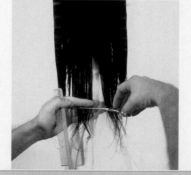
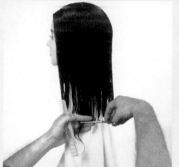

5. Continue cutting horizontally toward the front right, following the same procedure. Make sure to maintain the natural fall position as you cut. Note the scissor position.

6. Part off a section that moves from the center part in front, down to the sideburn area. Clip the remaining lengths out of the way. Hold this section of the hair downward and between the first and middle finger of your hand at the jaw-line level. Angle the fingers diagonally, with the tips of the fingers pointing toward the chin.

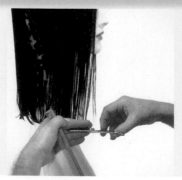
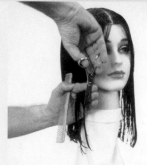

136

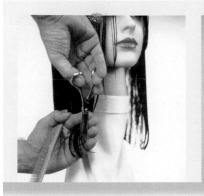
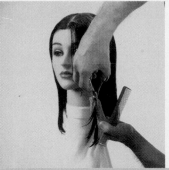

7. With your other hand, hold your scissors against the hand with the hair and begin to slide both hands down in unison as you open and close the blades along the hair to remove length. Continue moving steadily downward, making certain you maintain natural fall. Stop when you reach the bottom weight line, where you run out of hair.

8. Cut the opposite side in the same manner, layering the hair by sliding your scissors, as you open and close the blades, down the entire front perimeter. Note the holding, cutting, and scissor positions being used.

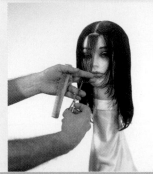
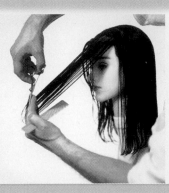

9. Cross-check the two sides for evenness, parting off a small, horizontal section at the front, combing it down, and making sure the two sides meet at the same point and blend.

10. Option: To create a looser, more highly textured effect, take the same partings as before, but comb and elevate the hair more forward. Cut the hair diagonally, slide cutting as before. More layers will result.

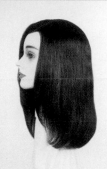

11. This shape is highly desirable for many clients. The possible variations with this slide cutting technique allow for the creation of a multitude of effects.

Success is a journey not a destination. The doing is usually more important than the outcome.

Arthur Ashe

$\mathcal{R}$ eflect

$\mathcal{E}$ xplore

Apply this technique to different lengths, colors, and textures for almost endless possibilities.

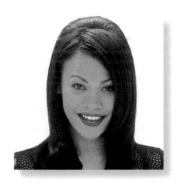

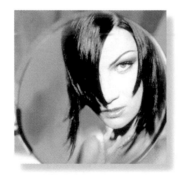

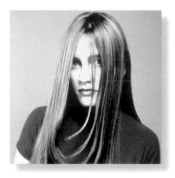

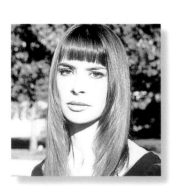

Avoiding Negative
People

The longer I live, the more I realize the impact of attitude on life.

Charles Swindoll

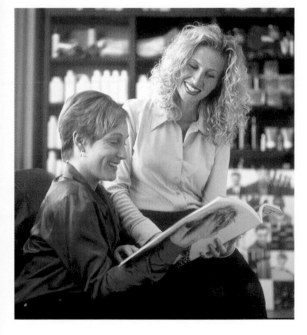

"Attitude, to me, is more important than facts. It is more important than the past, than education, than money, than circumstances, than failures, than successes, than what other people think or say or do. It is more important than appearance, giftedness, or skill. It will make or break a company . . . a church . . . a home. The remarkable thing is we have a choice every day regarding the attitude we will embrace for that day.—Charles Swindoll

In any business—and salons are no exception— attitudes, both good and bad, can be contagious. New employees often begin a new job with a positive attitude and high hopes, only to be taken down in no time by "veteran" coworkers who have gripes about everything from the salon manager to the kind of soft drinks sold in the break room vending machine. These people tend to want everyone else to be as unhappy as they are, and they find that newcomers are particularly vulnerable to their negativity virus.

If you go to work in a salon and discover that co-workers have negative attitudes, protect yourself! Just like you wash your hands to prevent infection from cold germs, keep your psyche and attitude free from the "bad attitude flu," which can be even more destructive.

Here's the prescription: Remind yourself that your career is what you make it. No matter what your co-workers think of the salon, its management, its clients, or their paychecks, you can learn something valuable from every experience, something that will help you build your career. You can keep a positive attitude in the face of others' negativity, and you can even triumph. Others just might discover it feels better to have a good attitude . . . and catch your positive attitude from you!

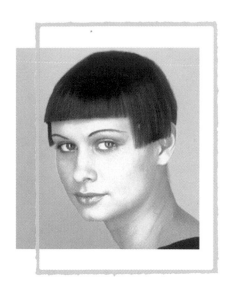

Light Layers

Overview

This shape is a true classic—and yet very contemporary, as well! Internal layers flow over the perimeter blunt cut. The longer layers in this cut are preplanned according to the initial guideline that you create around the front hairline; you'll bring all internal layers to this length. The use of this stable guide will make for shorter layers around the front hairline, increasing to longer layers at the crown and back areas of the head.

Connect
Layered Effect

When you layer the hair, your holding position is straight up from the curve of the head. When the hair returns to natural fall, it will then be distributed over the curve of the head, the ends progressively spreading out from the interior to the exterior. This effect diminishes weight and length. Adding texture to this cut or styling it for volume can create very voluminous and dimensional effects.

Because of the longer length of the first guideline you cut at the front fringe area, the layers will fall longer and farther away from the top of the head. This makes for a smooth, unbroken surface from the top of the head to where the first visible layers fall, hence the description "light layers."

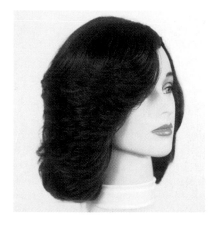

Focus

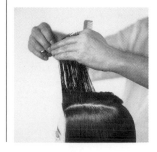

Pre-establishing the Perimeter—The layered technique in this style is performed over the horizontal blunt cut that you did earlier. Return to page 62 and cut this shape before you proceed with the layering.

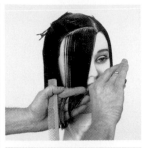

Creating the Guide—Next, cut the area framing the face to the desired length. Cut the front fringe to the lip-line area; you'll use this when you cut straight up from the top of the head through the interior. Blend the side hairline lengths from this lip-line fringe length down to the blunt cut's weight corner.

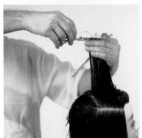

Holding Position—The holding position at the front fringe is at low elevation; direct the side hairline straight forward to blend from the fringe to the weight corner. In the interior, your holding position should be straight up from the head. Hold the side and back lengths straight up vertically.

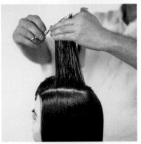

Cutting Position—Use a diagonal cutting position around the front hairline, as well as through the interior; bring all lengths up to the internal guide. The initial fringe line to which you cut the top is diagonal.

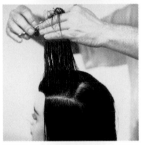

Scissor Position—Around the perimeter, use a palm-to-palm scissor position. Throughout the interior, position your scissors palm to knuckle.

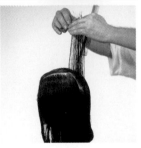

Radial Partings—Take radial partings through the central back area to bring these lengths up from the crown area. This way, you can blend and check these lengths from the top area.

Checking the Cut Response—When you've finished with the cut, ruffle your fingers through the hair to check the cut response (how the haircut responds after being ruffled), given its natural growth patterns and movement. This is the time to make any necessary adjustments in length, line, or shape. However, it's preferable to work through the haircut from the very beginning with as much precision as possible, so you don't have to repeat the cut. Subtle adjustments through texturizing or tapering will personalize the cut for your client.

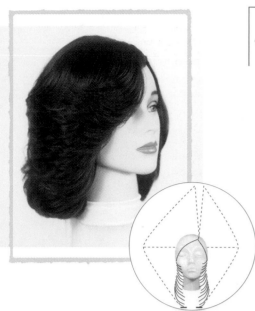

Apply *Light Layers*

With your clients, these technical steps will follow the consultation and shampoo.

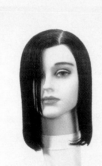

This haircut features long or "light" layers that flow over the perimeter blunt haircut. More layers frame the front area and move towards a lesser amount at the center back of the head.

1. Comb the hair in natural fall, and establish a side part on the left side. Create a blunt cut, following the steps for the horizontal blunt (page 60).

2. Locate the natural fringe area by parting a triangular section from the side part to the recession area, at the outside corner of the eyes. Part off a 1/2" (1.25 cm) horizontal section from the front and clip the remainder of the section out of the way. Use a point of reference on the face, such as the lip, for where you'll begin cutting diagonally back.

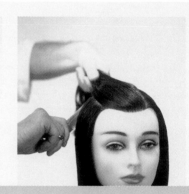

3. Direct the hair in natural fall and position your fingers diagonally; position the scissors to follow the same diagonal line your fingers form. Begin cutting near the lip and follow the angle of your fingers. Cut the entire fringe section to this guide.

4. Repeat this procedure on the opposite side of the part. Pick up the hair at the recession area of the right side. Cut diagonally from the lip line back, just as you did before.

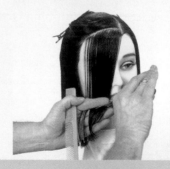

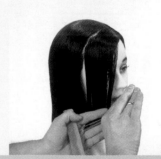

5. Section out a rectangle section through the interior of the head.

6. Begin at the front hairline area by taking a horizontal parting from the front of the section.

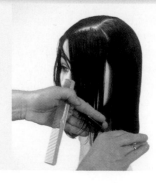

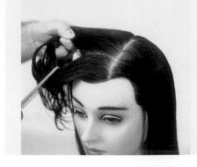

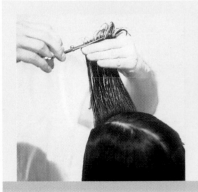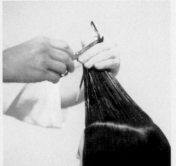

7. Hold this section straight up from the top of the head and begin cutting out diagonally about 6 inches from the scalp. This will be your stable guide.

8. Hold the stable guide straight up from the top of the head and bring partings to it as you cut on a slightly upward angle from the side part outward. Work from the front to the back of the section, taking partings and directing them to the initial stable guide until you complete the section. This technique will create a length increase.

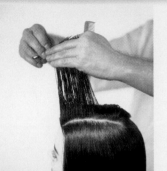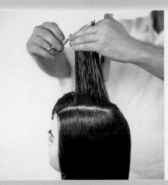

9. Cross-check these internal lengths by taking a vertical parting from the front to the crown. Note how the angle moves from shorter at the front . ..

10. . . . to longer at the crown area. Direct lengths straight up and check the line.

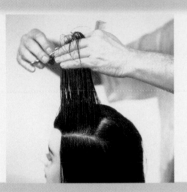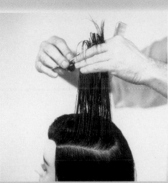

11. Use this internal length increase as your guideline for cutting the sides. Part vertically through the side. Using a section of hair from the top as the guideline, bring sections straight up, distributing the hair neatly to the stable guide, then cut to this guide along the diagonal line created.

12. Moving back, bring lengths straight up to the stable guide for cutting. Notice how the fingers of the holding hand are angled diagonally upward from front to back.

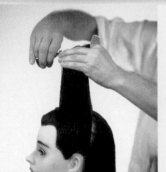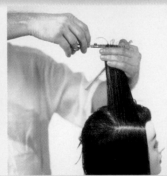

13. Continue layering one side until you run out of hair. This will be where you meet the lengths from the horizontal blunt.

14. Move to the opposite side and begin bringing sections to the stable guides and cutting diagonally.

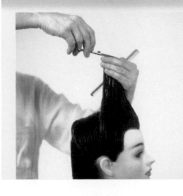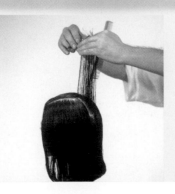

15. Continue layering that side until completed.

16. Blend the crown lengths into the top area. Use pivotal partings to work around the back crown area. Direct lengths straight up from the top of the head and begin cutting out diagonally using the predetermined length/guide from the top.

17. Continue this procedure through the crown to complete the layering procedure.

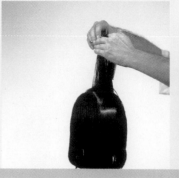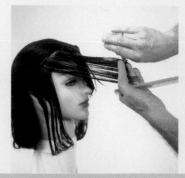

18. After completing the layering, check the cut response. Finish the cut by checking the line framing the face. Direct lengths forward and position the fingers outward from the fringe length cut earlier to refine the line.

19. Repeat the procedure on the other side.

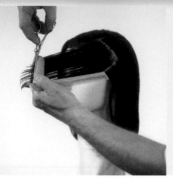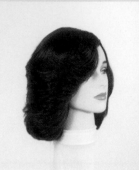

20. The finished silhouette shows the long layers that have been created. These layers will allow for movement, surface texture, and dimension to be achieved in the finished style. The cut is very versatile and can be styled a variety of ways, whether back from the face or forward onto the face.

If you can imagine it, you can achieve it. If you can dream it, you can become it.

William Arthur Ward

Explore

Apply this technique to different lengths, colors, and textures for almost endless possibilities.

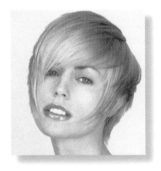

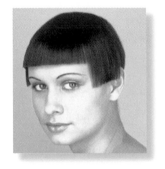

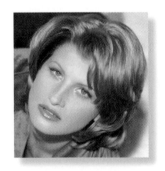

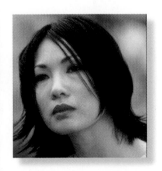

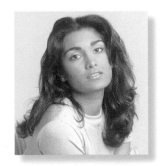

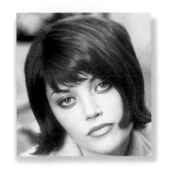

Building Your
Clientele

The best preparation for tomorrow is the right use of today.

Robert C. Savage

Look to this day, for it is life . . . the very life of life. Yesterday is but a dream and tomorrow only a vision . . . but today well lived will make all your tomorrows worthwhile.

—from the Sanskrit

That's a pretty intense opening for an essay on building a salon clientele, but there's a point here. Everything you do builds upon everything else to determine how successful you will be. That's the "today well lived makes every tomorrow worthwhile" point. As a stylist, you'll be successful when you have a loyal clientele who eagerly return to you time and again for service; so the time and effort you invest today to attract and retain clients will make tomorrow's paychecks worthwhile.

Later in this program you'll find more about how to satisfy clients, once they are in your chair, so they'll keep coming back. Here we discuss how to get those clients into your chair in the first place.

Many salons, because of their location in a mall or other high-traffic area, have a good amount of walk-in traffic that is assigned to new stylists. Others will advertise for new clients and offer a discount if they book with a new stylist. You may choose to work in such a salon for your first job simply because the "attracting" part is taken care of for you; all you have to do is provide top-notch service and personal attention to keep the clients coming back.

If, however, you choose to work in a salon because you like the work being done there, and that salon isn't in a high-traffic location or doesn't do a lot of advertising and promotion, then you'll need to do some yourself. The best way for a new stylist to create a clientele is to begin with who you know—and who they know. Here's a step-by-step plan.

1. Have business cards printed. A "quick print" shop can do it inexpensively. Talk to your new employer about sharing the expense, or at least letting you use the salon's logo and artwork to create your card. And remember, you're a designer. Your card should look good.

2. Make a list of everyone you know: your friends and family, their friends and family, neighbors, and the like. Send them your card with a simple letter that tells them where you're working, the address and phone number, and what your hours are and offer them a discount on their first service with you. Enclose extra cards for them to give to their friends.

3. When you service a client for the first time, make sure you ask her to rebook her next service before she leaves the salon. Give her your card and ask her to tell her friends about you. Tell her about your referral rewards program: She puts her name on the back of the card and gives it to a friend. If that friend books a service, you'll send the referring client a "thank-you for the referral" note with a gift certificate for a percentage off her next service. Or the incentive could be a free retail product or a free manicure or other "add-on" service. (Yes, you're spending a little money, but it's an investment that will pay off in the future.)

Stylists whose schedules are full every day will tell you that time flies, and work is something to look forward to. Use your time wisely and creatively to let people know about you, and do everything you can to encourage referrals.

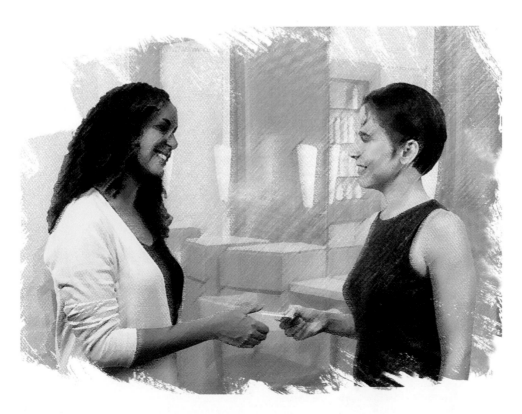

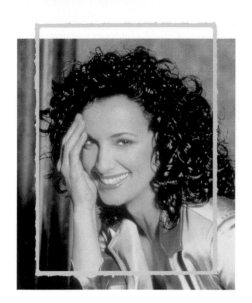

Heavy Layers

Overview

This shape's heavily layered or textured effect comes from the cutting technique used throughout the interior. It can be worn straight or in a full, voluminous look; it can be styled forward or back. It provides the client with great versatility.

Connect
Traveling Guide

Because you use a traveling guide throughout the interior of this cut—not a stable guide, which builds more length and weight—you'll end up with shorter layers through the top. This will give extra lift and volume to this interior area.

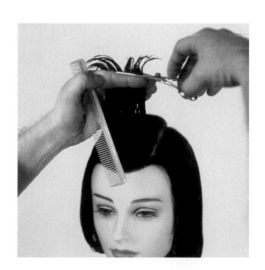

Cutting the Lengths

All lengths are brought straight up from the top of the head and cut horizontally.

All lengths through the crest of the head (curved region of the head) are brought straight out and cut outward along your fingers using the cutting out position, which should extend from the center top. You can adapt this cutting out position to cut a more extreme length increase by angling your fingers along a steeper diagonal. Another option is to bring these lengths straight up to blend the length to the top, rather than using a straight-out holding position. This would maximize length and weight.

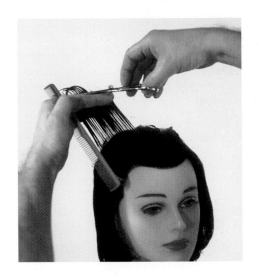

Focus

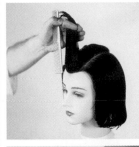
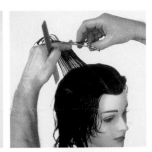

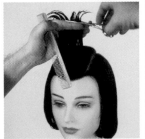
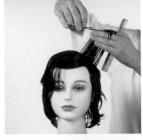

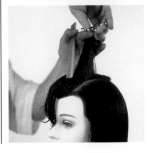
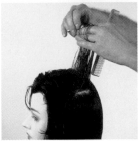

Holding Position—Through the top, use a straight-up or vertical holding position. Through the crest hold the hair straight out from the curve of the head.

Cutting Position—The cutting position through the top is horizontal. Use the cutting out position through the crest area to blend outward with the top length. Cut the hair through with your fingers aligned to blend outward with the top lengths.

Traveling Guide—Use a traveling guide throughout the top as well as around the crest.

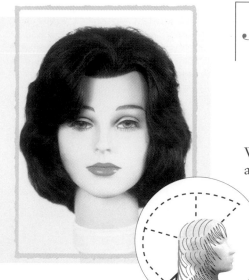

Apply Heavy Layers

With your clients, these technical steps will follow the consultation and shampoo.

In this heavily layered shape, lengths progress from short layers through the interior, to longer layers at the exterior. The layers provide textured volume.

1. On a client you may first need to establish the perimeter length and shape. Create a Diagonal Back Blunt off a center part, following the steps on page 76-77. Create a center part and take a 1/2″ (1.25 cm) section along the top front hairline.

2. Comb and hold the hair downward over the face at low elevation. Use a point of reference on the face, such as the lip, to establish the length, cutting horizontally.

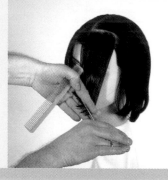
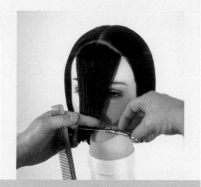

3. Section through the entire side hairline area. Direct and hold the hair with your fingers positioned diagonally. Cut the side lengths to blend from the fringe to the exterior length. Repeat on the other side, cutting diagonally.

4. Part out a rectangular section through the top from the front hairline to the crown.

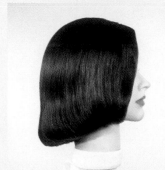
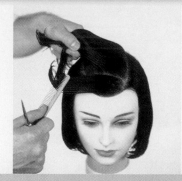

5. Part out a horizontal section at the front hairline. Hold the previously established front guide straight up from the top of the head.

6. Cut horizontally.

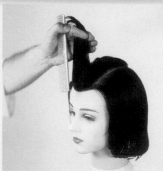
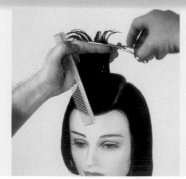

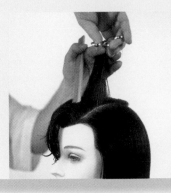
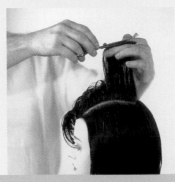

7. Use this section as a traveling guide. Pick up a small portion of it with each newly parted out section and cut horizontally, moving back toward the crown. Continue to use the same holding position, straight up from the top of the head, and horizontal cutting position throughout.

8. Cross-check your work through this top area by taking vertical sections and holding them straight up from the top of the head. Clean up any unevenness.

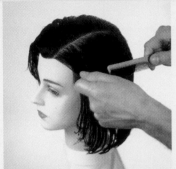
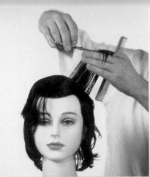

9. Section through the crest area. Part off a vertical section at the front hairline. Direct this section up and out from the crest area.

10. Begin cutting out with your fingers in the position shown. This connects to the length from the top.

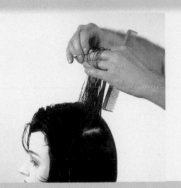
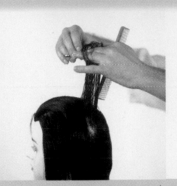

11. Use the first section as a traveling guide to cut the sections behind it. Angle the fingers diagonally and continue cutting out.

12. Take radial partings from the crown as you move from the side toward the center back, cutting out to the established guide line.

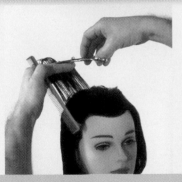
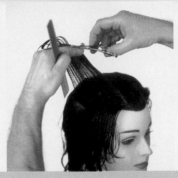

13., 14. Repeat the steps on the right side, starting with the establishment of the traveling guide.

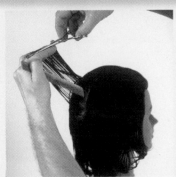
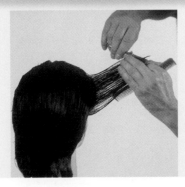

15. Work back and use radial partings as you move around the crown. Continue until you reach the center back.

16. In this technique you are cutting toward the perimeter. Continue this technique to the center back as a control measure for blending all lengths outward.

$\mathscr{R}$ eflect

$\mathscr{E}$ xplore

Apply this technique to different lengths, colors, and textures for almost endless possibilities

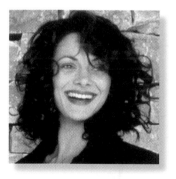

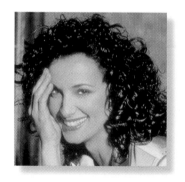

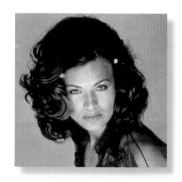

Establishing Your
Reputation

*E*verything you do that is witnessed by others becomes part of your reputation. In other words, people receive you as they perceive you. A reputation isn't who you are inside, it's what you demonstrate to others on the outside. That goes for your reputation as a person as well as a professional hairstylist.

The good news is that, with a little effort, you can control your reputation. You can manage the perceptions that others have of you. And that will benefit your career.

The most important thing to remember about reputation is: It's a lot easier to keep a good reputation than it is to lose a bad one. You can begin now to create a great reputation if you follow the list of do's and don'ts below.

Top Ten Ways to Create a Great Reputation ▼

1. Do come to work on time and give your best effort.
2. Do communicate easily and effectively with others.
3. Do react positively and receptively when a supervisor or senior stylist offers advice or instruction.
4. Do volunteer for a variety of work to develop your skills.
5. Do acknowledge when you've made a mistake and demonstrate that you've learned from it.
6. When a client appears dissatisfied with a service, don't ignore the problem.
7. Do ask what you can do to correct a problem and follow through until the client is satisfied.
8. Do observe salon time standards.
9. Don't get caught up in negative workplace politics.
10. Do continue your education and study new trends.

Perception is reality.

Immanuel Kant,

18th-century German philosopher

(paraphrased)

Reputations, both good and bad, last long after they are deserved.

Louann Werksma,

20th-century American writer

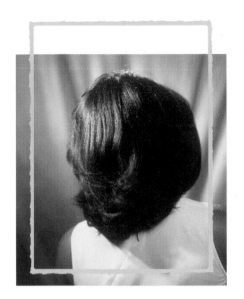

Heavy Layers

on pressed hair

Overview

A client who prefers to wear her curly hair in a smooth and straight finished style has two choices: Either chemically relax the hair or press the natural curl into a smooth texture. If the client chooses the nonchemical pressing alternative, you must first press the hair smooth and then cut it dry. This will ensure the creation of the most accurate, precise shape.

Techniques for straightening hair have come and gone through the years, but applying heat to dry curly or kinky hair along with pressure is a method that has endured. Pressing hair to straighten it will always be a popular technique, and it's important to know the proper method for cutting a pressed head of hair.

While many haircuts are performed on damp hair, hair that has been pressed will be cut dry. Not only does the dry method maintain the straightening achieved by pressing, but it permits greater precision in creating the shape, because you can perfectly predict where the hair will fall in the finished style. Whether dried straight and smooth or dried naturally, a precise shape is ensured.

Connect

Cutting Curly Hair

Determining the true length of very curly hair can be quite difficult. If you cut it wet, you run the risk of cutting too much hair length. When you cut hair dry, there is no second guessing as to how it will look because you're immediately seeing and creating the client's desired length and shape.

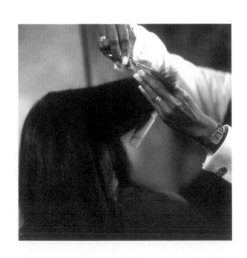

Cutting Pressed Hair Dry

The purpose of pressing hair is to remove the natural texture and achieve a smooth, glossy look. But pressed hair will regain its natural texture once it comes into contact with water. (Remember how all kinds of hair get frizzy on an extremely humid day?) Since the goal of pressing hair is to remove the natural texture, creating smoothness, wetting it for cutting defeats the purpose of pressing it. Always cut pressed hair dry.

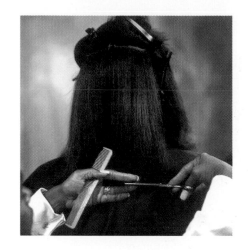

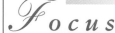

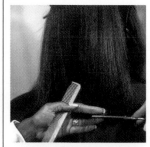

Dry Cutting—When you're dry cutting, keep in mind that the hair has no elasticity. This means it won't contract. Therefore, precision is the key to dry cutting.

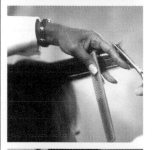

Holding Position—In the back and side perimeter, hold the hair in low elevation. In the fringe area, cut the hair in natural fall. Hold the hair straight out from the side while cutting the interior.

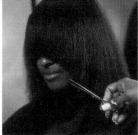

Cutting Position—The cutting position is horizontal in the back and in the fringe area. Around the sides of the face and through the interior, cut at a diagonal.

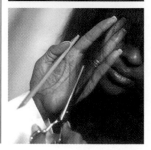

Scissor Position—In the back perimeter, fringe area, and interior, the scissor hand is palm down.

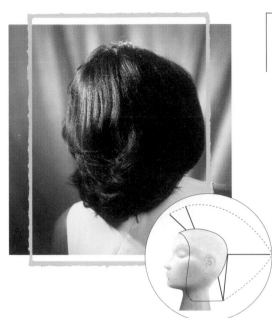

Apply *Heavy Layers*
on pressed hair

Before beginning this service, blow-dry the hair and press with a pressing iron. (Refer to the Hairstyling section, page 288 for more information.) After you complete the cut, curl the hair to add soft movement and body. (See page 292 for details.)

Heavy layers flow through the interior and along the perimeter frame that has been cut blunt.

1. Divide the hair into four sections: crown area, right side, left side, and back. Starting at the center back, hold the hair straight down and cut a horizontal line using a low (one-finger) elevation. Work toward the left side.

2. Release the hair in the crown area. Notice that the previously cut layers do not reach the blunt perimeter. These lengths will get cut during the layering process. Move to the right side of the back section, comb the hair down and cut.

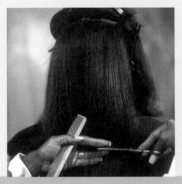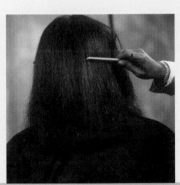

3. At the front of the head, comb the fringe section forward and, using the tip of the nose as a guide, cut straight across and adjacent to the outside corner of the eye. Repeat to cut the other half of the fringe.

4. Move to the side of the head. Comb the side and top sections slightly forward and, using the front fringe area as a guide, cut the side at a diagonal from the nose down, blending it with the fringe area framing the face.

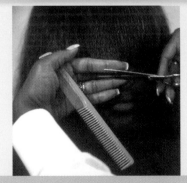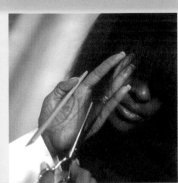

5. Move to the other side and continue framing the face, blending the hair at a diagonal with the fringe area.

6. Move to the top front area. Make partings so that they pivot around the crown. Part out a pie-shaped section from the top center crown to the front hairline. Hold the hair straight out from the front of the head and begin cutting out along the fingers to create a length increase.

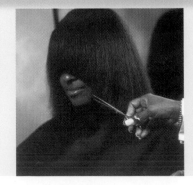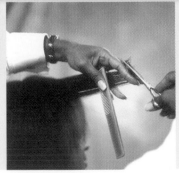

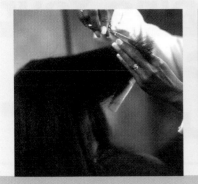
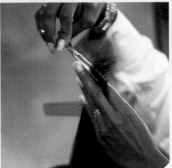

7. Move around the head, continuing to part out sections that radiate from the crown, holding them straight out from the side of the head and cutting out to the traveling guide that you've created.

8. Move through the crown of the head. Hold the hair straight out from the curve of the head and begin cutting out.

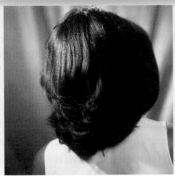

9. The haircut was curled to complete the style. (See page 292 in the Hairstyling section for more detail.) The completed style has fluid movement and frames the face with a soft fringe.

R eflect

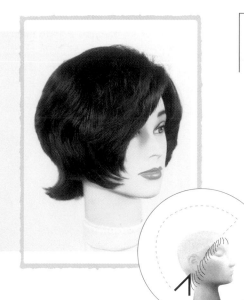

Apply
Full Layers

With your clients, these technical steps will follow the consultation and shampoo.

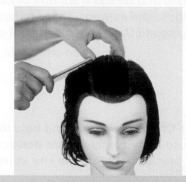

Shown here is the completely layered shape. Lengths move progressively from short layers in the interior to long at the exterior area.

1. Comb the hair in natural fall. Part out a rectangular section from the front hairline to the crown and upward from the center eye on either side.

2. Part a 1/2″ (1.25 cm) section from the front of the section at the hairline. Comb and hold at a low elevation and cut it horizontally to the tip of the nose.

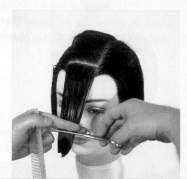

3. Holding the hair in natural fall, connect and blend this fringe length diagonally through the sides.

4. Release horizontal sections through the interior. Use the initially cut section to establish the traveling guide. Each section is held straight out from the curve of the head and cut horizontally.

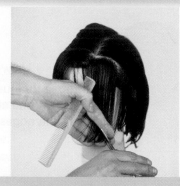
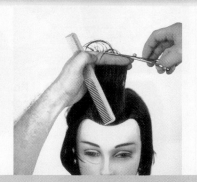

5. Work all the way back to the crown, picking up a portion of the previously cut section each time to act as a traveling guide. Comb and distribute the hair neatly out from the head and cut horizontally.

6. Having completed the top area, part out vertical partings through the crest area for layering through this panel. Direct the lengths straight up and out from the head and begin cutting out toward the perimeter area using a traveling guide.

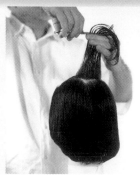
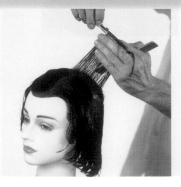

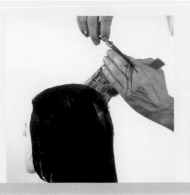
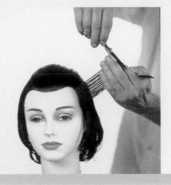

7. Continue this holding and cutting position to the center back. The partings radiate around the crown area.

8. Move to the next panel. Part off vertically, holding the hair straight and begin cutting out to blend to the perimeter frame.

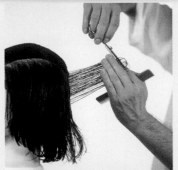
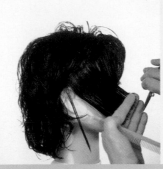

9. Using this section as a traveling guide, work toward the center back, cutting the side panels. The panels should be about 2" (5 cm) wide. Check through the nape lengths with vertical sections. Cross-check your work by pulling sections out horizontally. Work throughout the entire haircut in this manner.

10. To complete the cut, check and refine the entire perimeter frame area.

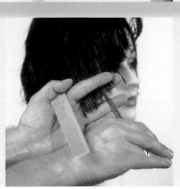
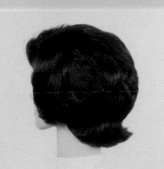

11. Detail the front perimeter to suit the face. Here, point cutting softens the look. Place the fingers according to the depth of pointing that will be made into the ends of the hair. Observe and check the softness as it's developing.

12. The layered cut gives the hair a lot of movement. The finished style shows the cut with a subtle flip in the nape area. This shape offers a multitude of styling options.

Wealth is not his that has it, but his that enjoys it.

Benjamin Franklin

Reflect

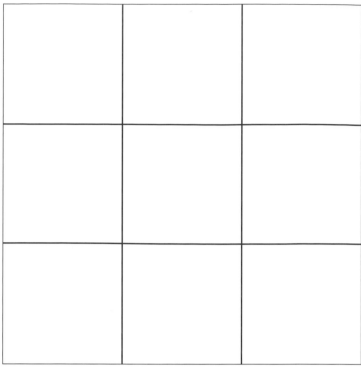

Explore

Apply this technique to different lengths, colors, and textures for almost endless possibilities.

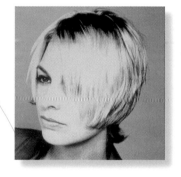
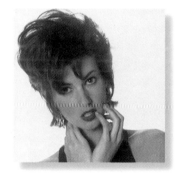
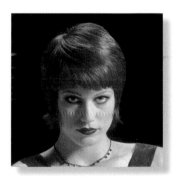

The 80/20 Rule

Here is a simple but powerful rule . . . always give people more than they expect to get.

Nelson Boswell

There's a rule that's often repeated in businesses the world over. It's called the 80/20 rule, and it has several variations, including this one: 80 percent of your success as a stylist comes from your nontechnical skills, while 20 percent of your success is based on your technical skills.

In other words, clients choose their stylists only partly because they like their cuts, colors, and texture services. Far more important than these technical skills, however, are their interpersonal skills. Below are some examples of the interpersonal skills that make some stylists top performers.

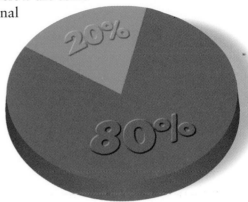

Traits of Top 20 Performers ▼

1. Showing genuine interest in clients and perceiving them as people, not just heads of hair
2. Listening to clients and learning about their image needs
3. Making every client visit a special time of personal attention and pampering
4. Looking to the future and creating a customized client service plan (see page 431) for each client
5. Following up with thank-you cards and calls, appointment reminders, and birthday and holiday remembrances
6. Finding the right way to communicate with each client to make her comfortable enough to develop trust
7. Educating clients about home-care products and styling techniques, and giving them an opportunity to purchase needed items before they leave the salon
8. Managing time wisely
9. Maintaining good health habits: proper exercise, nutrition, and rest
10. Ensuring that clients rebook for their next service before leaving the salon
11. Paying attention to their clients' patterns of visits and calling clients who have been away longer than expected
12. Encouraging clients to refer their friends and rewarding them when they do
13. Keeping their hairstyling skills and knowledge current

Keep a copy of this list handy so that you remember to practice these behaviors. In no time, you will be a top performer yourself.

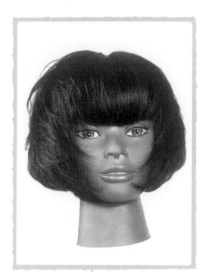

Layered Graduation

with clippers

Overview

Clipper cutting decreases cutting time—which means faster service. Using this free-form method will give you very accurate results because it offers precision in creating lines. Generally, when you use a clipper, the emphasis of the cut will be on the silhouette. For extra control, some stylists use both hands to hold the clipper. If you're holding the clipper with one hand and the hair or a comb with your other, remember that the more tension you use, the more precise the line your clipper will create. Before you begin any cut with your clipper, however, you must envision where you are going with it.

Connect
Choosing Clipper Blades

Be sure to select the proper clipper blade to create the desired look. Some blades—such as the kind with a diagonal cutting angle—produce a textured look by layering the hair as they cut. Straight blades create precision looks by cutting hair all one length.

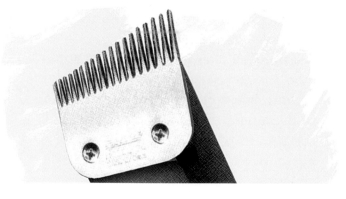

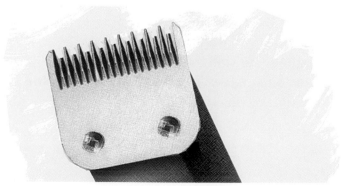

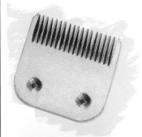

Clipper Care—Always make sure there are no nicks, broken metal, or sharpness on the blade that could injure skin. When you clipper cut against the skin in some areas, you will have to apply light pressure, and any irregular sharpness could cut the skin. Clean and oil your clipper unit and blades to maintain its condition.

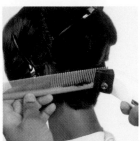

Beveling Comb—Beveling the comb involves turning it to angle outward away from the head while clippering the hair. The angle at which the comb is held and moved will determine the degree of graduation created.

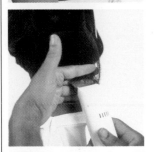

Free-Form Cutting—To use this style of cutting, comb the hair down on the face and cut without applying tension. Create the frame around the head and face, using the facial and head features as guides—for example, earlobe, cheek, or eyebrow. This technique uses no sectioning and no tension.

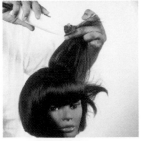

Condensed Cutting Technique—This technique allows you to cut large sections of hair at once, creating softness in the layered shape. Gather hair together at the front of the head, perhaps at the tip of the nose or the eyebrows or forehead; then make a single cut.

> ***Man alone can dream
> and make his dreams
> come true.***
>
> *Napoleon Hill*

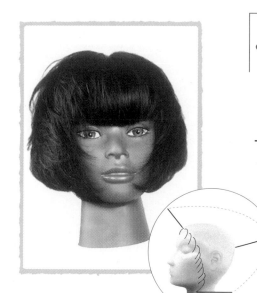

Apply
Layered Graduation
with clippers

With your clients, these technical steps will follow the consultation and pressing.

In this design, interior layers flow over the perimeter graduation. A blunt fringe adds dramatic flair. Precise lines are easily created using the clipper cutting technique.

1. Before beginning examine the clipper blade to ensure that it is in top notch condition. Clean and oil the clipper regularly. Begin by doing a rough cut through the back area to remove excess length. Work methodically with the blade inverted against the hair as shown.

2. Establish the perimeter frame through the back of the head. Point the clipper blade toward the neck and use the clipper to create the line from ear to ear.

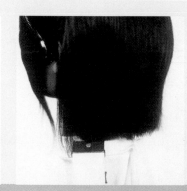

3. At the front of the head, section off the fringe area. For instructional purposes only, a piece of white cardboard has been clipped under the fringe. Cut first at the center of the forehead area, then extend the line outward on either side, to the outside corner of the eyes. Leave the fringe slightly longer if you intend to use an iron, which will make the fringe look shorter.

4. Move to the left side. Establish a new length for the side. This design length does not connect to the back section. From the tip of the earlobe to the jawline is the ideal length on the appropriate head shape.

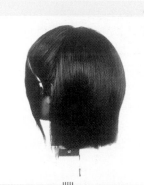

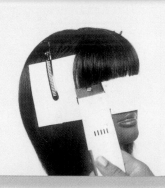

5. Note the new position used here to sweep the blade sideways along the line. Cut to refine.

6. Create the same perimeter line on the other side. This freehand inverted clipper position works well when cutting a line against the skin. If cutting away from the head, hold the hair between the fingers.

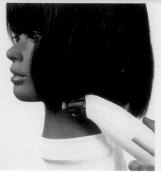

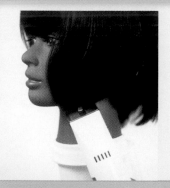

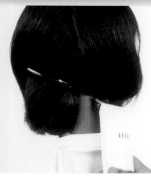

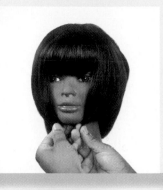
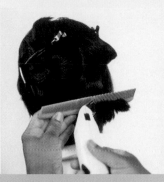

7. Using your mirror and standing directly in front of the head, check for balance in the length of your cut.

8. Using a clipper-over-comb technique, taper the neckline area. Hold a section of hair straight out from the curve of the head with the comb angled as shown. Establish your first cut with the clipper. Remember to envision where you are going with the cut.

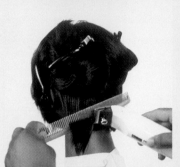
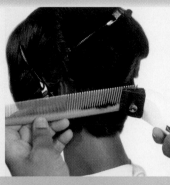

9. Continue to create graduation toward the outer edges of the nape, using the clipper-over-comb technique. As you work toward the occipital bone, allow your elevation to gradually move outward from the neckline

10. The comb here is slightly beveled—closer to the head along the back edge of the comb, and farther away from the head along its teeth. Note the high graduation developing through this area.

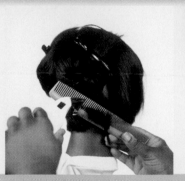
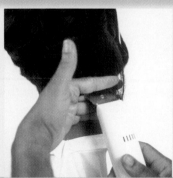

11. Consistency in angling the comb, hair length, and graduation are essential. Blend from the center area toward the area behind the ear.

12. When you're cutting to blend the remainder of the back to the graduated nape area, control the hair lengths for cutting between the fingers.

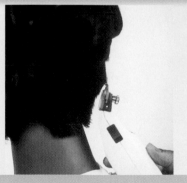
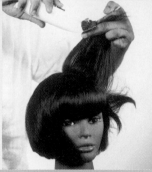

13. Refine the sculptured shape for softness and precision using the clipper.

14. Through the top of the head, you will use a condensed cutting technique with large sections that radiate around the curve of the head. Comb a large section up behind the fringe. Begin cutting out from the fringe to the crown lengths. You will use this as a guide to move around the head with radial sections cutting out.

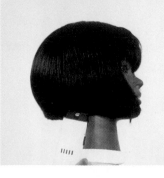
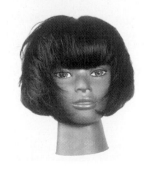

15. Comb and check the cut around the entire perimeter of the head for detail, trimming any uneven hair.

16. The finished style is smooth and voluminous, with graduation creating body at the nape.

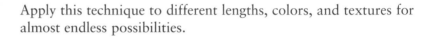

Reflect

Explore

Apply this technique to different lengths, colors, and textures for almost endless possibilities.

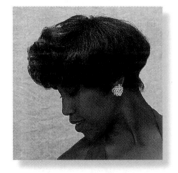

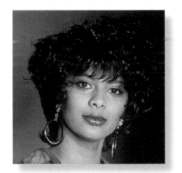

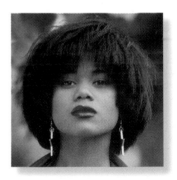

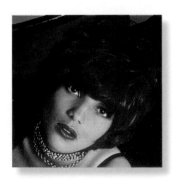

Continuing Education
and
Professional Development

Education is not filling a bucket, but lighting a fire.

William Yeats

There's only one corner of the universe you can be certain of improving, and that's yourself.

Aldous Huxley

After 13 years of public education and then one to two years of career education, many stylists have been heard to say, "I'm done with school!"

Well, you can be done with school, but you should never be done with education. Learning should be a lifelong habit, particularly for someone entering the fashion industry, where trends change and new skills and techniques are introduced daily.

One way to ensure your continuing education and professional development is to look for jobs at salons that make education a priority. When you're being interviewed, interview the owner right back. Ask, "What continuing education does the salon provide?"

Even if you don't work in a salon that makes ongoing education a priority (although today most good salons do), make it your responsibility to get to know what courses, workshops, and materials may be available from beauty supply distributors in your area, regional hair shows, and community colleges. Perhaps the school you're currently attending offers advanced education for alumni. At the very least, you can purchase videos and books, and practice, practice, practice. Join your local professional association for hairstylists; subscribe to professional magazines; keep on top of what's happening in your profession; learn what education is available in your area. Make lifelong learning your goal.

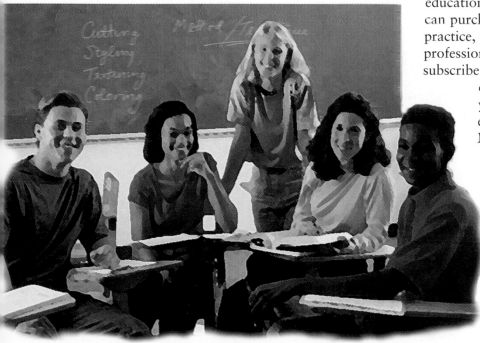

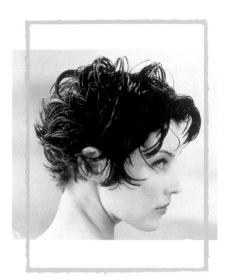

High Graduation

Overview

In this shape, you'll create high graduation throughout the entire back area of the cut to blend and harmonize with the layered shape that frames the face through the top and sides. This cut defines the head shape through the back area by the closer contours of the graduation; the layered lengths around the face frame it attractively, adding a soft feminine touch as well as versatility.

Connect Graduation

In this haircut, the entire back area is graduated, from shorter at the perimeter area at the nape toward longer at the crown. You'll continue graduating including the top and sides by bringing them back to a stable guide that runs from ear to ear.

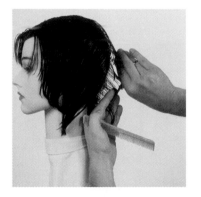

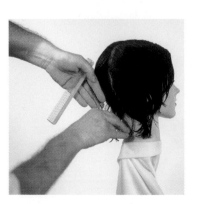

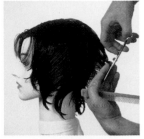

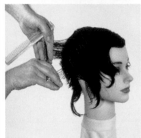

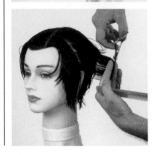

Holding Position and Guides—Throughout the entire back area, hold the hair straight out from the side of the head and use a traveling guide. Around the top and sides, use a stable guide, holding the hair straight out from the curve of the head from a vertical section taken ear to ear.

Cutting Position—To create the graduated effect, use the cutting in position along your fingers, which you should position diagonally to the head.

I have had dreams, and I have had nightmares. I overcame the nightmares because of my dreams.

Jonas Salk, MD

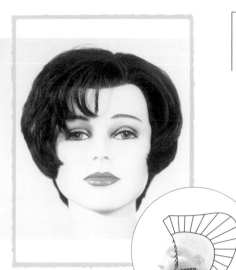

Apply
High Graduation

With your clients, these technical steps will follow the consultation and shampoo.

This versatile shape combines a high graduation through the back with soft layers that frame the face.

1. Comb the hair in natural fall. Create a side part. Distribute the hair around the curve of the head in natural fall.

2. Move to the back and part out a 1/2" (1.25 cm) section from crown to nape.

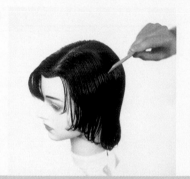
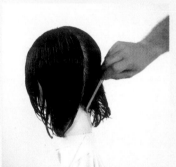

3. Starting at the top of the section, hold the hair straight back from the crown area, angling the fingers outward from the curve of the head. Begin cutting in along the section angling toward the nape.

4. Continue down the section, cutting in closer to the head as you approach the nape. This will be your traveling guide for the top and sides. Notice the holding position, straight out from the curve of the head, as you work from the crest area down.

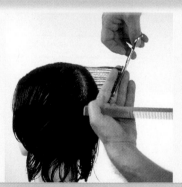

5. Finish cutting the traveling guide at the nape, directly below the section you just cut.

6. Part out the next vertical section and cut along the traveling guide, using the same holding position and cutting angle. Continue parting and cutting vertical sections. Take a small portion of the first section you cut, hold it with the next vertical section, and move from the back toward the sides, cutting sections to the same angle as the traveling guide. Let the guide travel slightly toward the new section being cut.

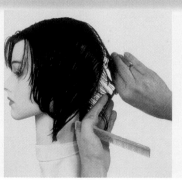
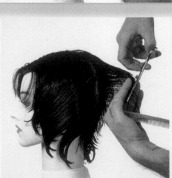

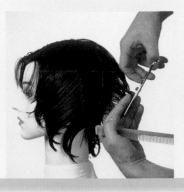
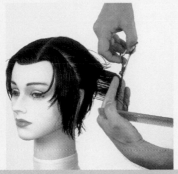

7. Part out vertically, pivoting around the crown. Follow the traveling guide forward, cutting from the top section toward the nape. Always pull the hair straight out from the curve of the head and use the cutting in position along the guide.

8. Continue cutting the back and sides until you reach the ear area.

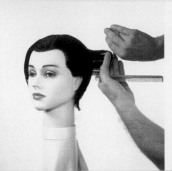
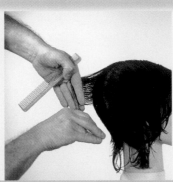

9. The last back section that you cut, which is behind the ear, will now serve as a stable guide to which you will bring all the side lengths. Hold the section above the ear straight out from the curve of the head. Direct all side lengths back to this guide, section by section, and use the cutting in position along the pre-established line. This will create the layered effect through the front.

10. Move to the opposite side. Pick up your traveling guide to follow.

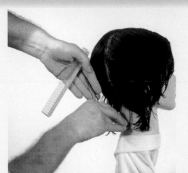
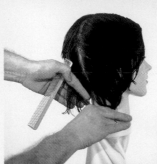

11. Complete each vertical section, using the same technique that you used on the left side.

12. The vertical sections that you are cutting radiate around the head. Make sure you follow your traveling guide, which should be visible at all times.

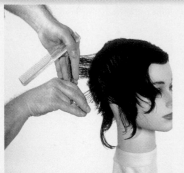
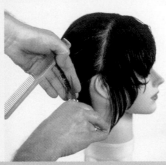

13. Stop using a traveling guide when you reach the ear area, as you did on the left side.

14. At this point, you'll switch to a stable guide, as you did before. Bring sections back to this guide.

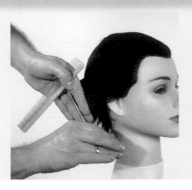
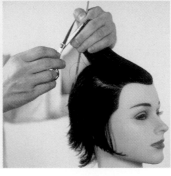

15. Continue using the stable guide to cut the remainder of the sides, bringing 1/2" (1.25 cm) sections back to it.

16. Bring top sections back to the crown to check in and blend internal lengths across the top of the head. Cross-check throughout the cut, cleaning up any unevenness.

17. In the finished cut, graduated effects make for much textural movement.

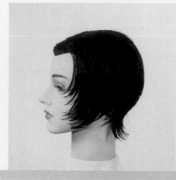

18. Refine the perimeter of the cut, working with the facial shape and hair texture. A slicing technique is used here to soften and variegate the perimeter line.

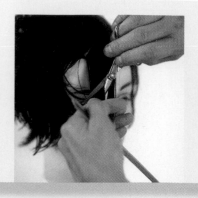
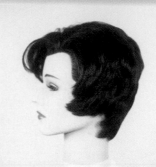

19. The finished shape has a diffused softness to it. The face-framing layers blend harmoniously with the graduated back area. This is a versatile and very desirable shape to suit a multitude of clients.

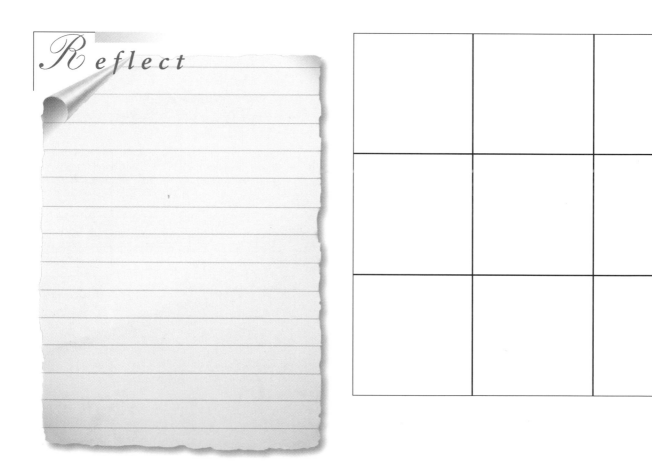

Reflect

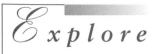

Explore

Apply this technique to different lengths, colors, and textures for almost endless possibilities.

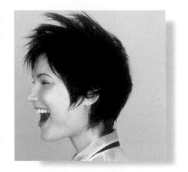
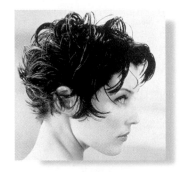
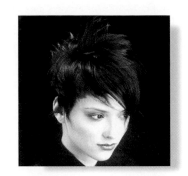

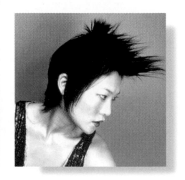
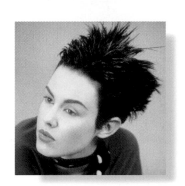

Destiny is not a matter of chance, it is a matter of choice; it is not a thing to be waited for, it is a thing to be achieved.

William Jennings Bryan

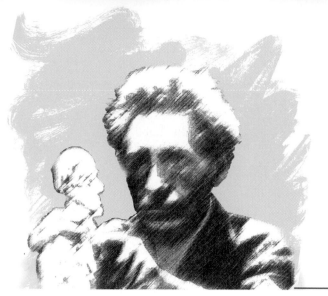

Razor Cutting

A sculptor using his tool

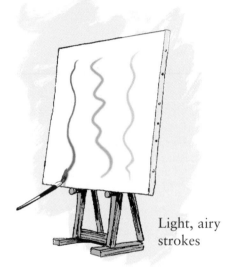

Light, airy strokes

The razor is a superb tool for making the hair fluid and supple. Using the razor may be equated to sculpting the hair in that it carves or etches into the hair to remove the desired lengths, much as a sculptor using a tool to cut into clay. Razor cutting tapers the lengths, creating a variety of lengths, and eliminates any angularity. This type of cutting is used to very good effect wherever a soft, diffused, wispy or fringy edge is desired.

Using the razor requires a light versus a heavy-handed approach. Think of razoring the hair as making brushstrokes on a canvas—delicate and measured, yet allowing great creativity, especially in the areas around the hairline, where a more freeform approach can be used. Using a razor to cut hair creates softly variegated texture along the edges as opposed to the blunt straight edge achieved with the shears.

It is very important to work with a sharp razor to make razoring quick and efficient as well as comfortable for the client.

Tool Position

Note the position of the tool as held in the hand. The handle is opened out to create a straight edge with the blade area.

Blade Position

When etching the hair with a razor, it is important that the blade is against the hair and the guard is facing toward you. Consider the angle of the blade against the hair for the amount of taper that you want to create. When the blade is flat against the hair, the taper along the strand is the most elongated; when the blade is angled toward the hair, you can adjust or adapt the amount of the taper at the edge.

There are some very interesting state-of-the-art razors available that you may want to seek out to progress your skills further in this area. This is also a frequently used tool and approach in men's cutting.

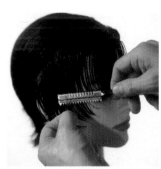

Blunt, straight edges

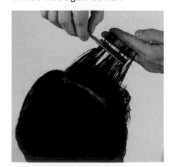

Blade flat against hair

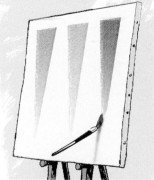

Etching as a tapering effect

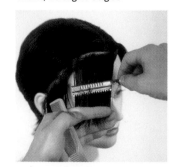

Blade angled toward hair.

layered razor cut

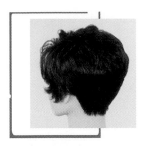

*T*he heavily layered shape will be very light and airy—rounded throughout the interior and contoured close through the nape.

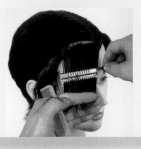 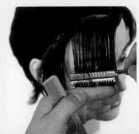

1. Comb the hair in natural fall. Take a 1/2" (1.25 cm) section at the front hairline, holding it at low elevation. Cut it to the desired length with the razor. Position the guard toward you and the blade against the hair. Place the razor at that point along the strand where you want to begin the tapering effect. Then etch the razor back and forth along the strand as shown.

2. Cut parallel to the hairline and taper toward your fingers.

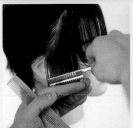 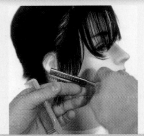

3. Continue cutting around the hairline, down the side.

4. Take 1/2" (1.25 cm) partings, position the razor where you want to start tapering the length, and angle it so the section will blend to one you previously cut.

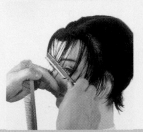 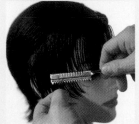

5. Complete the front perimeter on both sides, blending to your initial guide.

6. Refine the fringe all the way around as desired by taking small pieces and razoring them separately. The more pieces you cut, the more light and airy the finished look will be.

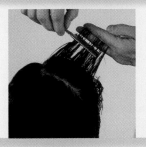 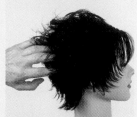

7. Using the previously cut hairline perimeter sections as your traveling guides, work from the front to the back, razoring the hair in 1/2" (1.25 cm) sections. Etch along the top of the hair to taper from the mid-shaft toward the ends, removing the length just above the fingers.

8. Move to the back and taper the nape. Hold the sections slightly outward, then etch along the top surface to create the desired length.

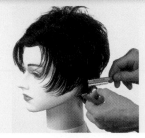 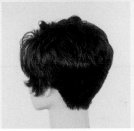

9. The variety of lengths throughout the silhouette creates volume without any hard edges. Personalize the nape area as required. Leave fringy and soft, or take short to contrast with the longer frame around the face.

10. The finished style is softly tapered throughout for movement and dimension.

Quality is the first thing seen, service is the first thing felt and price is the first thing forgotten.

Jay Goltz

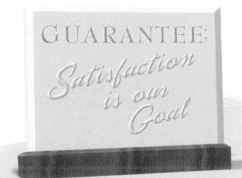

GUARANTEE: *Satisfaction is our Goal*

Another name for a policy is a rule, and a well-run business needs rules and policies to protect itself, employees, and customers. For example, policies regarding sanitation procedures and correct use of chemicals protect the health and safety of everyone inside the salon. At the same time, by creating a safe environment for both employees and customers, the salon business protects itself from expensive legal actions that could result if someone in the salon hurts herself because a floor wasn't clean and dry or a chemical wasn't mixed properly.

Other policies help resolve conflicts that sometimes arise among coworkers. They also can help solve problems and keep clients from leaving the salon. For example, if the manager is not in and a client complains that a perm was over-processed and her hair damaged, which of the salons described below will have a better reputation and be more successful?

The No-Policies Salon

Salon employee: "I'm sorry, ma'am, but my manager is out and we can't give refunds or do anything unless he's here. You'll just have to call him or come back."

The Customer-Satisfaction Salon

Salon employee: "Ms. Alexander, we're truly sorry. We took every precaution to ensure that the perm product we used would not damage your hair, but in rare instances the hair's chemistry combines with the chemicals in the perm solution in ways we cannot predict. But your satisfaction is our goal. Our customer service policy states that you will not have to pay for your service today, and we would also like to schedule a complimentary follow-up corrective appointment. In the meantime, I'd like to give you this special conditioner to use on your hair daily to condition it . . . no charge, of course. Do you have any questions?"

When a salon's management has taken the time to create policies that help employees and customers solve problems, that is a well-managed salon. When you're interviewing for your first salon job, find out if it's a good fit for you. Ask the interviewer, "What policies do you have concerning customer complaints?"

Employee Orientation
to the
Salon

The important thing is not to stop questioning.

Albert Einstein

Your introduction to how a salon operates, its rules, and its procedures will probably happen on your first day. Some salons take a whole day or several days to conduct a formal training program for all client service employees before they ever work with clients. The salons do this because they believe that if employees are given time to learn what is expected of them, they are more likely to have a positive experience working in the salon. Others put all the information in an employee manual and expect new employees to familiarize themselves with it.

A structured orientation is more likely to happen in chain salons and large, independent salons. Some of the things an employee orientation might include:

1. *A tour of the salon.* Introductions to employees and explanations of responsibilities. Information about where to find necessary equipment and products; how to care for equipment; policies regarding dispensary product safety and inventory control; what to do when something needs repair.

2. *Booking procedures and time standards.* What to expect in terms of time allowed for each service; what to do when you are running late; how to communicate with a client who has arrived late for an appointment; how to fill out a service ticket and maintain client records; procedures for rebooking and reminding clients of appointments.

3. *Retail product inventory.* Features, ingredients, and benefits of all the professional products carried by the salon. Information about pricing and techniques for recommending products during consultation. Discounts offered to employees. What manufacturer and distributor training will be provided to help stylists learn how to recommend appropriate products.

When you are being introduced to the salon, its people, policies, and procedures, don't be embarrassed if you don't understand something. It's a new environment, and you'll have a lot to learn at once. Take notes to review later, and don't be afraid to ask questions.

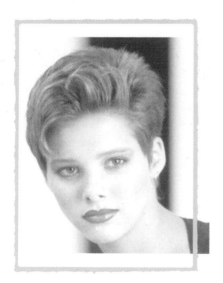

Uniform Layers

Overview

In the Short Uniform Cut the layers you create will echo the curves of the head. The resulting shape is quite sculptural and head hugging. This cut is generally an easy-care, easy-wear design that many of your clients will appreciate.

Connect

Roundness

To master the Uniform Cut, you must develop a sensitivity to head shape—its roundness and the various planes that its bone structure gives it. Think about the globe. It's round, yet there is dimension—hills and planes that you travel over as you travel the globe. In this cut, you'll circumnavigate the head—travel around it—using the method that allows you to cut to the curves effectively while adapting for the different side-to-side planes.

Feel the client's head shape before you begin any haircut. This will let you know the shape that you're working with; tell you how short you may cut; and tell you if you need to adjust the uniform cut in any way to create a weight buildup in a certain area—like the occipital, for instance.

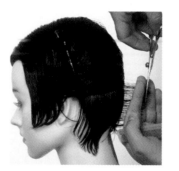
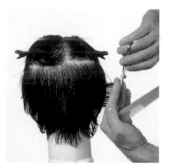
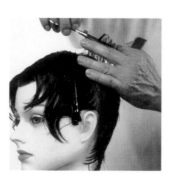

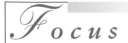

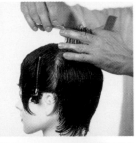

Sub-Division of the Head —You'll subdivide head into panels throughout the cut. This will enable you to easily control the differing planes of the head and cut them to uniform lengths.

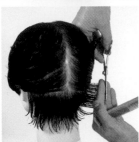

Holding Position—The holding position throughout this haircut is straight out from the curve of the head.

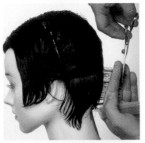

Cutting Position—The cutting position throughout this haircut is parallel to the curve of the head shape.

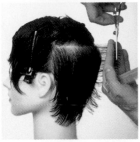

Traveling Guide—The guide that you create initially in the nape area will travel from section to section to serve as your length guide throughout the cut. As you move from one parted-out section to the next, bring a small amount of the previously cut hair to the new section to be cut.

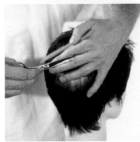

Cross-Checking—Cross-check your work throughout the haircut by taking partings opposite those that you used to cut. Check for any irregularities and refine as needed.

Hitch your wagon to a star.

Ralph Waldo Emerson

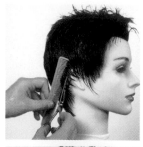

Refinement Perimeter—After you complete all uniform layers throughout the cut, refine and define the line around the perimeter. Here, this was done by holding the hair at the desired line and, at a low elevation, then pointing into to create softness.

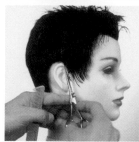

Refinement Around the Ear—The hairline area around the ear is refined and cut shorter by working from the nape upward. Control the hair lengths with your comb as you cut. Cut the area above and in front of the ear freehand, with the hair combed into natural fall to allow for its natural growth patterns.

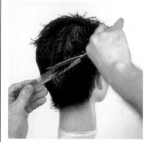

Scissors Over Comb—Use the scissors-over-comb technique from the nape to the occipital to tighten and shorten the lengths in this area. Work your comb and scissors together as a unit to move from the hairline upward in a smooth, fluid motion. Let your comb follow the curve of the head and at the occipital area, working into the previously established shape and length.

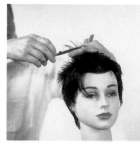

Tapering Technique—Use tapering scissors throughout the interior along the ends of the hair to accentuate the softness, mobility, and blending of the ends. Use your comb to lift the hair away from the head, then move smoothly and evenly throughout the top with your tapering scissors, opening and closing these scissors along the top of the comb to create the texturized ends. Place the comb at the hair length at which you want the scissors to cut.

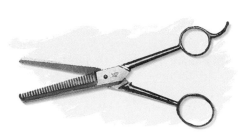

The only place where success comes before work is in the dictionary.

Vidal Sassoon

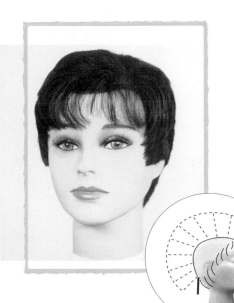

Apply *Uniform Layers*

With your clients, these technical steps will follow the consultation and shampoo.

The uniform layered shape consists of equal lengths throughout the entire head. This allows for exceptional movement and volume. You may personalize this cut by the type of frame that you create around the perimeter.

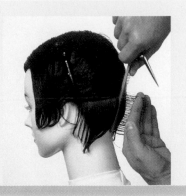
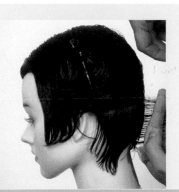

1. Comb the hair in natural fall. Part vertically down the center back. Comb out a wide section in the nape with a horizontal part that moves from ear to ear. Starting in the center of the nape, direct and hold a vertical section straight out from the curve of the head and cut it parallel to the curve of the head. This will become your traveling guide.

2. Continue cutting toward the side, using the traveling guide to cut vertical sections. Hold the sections straight out from the curve of the head and cut them parallel to the curve of the head.

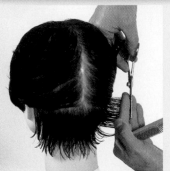
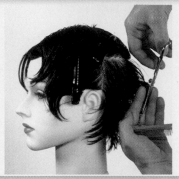

3. Cut from the center to the side, then move to the opposite side and cut in the same manner, using a traveling guide, until you reach the perimeter.

4. Move up and release the next horizontal panel. Establish the length by cutting a vertical section at the center, as you did before with the same holding and cutting positions.

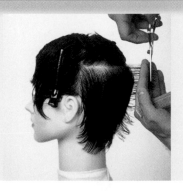
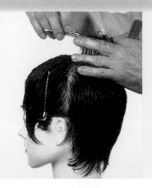

5. Move from the center to the left side, then cut from the center to the right side, completing the horizontal section on both sides. Use the traveling guide throughout.

6. Move up to the crown. Part a 1/2" (1.25 cm) vertical section at the center, hold it straight out from the curve of the head, and cut it parallel to the curve of the head to establish the guide for the crown area.

7. From the guide, take radial partings on either side and complete the top, using your initially cut section as a traveling guide. Stop when you reach the point above the ear on each side. Cross-check the back by holding out sections horizontally—the opposite of how you cut them. Clean up any unevenness.

8. Move to the side sections above and in front of the ear. Cut a section at the front sides to the same length as the back section. Cut parallel to the curve of the head as you work toward the hairline.

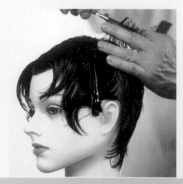 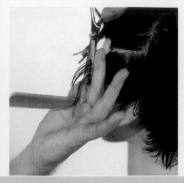

9. Work from just above the ear to the front hairline, then move up to the next section. Cut it in the same manner, holding the hair straight out from the curve of the head.

10. Next, move to the panel along one side of the top. Beginning at the crown area, you now have two guides to follow and blend with—the one from the side crest area and the one from the crown. Part horizontally, direct lengths straight out from the curve of the head, and cut parallel to the head shape.

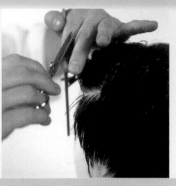 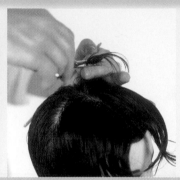

11. Work all the way to the front hairline using the traveling guide. Direct lengths straight out from the curve of the head and cut parallel to the head.

12. Continue in this manner to the front hairline.

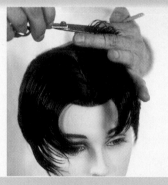 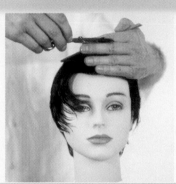

13. Repeat the entire procedure on the other side and top of the head. Work through the center top to blend and ensure balance between the two top panels.

14. Cross-check the hair in every direction, taking partings in the direction opposite to how they were cut.

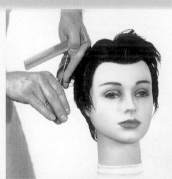 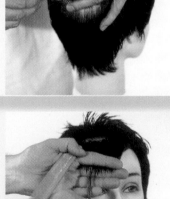

15. Refine the top and the perimeter as desired.

16. To cut the fringe into a soft, pleasing shape, hold the section out and point cut into the ends with the tips of your scissors. Leave some pieces longer than others.

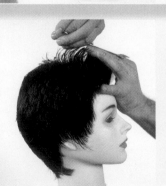 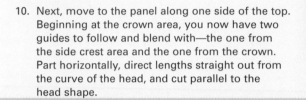 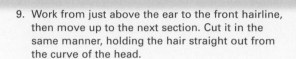

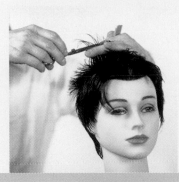
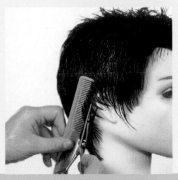

17. Tapering scissors, can be used to create longer and shorter lengths along the ends of the hair. Work from the crown area forward to the front hairline. Place the blades into the ends of the hair as controlled by the comb, then methodically work section by section. This will create a well-blended effect.

18. Direct the teeth of the comb downward to hold the hair just behind the ear. Cut around the ear carefully to shape the back hairline.

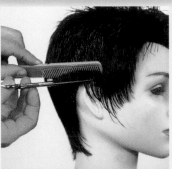
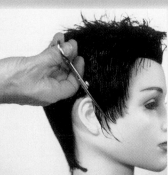

19. Holding the hair with the comb, cut around the ear from the back, up to the top of the ear.

20. When you reach the top, cut the hair in front of the ear by angling your scissors downward.

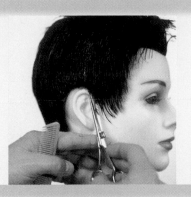
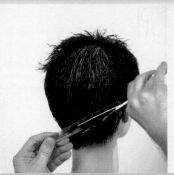

21. Refine the line around the ear and in front of it.

22. Use a scissors-over-comb technique to diagonally work upward from the perimeter hairline toward the center back.

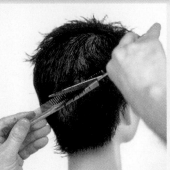
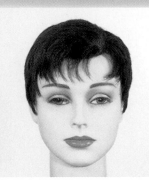

23. Then reverse and work diagonally from the center back to the area behind the ear to blend and cross-check lengths while creating the shape.

24. To taper in the nape area, comb the hair at a diagonal and cut, using the scissors-over-comb technique. Then move in the opposite diagonal direction upward from the center back toward the ear area to blend and cross-check lengths. The finished cut provides a soft, wispy perimeter frame around the face, and the extra length through the crown complements and harmonizes with the short nape area.

$\mathcal{R}$eflect

$\mathcal{E}$xplore

Apply this technique to different lengths, colors, and textures for almost endless possibilities.

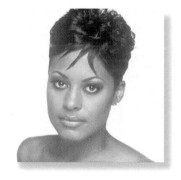

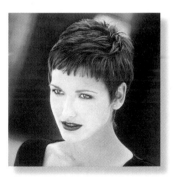

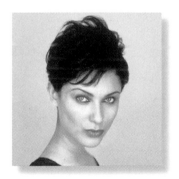

Employee
Manual

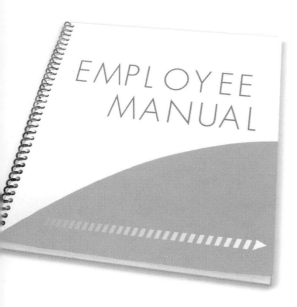

During your new-employee orientation, you may receive an employee manual that gives you information about important aspects of the business, such as those below.

Payroll Policies and Procedures

◆ How stylist hours and/or service and retail sales are recorded
◆ How salaries/commissions are calculated
◆ When pay periods begin and end
◆ When paychecks are issued

Employee Benefits

◆ What fringe benefits (such as health and life insurance premiums) are paid by the salon, when you are eligible to receive them, and what amount, if any, will be deducted from your paycheck to pay your portion of them
◆ Paid holidays and vacation benefits; continuing education benefits

Attendance Policies

◆ Sick days, personal time off, and late arrivals: how many are permitted
◆ What you should do if you know you will be late or absent
◆ What time employees are expected to report to work (A good rule of thumb is to be at work and ready to work before your first appointment is scheduled; typically you should arrive at least 15 minutes before the salon is open.)

Employee Evaluations

◆ When they will occur
◆ What standards you will be evaluated by (Often, a blank copy of an evaluation is included.)
◆ Reasons for employee dismissal and dismissal procedures

Other topics covered could be customer service policies, salon time standards, and job descriptions.

STYLIST **1:** "This break room is a mess! There's leftover take-out food in the refrigerator that's about to get up and walk. And look at these sticky coffee cups and soda bottles everywhere. Why doesn't anyone clean this up?"

STYLIST **2:** "I don't know. It's not my job."

To be successful, you don't have to do extraordinary things. Just do ordinary things extraordinarily well.

John Rohn

Job Title: Salon
Assistant

Job descriptions are used in many businesses to help employees understand their job duties as well as the job duties of others. When someone says, "That's not my job!" a written job description helps a manager show her that it is indeed part of her job—it's right there in black and white. Here's what a salon job description might look like:

▶ Client Service

- ◆ **Introduce yourself and show clients to dressing room; when they come out, escort them to shampoo bowl.**

- ◆ **Explain to clients what products are being used during the shampoo and inform them the stylist will recommend specific products for home use.**

- ◆ **Test water for proper temperature; shampoo clients' hair and show them to stylists' stations; ask if they'd like something to read or drink while waiting.**

- ◆ **Remove hair from basins after each shampoo per health department regulations; dry and wipe basins and chair, mop up water on floor.**

- ◆ **Assist in chemical services when requested by rinsing color, texture, and conditioning services according to directions on each client's service card.**

- ◆ **Show genuine concern and interest in the salon's clients. If you notice a client having a problem, ask to speak with the stylist privately and discuss your concerns. Never suggest to a stylist that something is wrong with a client's hair or that you think there is a problem with the way a chemical service is processing in the client's presence.**

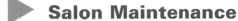

▶ Salon Maintenance

- ◆ Launder, dry, and fold towels and smocks and put away in designated cabinets; make sure supplies are adequate throughout the day.
- ◆ Keep mirrors, counters, and windows clean.
- ◆ Keep combs and brushes washed and clean.
- ◆ Keep shampoo area clean and back-bar products stocked.
- ◆ Monitor dispensary product inventory levels and enter needed items on reorder sheet, according to minimums stated there.
- ◆ Remove soiled glasses, cups, and other debris from around salon; wash and put away glasses; keep break room tidy.

▶ Appearance, Work Habits, Communication

- ◆ Arrive at work on time, with hair styled and appropriate makeup (if applicable) applied.
- ◆ Wear clean, fashionable, well-fitting garments and shoes; wear a laundered and pressed salon lab coat over street clothes and have a clean, spare lab coat available in case of spills.
- ◆ Present a cheerful but respectful demeanor to clients; no smoking, gum chewing, or profane language in the salon at any time.
- ◆ Help promote salon harmony by avoiding confrontation with co-workers or allowing personal feelings to interfere with your professional conduct.
- ◆ Do not make or receive unnecessary personal telephone calls while working on the salon floor. Use the telephone in the break room during your scheduled breaks, and do not charge long-distance telephone calls to the salon.

Hairstyling
Creating an Image

"One step at a time" is the formula for achieving a perfect finish to a hairstyle. There really is no mystery to styling hair. Every style starts off the same: with the cut. Styling enhances the cut's purest form, and the next day, when the client works with it at home, she should be able to achieve the same look with ease.

In this section, you'll learn the importance of investing in the right tools to help you achieve a specific look; how to use the tools most effectively; and how to enhance the fundamental skills you learn here by using the tools creatively. The use of liquid styling products will be discussed. These products are integral in the finished style—whether using the lightest hold to the firmest hold formulas to accentuate/add control, body, hold texture, and shine to the hairstyle. You'll learn, too, how to approach each client's cut with a "what if" mentality, exploring many styling possibilities to give your clients a finish with finesse. Remember that the styling techniques shown here to finish the haircuts are one interpretation. When it comes to hairstyling, this is where individuality and creativity can come forward.

You can indeed make positive changes in your clients' appearance and sense of well-being through the proper use of hairstyling techniques. But to create the most attractive style for a client, you must understand and consider a few basic concepts.

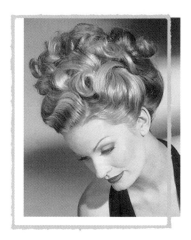

French twist style

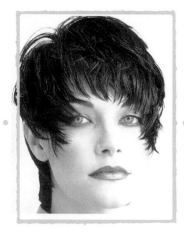

Styling a razor cut

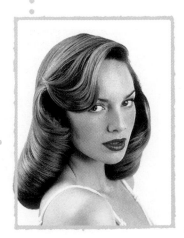

Style with hot rollers

Shape

Everything that can be seen or touched has a shape, or form. Look around you: Most rooms are either square or rectangular, and most furniture is a combination of rectangular and oval shapes.

In nature, the same shapes are repeated in an infinite variety of combinations. Open your eyes to these patterns and shapes all around you – the branching of a tree, the petals of a flower, and the billowing roundness of the clouds.

Shapes have dimension, meaning that hair cuts and styles are three-dimensional in nature, having length, width, and depth. In hair design, shape and volume are created by moving hair into different positions, using tools and techniques in various combinations. There are endless numbers of possibilities for shape. The challenge is to decide which one will best suit a client's physical makeup and lifestyle needs.

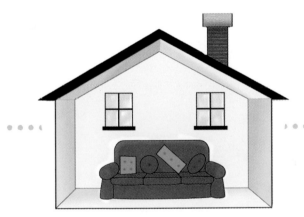

Various forms

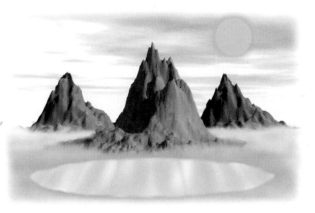

Shape in nature

Face Shape

Before determining which shape to create, you need to consider the shape of the client's face. Notice how the same hair shape—in this case a rounded shape—looks on different face shapes.

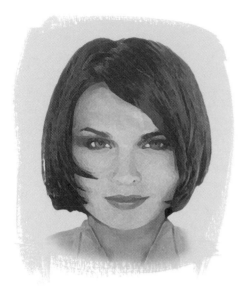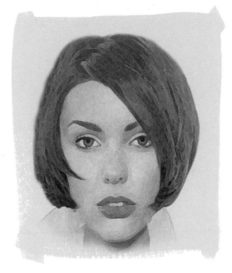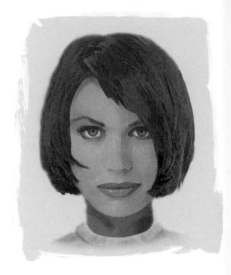

Proportion

Another factor to consider is the proportion of the style in relation to the head shape and body size. A small head and face might be overwhelmed by large hair, while a small head with a large body would look even smaller without adequate volume, regardless of shape. You may control and adapt the cut shape to create a variety of illusions that will compliment the client.

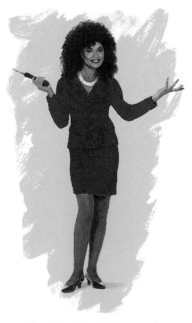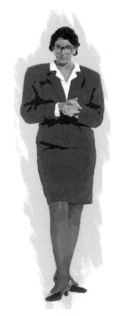

Small body with large hair   Large body with small hair

Basic Shapes from Basic Cuts

The final form of a style depends on a combination of basic shapes. The process of creating shape begins with the cut and is then emphasized or enhanced in the styling phase. Remember that there is the cut shape and the style shape. They may be different. Study the following often created hairstyle shapes:

Rounded or Spherical. A round shape has equal width and height with no corners. This shape can be created with a uniform layered cut shape.

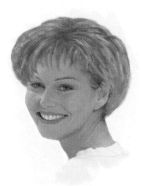

Oval. An oval or elliptical shape has more width than length, and the resulting hairstyle has more volume at the sides. The oval shape may also be an elongated shape that has more length than width. It can be created with a blunt or layered cut shape.

Squared. A squared shape has weight corners that add a uniquely different dimension to the silhouette.

Triangular. A triangular shape is usually wider at the sides and narrower toward the crown. The graduated cut shape or wedge as well as blunt cut can create this styled shape.

Rounded or Spherical

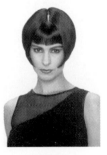

Oval

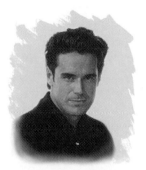

Squared

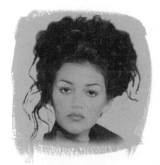

Triangular

Color

The element of color can enhance the finished appearance of a shape as well as create the illusion of movement and change. The way that light responds to movement of hair alters with color change, and the finished appearance of a style can differ considerably on blonde and brunette heads. Blonde hair appears lighter and airier, particularly around the perimeter frame – while dark colors appear weighty and more solid around the perimeter frame. Good stylists will take the client's color into consideration as a variable when suggesting a style.

Darker colors feature the shape of the style by drawing the eye to the outline of the form.

Lighter colors reflect more light, making texture patterns more apparent than they are on darker hair.

Line and Directional Movement

Movement can best be defined as the direction that hair travels, whether curved or straight, horizontal, vertical, or diagonal. As examples, blunt cuts styled into the natural lines of the cut without texture travel straight downward into the natural fall, while uniformly layered shapes may have movement that is directed back, forward, up, or down.

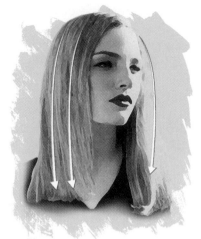

Blunt cut traveling downward

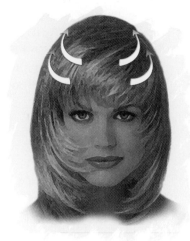

Layered cut with movement

Hair movement can travel in several directions:

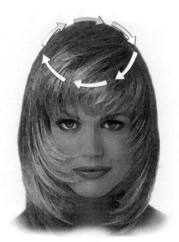

Clockwise

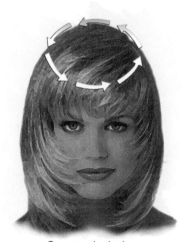

Counterclockwise

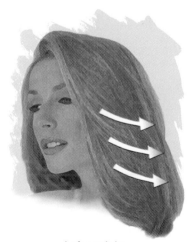

Left or right

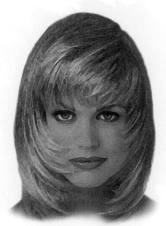

Toward the face

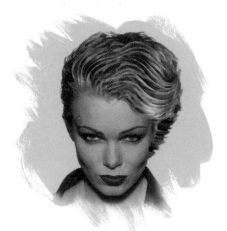

Away from the face

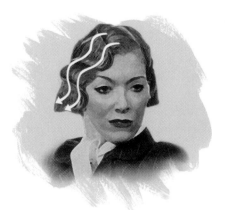

Repeated Lines

Distribution

Hair can be moved in any direction from its base or scalp area. Where and how hair is moved over the head is called its distribution.

Radial Distribution. Hair is distributed from one point or area on the head, moving outward in each direction.

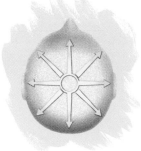
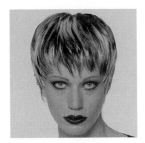

Parallel Distribution. Hair is distributed from a part or from the hairline in one direction, usually moving away from the face or on either side of the part.

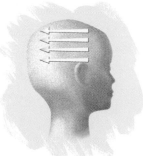
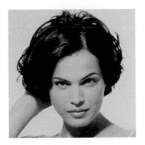

Base Controls. This relates to how the hair is directed out from the scalp aria. It determines how much lift the hair will have. A blow-dry along the top surface of the hair for the closest contour. Use directional influence for lifting hair outward from the base area when drying. Overdirected, on-base, half off-base and off-base tool positioning may be used for blow-drying with brushes and when using curling irons and setting tools.

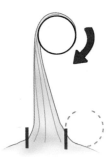
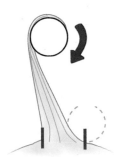
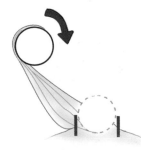

Texture

It's important to consider the texture of the hair when making styline decisions. Traditionally, texture has referred to the quality and feel of hair, such as coarse, normal or fine. Today, it has come to mean that and more. Now, it is also used to refer to the surface quality of hair, texture includes how it looks—straight, wavy or curly, for instance—as well as how it feels—smooth, rough, grainy, or silky. Texture can be given long-term change through cutting and chemical treatments; texture change can be achieved on a temporary basis by using styling techniques and tools.

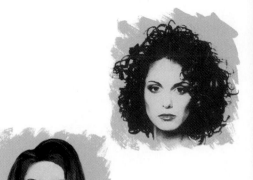

Different texture looks

Texture Type. The main types of texture that we'll identify and create in hair are sleek or straight, wavy, curly, or crimped. Each of these can be combined to create almost endless variations, especially when hair length, and color are factored in. These texture types are the basic components from which you can mix and match for a creative array of looks.

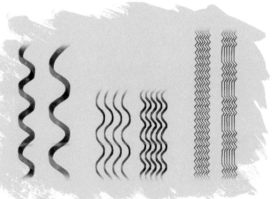

Various texture types

Texture Movement. This is the amount of movement from slow languid wave patterns, to highly activated curl patterns. Hair with slow movement has less change, as with loose curls, for instance, or waves with slight curves. Hair with highly active movement changes direction frequently in a relatively short space and may include tight waves, curls, and angular texture.

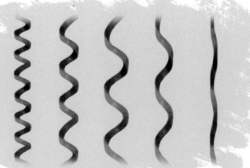

Range of curl patterns

STUDENT COURSE BOOK

Styling Tools

Combs and Picks. Used for distributing and parting hair, combs come in a wide variety of sizes and shapes to adapt to many styling options. The length and spacing of the teeth is the most significant variable: teeth closely spaced will remove definition from curl and create a smooth surface, while widely spaced teeth shape larger sections of hair for more surface texture.

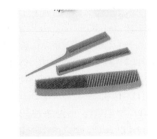

Brushes. Brushes come in many sizes, shapes, and materials. The cushion brush is designed to smooth dry hair, while round brushes and vent brushes are used with a blow dryer to create movement and shape damp hair. Metal brushes conduct the dryer's heat to speed styling.

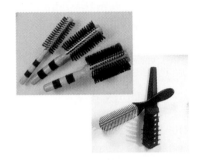

Blow-dryers. The directional feature of blow-dryers helps to target the air stream. Use a dryer attachment called a concentrator to create a more intense air flow; use a diffuser to accentuate or retain textural definition.

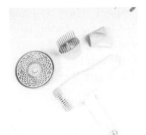

Rollers. Rollers are used with wet hair to mold hair as it dries and used on dry hair to add body and dimension to the hair. Available in a wide variety of sizes and materials, some are self-gripping while others require the use of pins or picks to stay in place.

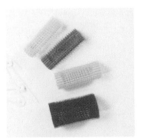

Curling Irons. Used with dry hair, curling irons focus heat to a small section of hair to create curves and curl. Available in different diameters (1/2 inch, 3/4 inch, jumbo) and styles, they are an indispensable styling tool.

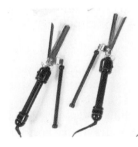

Lifestyle and Fashion Considerations

Today's women desire hairstyles that require minimum time and effort to maintain. The selection of styling tools, techniques, and products must relate to the client's lifestyle, which includes her ability to syle her own hair and how much time she has available to do it. A client who wants a carefree hairstyle will be unhappy with a perfectly cut and designed style if the shape depends on the use of a curling iron or a blow dryer with a round brush. You also need to learn whether the client is willing to use any of the wide variety of liquid styling tools (i.e., gel, mousse, shiner, spray, etc).

The importance of the client consultation can't be stressed enough when personalizing a cut and style for a client. Some clients are strongly influenced by current trends, while others know what they like and don't like, and no stylist is going to change their minds. It's your job to find out where your client falls on the yardstick of trend-setting fashion and then accommodate her wishes. You may have suggestions based on current trends, but the client will have to live with the style, and her wishes must be honored first.

Choosing the Right Styling Products

With the many liquid styling tools on the market, you need to take into account several things before choosing one. First, how long does the style need to hold? Under what environmental conditions—dryness, humidity, wind, sun—will the client be wearing the style? You also must consider the type of hair—fine, coarse, straight, curly—when deciding on a product to use and recommend. Heavier products work by causing strands of hair to cling together, adding more pronounced definition, but they can also weigh hair down, especially fine hair. The resins in liquid styling products may range from the lightest all the way to the firmest hold. Choose accordingly for the amount of support that is desired.

Foam or Mousse. Foam builds moderate body and volume into the hair. Applied to damp hair, it can be dried by massaging and diffusing to accentuate textural movement in the hair or blow dry straight for styles where body without texture is desired. Foam is good for fine hair because it doesn't weigh hair down. It will hold for six to eight hours in dry conditions. Conditioning foams are excellent for drier, more porous hair.

Styling Products (continued)

Gel. Usually clear or transparent, gel comes in a tube or can and is firm bodied. It is probably the strongest holding of all products, other than a finishing spritz. It creates the strongest control for slicked or molded styles and distinct texture definition when diffused with the fingers; when brushed out it creates long-lasting body and "set memory" according to how the hair was styled, regardless of conditions. The firmness that produces the longest hold may overwhelm fine hair because of its intense resin level. This wouldn't be a concern however, if fine hair was molded into the lines of the style and did not get brushed through when dry.

Liquid Gels or Texturizers. Similar in function to firm hold gels, these products are lighter and more viscous, or liquid, in form. They allow for easy styling, defining, and molding as well as diffusing of curl definition. With brushing, they add volume and body to the style. Good for all hair types, they offer firmer, longer hold for fine hair with minimal heaviness, and a lighter, moderate hold to normal, or coarse hair types. Pomades. Similar to an ointment, pomades add considerable body and weight to the hair, by causing strands to join together. Used on dry hair, this makes the hair very malleable and moldable. It allows greater manageability but use sparingly on fine hair, because of weight.

Hairspray or Spritz. These products are the most widely used and most versatile. Available in a wide variety of holding strengths, in aerosol or nonaerosol sprays, they are useful for all hair types and are effective in dry or damp weather to hold the style in place. Sprays generally may be easily combed or brushed through while the spritz is used for the firmest possible hold where the style will not be disturbed.

Silicone Shiner. Shiners add gloss and sheen to the hair while creating texture definition. Non-oily silicone shine products are excellent for all hair types, for either finishing the style at the very end or even put on before drying to provide lubrication and protection to the hair while blow-drying.

Spray Shine. Applied like hair spray, this product adds shine without weight, making it good for all hair types.

Regardless of which product you use, always apply the product according to the manufacturer's instructions for best results. Guide the client on the amount of product used, and the technique for styling to ensure their happiness and success with the style.

Joel Moore

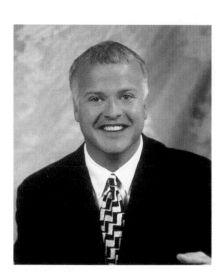

Growing up in Savannah, Georgia, Joel Moore, top international hair designer and the author of the hairstyling section in this program, watched his older sister become a hairstylist without thinking that he would want to do the same with his life. "I wasn't exposed to all the opportunities in this business," he said. After high school, he went to college to become a respiratory therapist but, "As fate would have it, I got ill and had to take time off school. During that time, I found myself asking, 'What do I really want to do?'"

Joel decided to quit college and go to cosmetology school, where he discovered his innate flair for hairstyling. In spite of his success in school, however, when he got to his first salon job as a stylist, he said, "I was in way over my head. The stylist who worked the station on the other side of my mirror would literally come over and take the scissors out of my hand and show me what to do." That same stylist became Joel Moore's hair model several years later as he won countless major hair competitions in Europe and the United States, including the National Coiffure Championship, the European Championship, the Rose D'Or in Paris, and the Golden Curl in Brussels.

He opened his Savannah salon, Joel and Company, in 1979, which today employs 40 stylists. He opened a cosmetology school in 1984, and he is actively involved in both. He also found time to be Revlon's Artistic Director for six years and to coach the Ladies' Professional Hair Design Team in the '96 Hair Olympics.

Of the competition stage, Joel says, "I love the thrill of competing, but more than that, it has given me the confidence to believe in my skills. You learn to think on your feet, to get better faster. Because of my competition experience, I can look at a hair design and right away see what it needs."

Joel thinks he has been successful because, as he says, "I could do many things. In addition to being a good stylist, I was a strong communicator, a teacher, a business person. I brought a full plate to the table in any negotiation."

And as for his advice to the up and coming stars of tomorrow, Joel cautions: "Think long term. Realize the importance of a good educational foundation, and work hard to develop your skills for the long term. Observe how classic design and technique have endured over the years and continue to be valued through all the trends and sensations."

And to succeed in your career, Joel advises, be three dimensional. In addition to a strong skill foundation, look the part and communicate well. Show enthusiasm. Says Joel, "When I hire a new stylist, I look for someone who gets what this business is all about."

Because "without the style being there, it doesn't matter what the cut or color is, you will be judged on the finished product."

Charlene Carroll

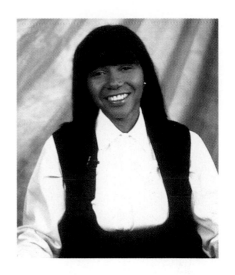

Charlene Carroll—top salon owner, educator, platform artist, stylist to celebrities, and co-creator (with colleague Floyd Kenyatta) of the black hair care and styling segment of this course—was 19 and fresh out of high school when her mother died, leaving Charlene on her own in the world. "I knew I wanted to learn hairstyling, fashion design, or interior design," she recalled, adding, "There was a hair school within walking distance of where I was living, so that's where I went."

Charlene remembers her first job at a suburban Boston salon that catered to a conservative, older suburban clientele. For two years she did nothing but shampoo hair. "I was always loyal and patient," Charlene explained, adding that, because such loyalty in young people is rare, her employers appreciated and encouraged her. But she also was motivated to succeed in this industry, so—with the blessing of her first employers—Charlene left for a position in a hip downtown Boston salon owned by Olive Benson, one of the country's top hairstylists and educators. "Olive pushed me to excel," said Charlene, who saved her tips and traveled whenever she could to top trainers for advanced education—well known schools such as Sassoon, Jingles, Chadwick's, Bruno's, and John Delleria. She became one of the salon's top haircutters and, after seven years, opened her own salon—Charlene's—in Boston's Dorchester section, which she has owned for 20 years. Charlene and her 12 stylists are in demand by clients such as Boston television news anchors and other television personalities and celebrities.

In those 20 years, Charlene has also made a name for herself worldwide as a gifted educator and platform artist. She has been the President of the Black Hair Olympics; a platform artist for major manufacturers including Revlon, Soft Sheen, and American Beauty Products; is a member of the prestigious Hair America; and her work and words have appeared in Black Hair, Shop Talk, Essence, and Black Enterprise magazines, among others.

So how did a young woman, alone in the world at the tender age of 19, achieve success? Charlene smiles patiently. "Faith in God and faith in myself," she answers, displaying some of the calm strength that has always been her hallmark. She urges beginning stylists to do the same. "You must really know who you are and what you want from life," she adds, "before you can set about getting it. If you don't know yourself, you won't be able to find space anyplace else."

"I always knew I had to be good, and that I had to do it myself. No one else was there to do it for me. In a way, that was a gift. I was blessed."

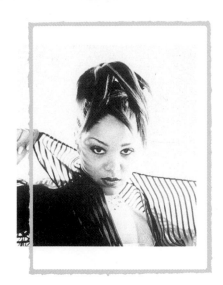

Creating a Chignon

Overview

The chignon is a classic hair design that has been popular for centuries. It can be dressed up with ornamentation or worn casually with equal grace.

Focus

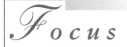

Bobby vs. Hair Pins—Use bobby pins where a firm support is needed, generally pinning large areas to each other, internally. Hair pins will support and hold more delicate areas together, usually external.

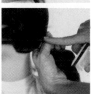

Locking Bobby Pins—Overlap bobby pins to secure their position.

Back Brushing—Back brush along the bottom of the ponytail lengths to create and support volume.

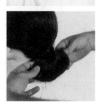

Forming a Chignon—Roll the lengths of hair, pin, then fan out to form the chignon.

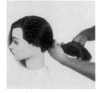

Twist-over-hand Technique—With your palm up, comb the hair over your hand. Grasp hair as in a ponytail and twist your hand over, fist down. Push the hair forward and pin. This creates volume in the formation.

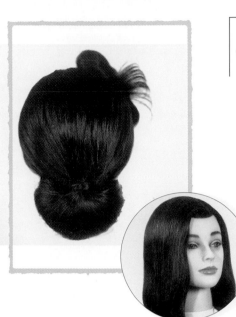

Apply

Creating a Chignon

With your clients, these technical steps will follow consultation, shampoo, and power or towel drying.

1. Work with a bristle brush. The top and right side are left out. Comb the remaining hair over your hand into a ponytail, smoothing as you do so.

2. Place two bobby pins onto a rubber band. Place one of these bobby pins into the base of the ponytail.

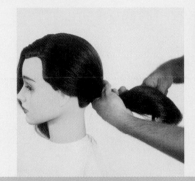
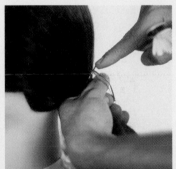

3. Stretch the rubber band around the ponytail's base.

4. Place the second bobby pin into the base of the ponytail.

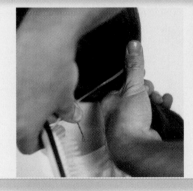
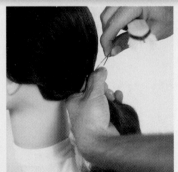

5. Lock the two pins together.

6. Part out a small section of hair from the underside of the ponytail.

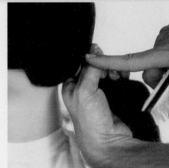
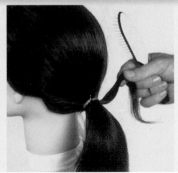

7. Wrap it around the banded base of the ponytail.

8. Pin on the underside to secure.

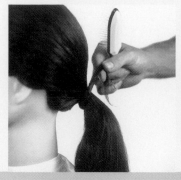 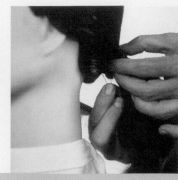

9. Brush through the ponytail to smooth and control.

10. Back brush from underneath for added volume. Rotate the wrist as back brushing from near the base of the ponytail out to the ends.

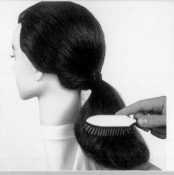 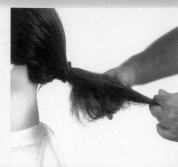

11. Gently skim the brush over the outside surface of the hair lengths to shape and form the hair.

12. Begin rolling the ends toward the head to form the chignon. Fold in close to the nape area.

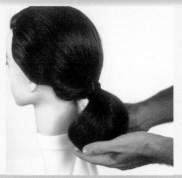 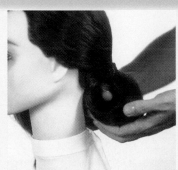

13. Using bobby pins, pin the rolled area from the left.

14. Repeat this pinning on the right side.

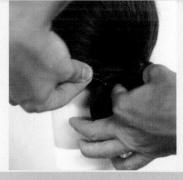 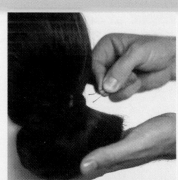

15. Fan out to spread and shape the hair.

16. Pin tight and close to the nape using a hair pin.

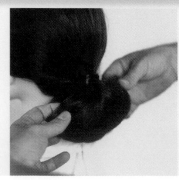 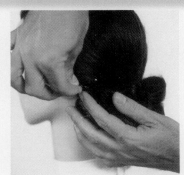

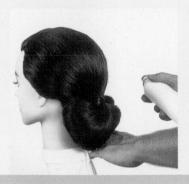

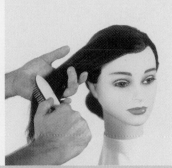

17. Spray the hair. Use spray according to the type of hold desired—soft to firm.

18. This front area as styled into a twist is an option—you may choose to incorporate this hair into the chignon. Comb the front section over your hand.

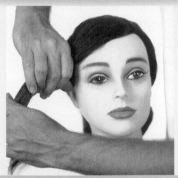

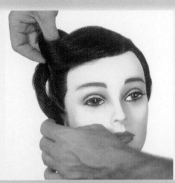

19. Use a twist-over-hand technique as shown to twist the hair lengths upward to form a looped shape at the top of the head.

20. Twist around with your thumb and pin.

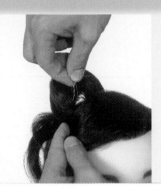

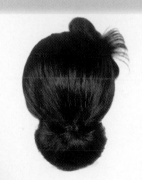

21. Note where the bobby pin is secured. The ends are left free.

22. The finished style is definitely for special occasions. Add ornamentation, i.e., flowers, ribbons, etc., as the occasion requires. Given your expertise, a large segment of your clientele may require long hair designing services—particularly for special occasions—such as weddings, proms, graduations, etc.

It takes guts to get out of the ruts.

Robert Schuller

*R*eflect

*E*xplore

Apply this technique to different lengths, colors, and cuts for almost endless possibilities.

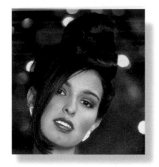

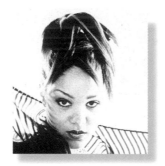

Salon Service
Menu

"What are we going to do today?"

Those are the seven words most often spoken by stylists, and seven words you should erase from your vocabulary right now if you want to be a successful stylist whose clients are satisfied with your services. Why? Think about this: You are seated in a restaurant, and the waiter appears with a pad in hand, but there's no menu in sight. No chalkboard with listings. Nothing. The waiter asks, "What will you have?" You answer, "What do you serve?" He replies, "Whatever you'd like."

Would that seem a little odd to you? Would you be confused, uncertain? How do you know that what you like would be something the chef can prepare?

Well, it also seems odd to clients when salons do not have printed "menus" of their services. A service menu, with prices, helps clients select services without having to ask "How much is that?" In many cases, when clients don't know if a service is available or at what price, they simply won't ask about it.

A service menu also helps to promote services that clients may never have tried or weren't aware even existed. (As in, "Hmm . . . color highlights . . . tell me about those.")

Every new client consultation should include a review of the service menu and an explanation of each item, how long it takes, what it involves, and so on. If your salon has printed brochures that list services (with or without prices), keep a supply at your station for clients to read. Even regular clients need to be reminded of what's available.

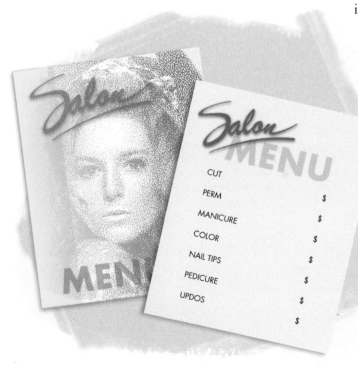

Salon MENU

CUT

PERM $

MANICURE $

COLOR $

NAIL TIPS $

PEDICURE $

UPDOS $

                            $

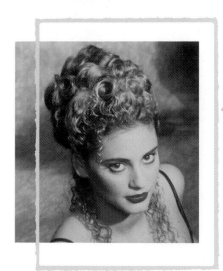

Traditional French Twist

Overview

The French twist is easy to create and can dramatically transform long hair in a relatively short time. The French twist is very adaptable from casual wear to an evening style. You can create the style for clients who have extremely curly hair by blow-drying the hair straight. If your client has a medium curl pattern, you can create the style using her natural curl. Let esthetics (judgments about beauty) and the final effect be your guide. The only time that this style is not advisable is when the client's hair is too fine (fine hair may need to be prepped by blow-drying product into the hair and thermal setting), or when it's shorter than four to five inches (10 to 12.5 cm).

Connect

Back Combing for Volume

The use of back combing is important for the connection of lines, and for adding fullness to the hair. Think of the exaggerated bouffant styles of the 1960s, in which the hair was teased to new heights. However, today's use of back combing is much more subdued. The art to this technique is to push the hair lengths from along the strand toward the scalp area. This creates a cushion of support at the scalp or base area and causes the hair to spread out, creating more volume.

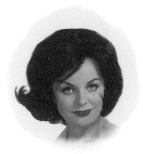

Securing with Pins

By using bobby or hair pins to secure an updo, you are providing lasting support, just as the iron girders in a building invisibly secure the rest of the wall. Use bobby pins where dynamic, firm support is needed, given the pressure exerted by the pin. And, use hair pins where a more delicate, gentle support is needed.

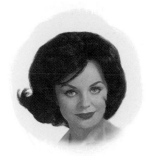

Focus

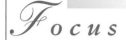

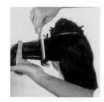**Back Combing** — Back combing locks hair together to form height, fullness, and control. This is done by using a comb to push the hair repeatedly from along the hair strand toward the base area or scalp.

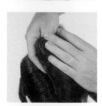**Invisible Pin Placement** — For a desirable and professional salon look, remember to place pins as invisibly as possible.

Seam Line — The interlocking row of pins through the center back is used to secure the hair before twisting.

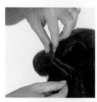**Back Brushing** — While holding the ends of hair strands up and outward, brush the strands back toward the scalp to create a look of softness and bulk.

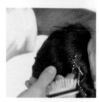**Molding the H a i r** — Molding the hair is the art of forming or directing hair into a desired pattern. Molding of hair may be done on dry or damp hair. In this design, hair is molded dry.

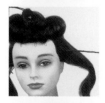**Slicing** — Carefully removing a small section of hair from a larger section.

Spraying for Hol d — Whenever necessary during the procedure, remember to use spray for holding the hair in place. Use sparingly and spray specific areas as required.

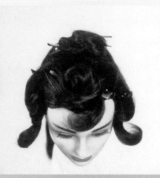

A pply
Traditional French Twist

With your clients, these technical steps will follow consultation, shampoo, and power or towel drying. This can also be done on hair that has been prepped with a wet set, or any form of thermal setting such as electric curler set, curling iron set, etc.

1., 2. Part the front half of the head into four sections (two top sections and two side sections).

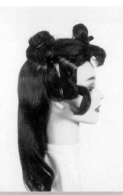

3. Leave the back section loose for the traditional French twist area to be formed.

4. Back comb the hair in the back section. Back combing is used for control and fullness. Part off a vertical section. Hold the hair out from the base area and begin working the comb through the lengths, back combing along the hair strand, from the base area outward.

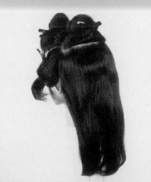

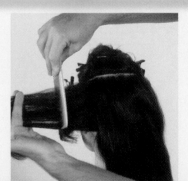

5. Hold the hair together to connect it as one unit, as well as for fullness. Take small sections, blending the ends together. Continue this technique to the center back. Repeat on the other side.

6. Brush the hair to one side of a center line. Brush the hair until smooth and controlled. Note how the other hand supports the hair as it is being brushed.

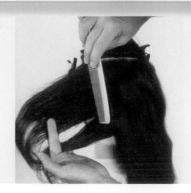

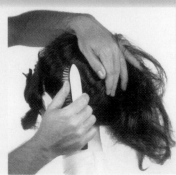

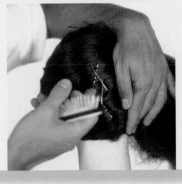
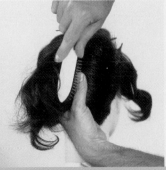

7. Pin the hair, overlapping the pins. Place the pins upward, starting at the center nape area.

8. Brush and bring the opposite side over the pinned area to begin the twist.

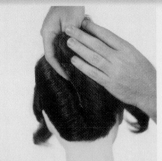
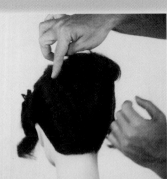

9. Smooth the hair, then grasp the lengths and turn inward and upward as forming a twist with your hand.

10. Unless you're using ornamental pins, place all pins as invisibly as possible.

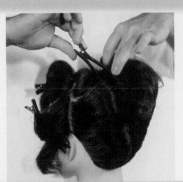
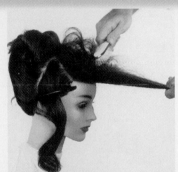

11. Unclip the crown section and lay back out of the way.

12. Backbrush along the surface of the top front section. Spray the lengths to provide hold and control. Brush as needed to refine and smooth the surface. Twist the lengths and turn the twisted area down towards the scalp.

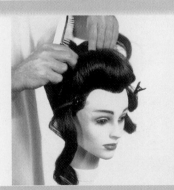
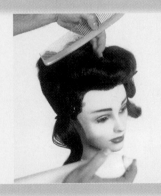

13. Push the hair slightly forward into a volume shape in the fringe area to create fullness. Fan out the outer edges and pin. Use a bobby pin to secure where the twist is being held at the scalp.

14. Use a hair pin to adjust the shape, pin for control, and hold, these pins will be removed after spraying.

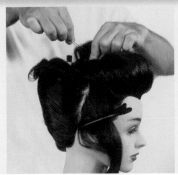
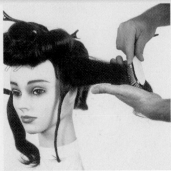

15. Place additional pins for control.

16. Through the side, an interesting mix of techniques will create unique texture. Back brush a portion of the hair and spray as needed. Lay this section out of the way.

18. Slice out a small front section and twist this section with your hands from the base out to the ends. Spray to control.

19. Wrap the twisted hair around the other section.

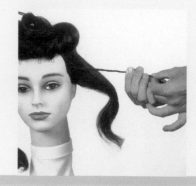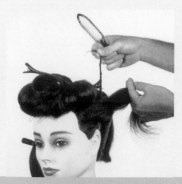

20. Hold in place at the top of the head, and pin to secure.

21. Move to the other side section.

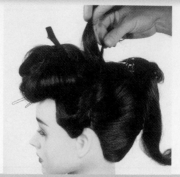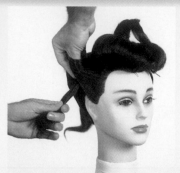

22. Reaching over the hair, turn and slide the hair up. A twist will form around the base of a loop. Leave the ends loose for now. Secure with bobby pins as required.

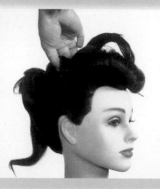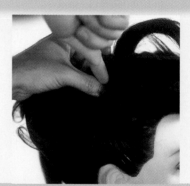

23. Proceed to the top section. Comb the ends of the hair left from the top front section. Brush and mold this hair into a curl. With your thumb on the curl, smooth it with a wide-toothed comb and a very light touch. Secure the hair with a hair pin and spray in place. Make any adjustments as needed to the shape.

24. Move to the back area. Form a curl with the ends left from the twisted left side. Delicately form, place, and pin the curl.

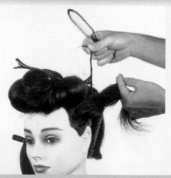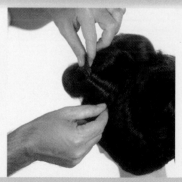

25. Brush the lengths from the crown area forward and pin this section on either side to firmly hold in place. It is pinned directly behind the top front section.

26. Divide this section into two strands at the top of the head. Place one strand out of the way.

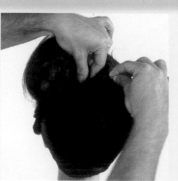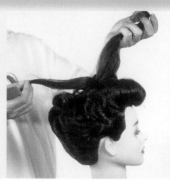

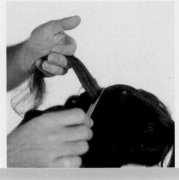
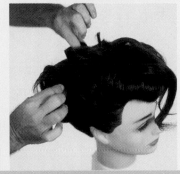

27. Back comb through each strand with the comb. Smooth with the brush. Note how delicately the hair is smoothed into place.

28. Roll over your hand. Twist and mold the hair into a curl.

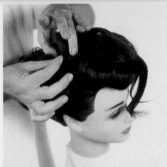
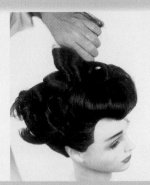

29. Secure with a hair pin and spray for hold.

30. Repeat the process on the other strand. Back comb to create support. Then smooth through the section.

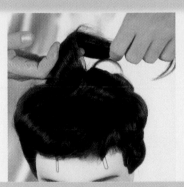
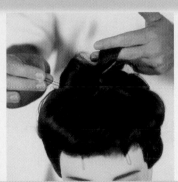

31. Begin to form the curl and place.

32. Spray as needed.

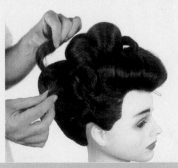
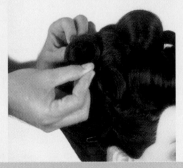

33. Finish off the ends to balance the style. This is where each stylist brings their own artistry and creativity to designing hair.

34. Back comb, smooth, and mold a small curl, then pin to secure.

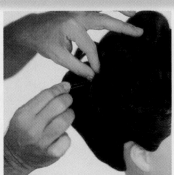
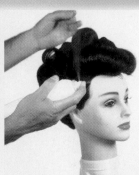

35. Mold a second curl and secure with a pin.

36. Spray for hold.

37. Adjust and balance the shapes as needed. Refine the finish with a hairpin and adjust the curl for continuity.

38. The finished style shows a combination of the classic French twist through the back with smooth, looping sections of hair molded into an elegant shape.

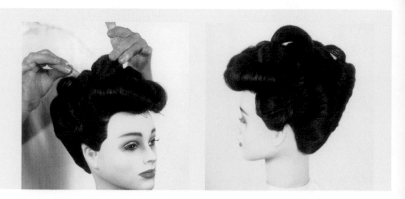

The difference between school and life? In school, you're taught a lesson and then given a test. In life, you're given a test that teaches you a lesson.

Tom Bodett

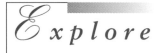
Explore

Apply this technique to different lengths, colors, and cuts for almost endless possibilities.

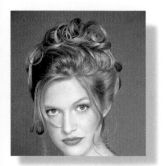

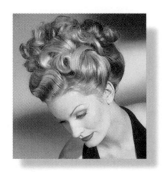

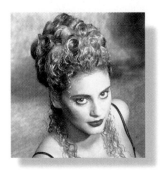

simplified french twist

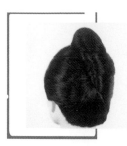

A traditional French twist requiring only a few steps, this timeless style creates a sleek shape that is simply elegant.

1. Grasping all of the hair, brush the hair back over your hand. Reach over the hair with the hand facing the client's body. Begin to twist the hair inward and upward. Holding all of the hair back, twist it in a clockwise direction.

2. Make a pocket at the base of the twisted hair and feed the hair into it. Tuck away all of the ends into the twist area. Reach into the pocket and ribbon the hair up.

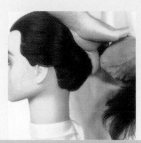
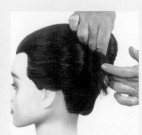

3. After folding the twisted hair into the pocket, begin to shape. Pin in place.

4. Brush and smooth any loose hairs. Check for balance and proportion. Adjust the shape of the twist as needed. If additional security is needed place more pins. Spray and smooth as needed.

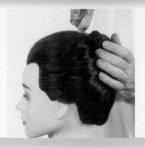
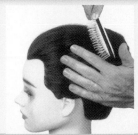

5. This simple interpretation of the French Twist may go from casual to special occasion. In this style variation, height is created in the crown area using essentially the same approach as before, however, with a few adjustments.

6. Brush all hair smoothly into a ponytail coming out from just above the occipital area. Note how the hair stays stationary against the head here as brushing to maintain control. Holding all of the hair back, twist it in a clockwise direction.

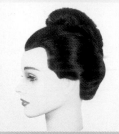
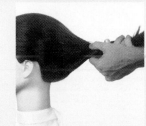

7. Bring the hair up and lay the twisted hair on top of the head. Fan the twisted area upward.

8. Adjust and balance the volume as desired and pin the twisted hair with a bobby pin to the hair underneath it. Place a second or even third pin if the texture and density of the hair requires it. Use a brush to clean and smooth any loose ends. Spray to hold and control the lengths.

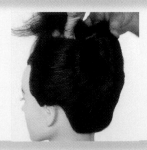
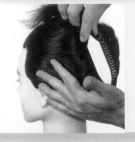

9. Take the ends and loop them over. Fan the looped ends out to create an enclosed continuation of the twist shape. If desired, you can add dimension—curls, loops, knots—at this point. Pin the shape in place around the edges to secure. Spray as needed for support and hold.

10. The finished style creates height in the crown with a smooth texture.

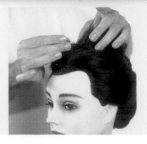
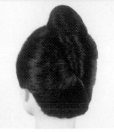

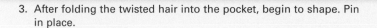

Personal Service Checklist

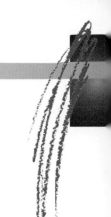

Ensuring Customer Satisfaction

Fix your eyes on perfection and you make almost everything speed towards it.

W.E. Channing

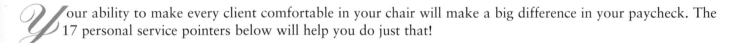

Your ability to make every client comfortable in your chair will make a big difference in your paycheck. The 17 personal service pointers below will help you do just that!

Personal Service Pointers ▼

1. Smile.
2. Make eye contact, face to face and in the mirror.
3. Hang up the client's coat when she arrives; and ask if she'd like a beverage or something to read.
4. Be friendly, courteous, and attentive at all times.
5. Before you begin the service, confirm that you and she are in agreement about what she wants and expects.
6. As you perform the service, explain what you are doing as you are doing it; reassure. Invite the client to ask questions.
7. Educate the client about home styling and maintenance; recommend appropriate products from the salon's retail display for home care of hair.
8. Choose appropriate–not intimate–topics of conversation for small talk; do not ask personal questions; avoid gossip; never discuss one client with another. Avoid chatter with co-workers; focus on your client.
9. Be on the lookout for signs that the client is physically or emotionally uncomfortable.
10. Watch for "drips and runs" when applying chemicals. Make sure the water temperature is neither too hot nor too cold.
11. If you are running late, inform the client and give her the option of rescheduling if this will inconvenience her.
12. Display confidence in your abilities.
13. Help the client select her home hair care products and schedule her next visit before she leaves the salon.
14. Remind the client of the home styling and maintenance tips that you discussed during the service.
15. Thank each client warmly and sincerely at the end of each visit.
16. Never take a client for granted. Treat each client as your favorite, the way you would want to be treated.
17. Follow up with each new client, and with each existing client who has just received a service from you for the first time. Write a note or make a telephone call between visits to see how each client is doing, and to reconfirm her next appointment.

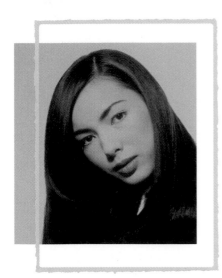

Blow-drying Horizontal Blunt

Overview

This style begins with the shoulder length horizontal blunt cut. The style shown here will maintain and show off that classic cut; you'll use a blow dryer and heat-resistant rubber-based brush to create a full, even line. It is important that you take the time to section the head properly, and to dry each section thoroughly with the brush and dryer. This will create a smooth shape that will highlight the exactness of the cut.

Connect

Blow-Drying

The purpose of blow-drying the hair is first to remove moisture from it, and then to create a finish to the blunt cut that emphasizes its line and creates smoothness. The other important tool in this finishing process is your brush. To see how important the brush is to the process of creating smooth hair, try blow-drying a finished cut without the brush. The result will be hair that is textured, perhaps unruly and out of shape, without any emphasis to the line of the cut. Next, blow-dry a section of hair while you run a brush through it. The result will be a neater finish. Finally, grip the hair with your brush, applying more tension, and you will create an even smoother finish.

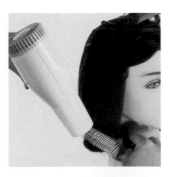

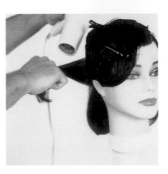

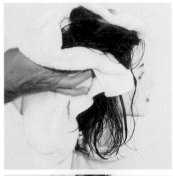

Towel and Power Drying the Hair Prior to Styling—Towel or power drying is the quickest way to remove excess moisture from the hair. This will lessen blow-drying time and effort required and will actually prove to be healthier for the hair. This will also give you more control when you direct your dryer and the brush through the hair for an even, full finish.

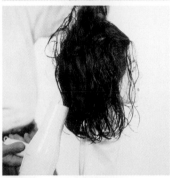

Styling Product—Apply the product for this style throughout the lengths concentrating on to the base area (near the scalp) of the hair. This will help achieve lift and height.

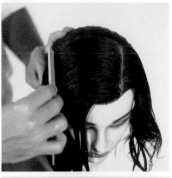

Natural or Artificial Part—Finding the natural part or creating an artificial part will help you maintain evenness in the ends of the design.

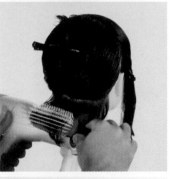

Heat-Resistant Rubber-based Brush (Denman brush)—A brush with a hard rubber base and rubber bristles is an important tool that you will use in this and a variety of style finishes. It is anti-static, and provides superb air flow through the brush.

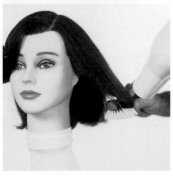

Curvature Shape—Use the brush to create roundness in the hair ends.

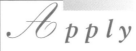

Apply

Blow-drying Horizontal Blunt

With your clients, these technical steps will follow consultation, shampoo, and power or towel drying.

1. Towel dry, then power dry the hair to remove excess moisture. Apply a styling product of your choice and work it through the hair, paying particular attention to the base area.

2. Find the natural part in the hair, or determine the artificial part if this will be different from the hair's natural part. Section off the sides from the back—clip out of the way to control.

3. Divide the back into two sections by parting from ear to ear. Control and comb the top lengths to clip out of the way.

4. Beginning at the nape, use a heat-resistant, rubber-based brush (Denman brush) to hold the hair initially at a low elevation. Follow the brush with a dryer at a medium setting while bending the ends in the preferred direction. Note how the nozzle of the blow-dryer is used when positioning for hair lengths for brush work.

5., 6. Continue, using the same technique with 1" to 1/2" (2.5 to 3.75 cm) sections, up to the occipital area. Note the angle of the hair from the scalp when blow-drying—this accentuates the base lift.

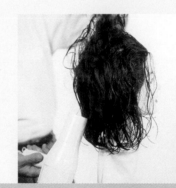
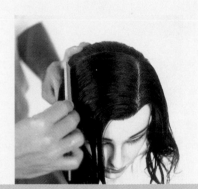
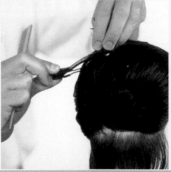

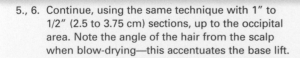
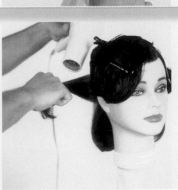

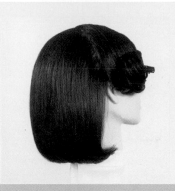

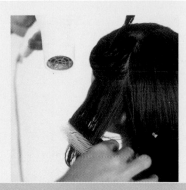

7. Here you see the results developing on the back section—a smooth rounded shape with a minimum of movement at the ends.

8. Continue with the style by subdividing the side section. Hold the hair at a low elevation with the brush and follow with the dryer, remembering to turn the edge of the brush to create a rounded edge or bend.

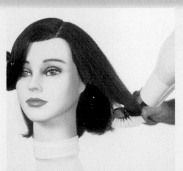

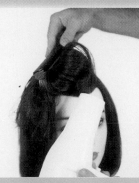

9. Continue in the same way through the rest of the side section. Turn the brush through the ends to accentuate roundness.

10. Starting with the front section, hold the hair straight up from the head. Dry the base or scalp area of the hair. At the fringe area, push the hair into a curvature shape, drying a wave formation into place. As the wave begins to form, roll the brush back to encourage a deeper wave. Work through the top with vertical sections.

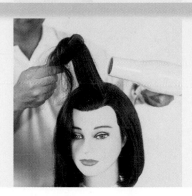

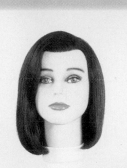

11. Next work through the top as shown. Continue drying from mid-shaft to the hair ends in the manner as outlined.

12. The finished style shows smooth sleek lines that accentuate the horizontal blunt cut.

They can because they think they can.

Virrgil

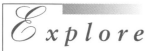

Reflect

Explore

Apply this technique to different lengths, colors, and cuts for almost endless possibilities.

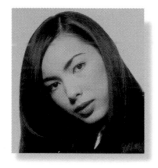

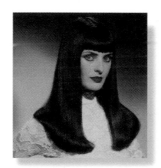

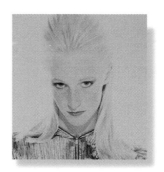

The Salon
Staff Chart

One trend that's happening in the salon business today is a trend toward "salon specialists." Rather than expecting every stylist to perform every service, these salons create specialized positions and fill them according to the talents and interests of the people on their staff. Besides giving the clients top-quality service, these salons also give their employees an opportunity to try new jobs and advance to higher pay and more responsibility. Let's look at some brief job descriptions for several different job titles in the new, "specialized" salon:

Junior Stylist: A newly licensed stylist or someone without a great deal of experience. This person might do a lot of assisting, or be limited to certain client services, until she qualifies to move up.

Stylist: An experienced, qualified generalist who can work independently when servicing clients.

Senior Stylist: Usually a veteran salon employee with a strong client following and a high rate of requests. This position sometimes includes supervision and salon management responsibilities.

Specialist (Color, Texture Services): A stylist who has really honed her skills in a specific area, such as color, texture services (waves or relaxers), or design finishes, and who works as part of a team of stylists for each client. For example, the colorist may only color the hair, while the client's regular stylist performs the cut and style finish.

Styles Director: A stylist who spends part of the salon day servicing clients, and the rest of her time hiring and supervising stylists, conducting training programs, and overseeing the salon's "image."

Salon Manager: The person responsible for making sure everything is in working order, the shelves are stocked, the employees and suppliers are paid, the tax forms are filled out. Depending on how sophisticated the salon business is, this person may also set goals for salon sales, develop a marketing program and budget, conduct staff meetings, and perform employee evaluations.

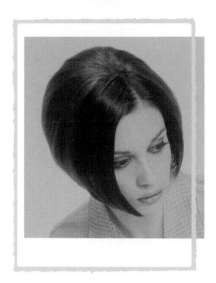

Blow-drying Diagonal Forward Blunt

Overview

This style begins with the diagonal forward blunt cut. As when you styled the horizontal blunt cut, you'll maintain the neat lines of the classic blunt cut while directing more hair forward, toward the face. It's a classic look with a contemporary twist that will work for a variety of clients' face shapes, ages, and lifestyles.

Connect

Blow-drying with the Round Brush

To create this style, the key is the use of a round brush. Roll the side hair around the face over the brush while moving it back-and-forth as you direct the heat from the dryer onto it. Be sure that the heat source moves in the same direction as the hair you're drying (especially on the surface) in order to maintain control and smoothness. Switch to a smaller brush to redefine the ends of the cut. Set the dryer first on hot, then on cool to create an evenly rolled effect toward the face. The cool air of the dryer adds strength to the design.

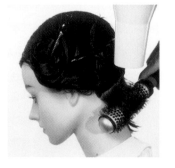 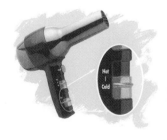

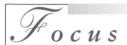

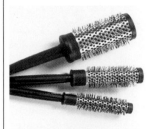

Round Brush—This cylinder-shaped brush is available in many sizes and is used to add shape or body to the hair. Using a metal cylinder brush contributes to a smoother style. The heat from the-blow dryer is transferred to the metal brush, which then smoothes the hair. ((JMB-F1))

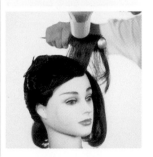

Base Area—It is important to dry the hair in the base area, the area closest to the scalp. This gives an even fullness to the design at the top of the head. Using air under the strand at the base area can strengthen and lift the motion.

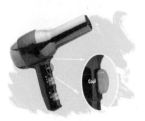

Cool Setting—Remember to set your dryer on cool to create a flip in the front of the hair. Direct the cool air from underneath for added strength. The cool air will also help lock in the style.

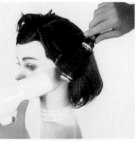

Tension—The more tension, or grip, on the hair that a tool creates, the smoother the finish will be in the final style.

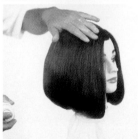

Finishing—Spray the top surface of the hair and smooth with the hand.

There is nothing permanent except change.

Heraclitus

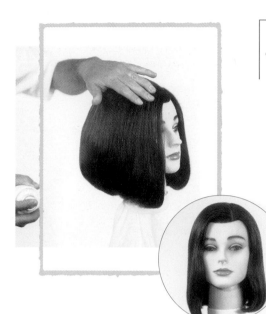

$\mathcal{A}pply$

Blow-drying Diagonal Forward Blunt

With your clients, these technical steps will follow consultation, shampoo, and power or towel drying.

1. Part the hair from the top of the ear, over the top of the head, to the other ear. Subdivide the back section, first down the center back, then the nape area. Part off diagonally on either side then comb and clip the upper lengths out of the way.

2. Starting at the nape and, using a round brush, roll the hair over the brush and raise and lower the brush while following it with a dryer.

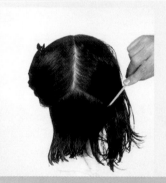
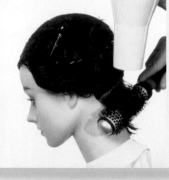

3. Continue this procedure up the back area in 1" to 1 1/2" (2.5 cm to 3.75 cm) sections. Revolve the round brush along the lengths of the hair to create the end fullness. Use tension for the ultimate smoothing effect.

4. Continue through to the side section; starting with the section over the ear, then moving up toward the side part.

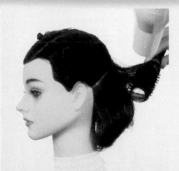
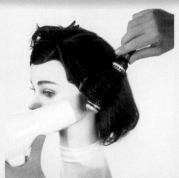

5. At the side part area, hold the section straight out while you dry the base area, and continue through to the ends.

6. Switch to a smaller brush and redefine the ends by first adding heat, then pressing the cooling button. Continue through the perimeter area following the lines of the cut. This will give a tremendous amount of extra fullness on the ends.

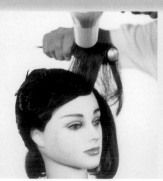
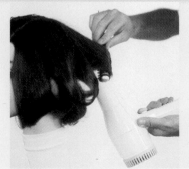
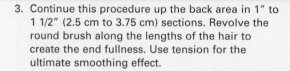

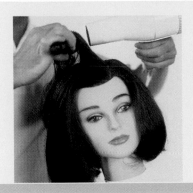

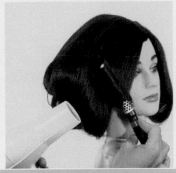

7. To create more height in the top area, hold the hair straight out from the base. First dry the base, then continue outward through the hair lengths for added strength.

8. To create a flipped under effect, roll the hair toward the face while drying, then cooling, from underneath (for added strength).

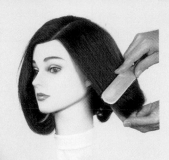

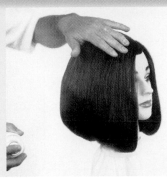

9. Again, use a small brush to accentuate the ends. Brush and loosen the entire design.

10. To finish the design, spray the top surface of the hair, and smooth with your hand. The diagonal forward blunt cut with swingy voluminous movement—a modern classic!

Genius is 99 perspiration and 1 percent inspiration.

Thomas Edison

Reflect

Explore

Apply this technique to different lengths, colors, and cuts for almost endless possibilities.

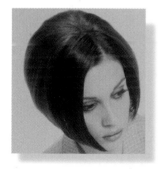
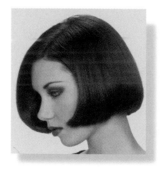
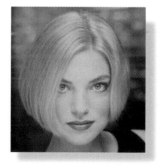

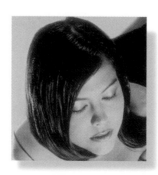

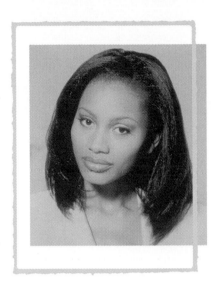

Blow-drying Textured Diagonal Back Blunt

Overview

One of the most requested services in the salon is blow-drying hair with texture into a straight shape. This style is relatively easy—but it takes patience, the right tools, and the right styling products. Focusing on one section at a time is the key to a straight finished design.

Focus

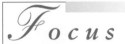

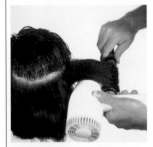

Blow-Dryer/ Brush Rotation—Using the dryer and the brush, grip the hair and stretch the brush through to its ends, letting it fall onto the side of the dryer nozzle for control. Reinsert the brush into the hair at the scalp and repeat the procedure. This constant action is the key to success with this style.

Heat and Air Settings—A higher heat and air setting will assist in drying the hair faster, given that curly hair is generally more porous and holds moisture.

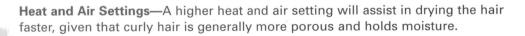

231

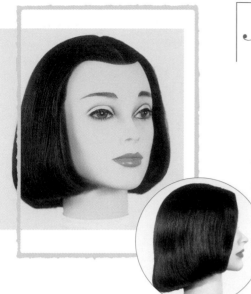

Apply

Blow-drying Textured Diagonal Back Blunt

With your clients, these technical steps will follow consultation, shampoo, and power or towel drying.

1. These are some of the styling products that you can choose from—liquid gel, conditioning foam, and silicone shiner. You may even choose to combine them.

2. Apply the product of your choice and work it through the hair.

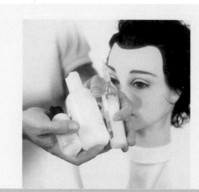
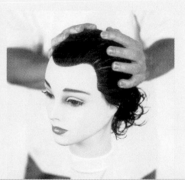

3. The hair will be divided into 1″ (2.5 cm) sections throughout the entire head for blow-drying. Clip the upper hair neatly out of the way. Start drying at the nape area. Use a large, round bristled brush to stretch and dry the hair. This type of brush allows for extra tension.

4. Use the side of the nozzle to maintain control of the section you're drying. This nozzle is inserted under the strand of hair to hold in place as repositioning the brush.

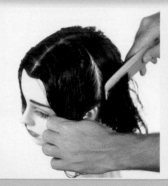
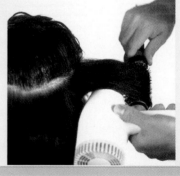

5. Follow the round brush with the dryer. Keep the brush and air flow moving through the hair.

6. Use tension to stretch the top surface of the hair for a smoother finish. Move the heat over the surface of the hair more slowly than normal, since it takes more heat to straighten.

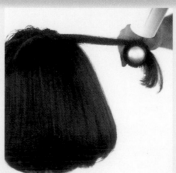
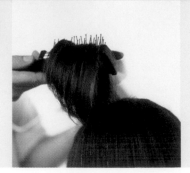

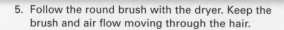

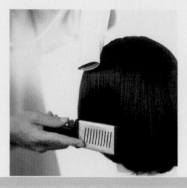

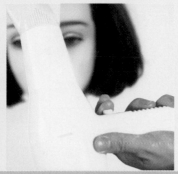

7. Holding the hair tightly, add heat to the surface of the finished style.

8. Use the cooling button on the blow-dryer to help set in movement or smoothness.

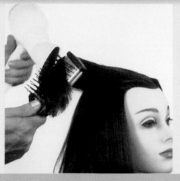

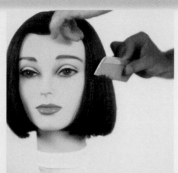

9. Use the curve of the brush to add bend to the ends of the hair.

10. Smooth the hair with a wide-toothed comb. Lightly spray the shape for hold and/or work a shiner product through the top surface.

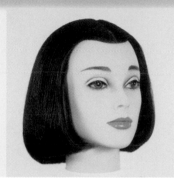

11. The finished style has a smooth texture, which defines the diagonal back blunt shape. Curly hair has been transformed through the blow-drying technique.

It is better to light a candle than curse the darkness.

Chinese Proverb

Reflect

Explore

Apply this technique to different lengths, colors, and cuts for almost endless possibilities.

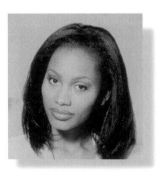

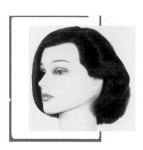

*Y*ou may use the technique featured in this style, waving the hair into an alternating wave pattern, quite effectively on a variety of different hair lengths. Practice this technique on the side area as featured here, and consider the possibilities!

1. In this style the diagonal back blunt cut will be styled on the lighter side of the part using a blow-dry waving technique to create an asymmetrical shape.

2. A vent brush is used here. A comb may also be used particularly when working on shorter lengths or wanting the waves to be smaller.

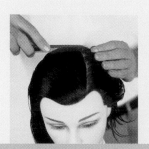
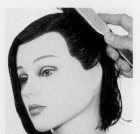

3. Direct the vent brush through the hair to create a wave pattern or "C" shaping. Direct the air flow into the trough of the wave. This is the middle of the "C" shaping.

4. Direct the brush through the first wave and into the second wave.

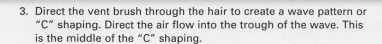
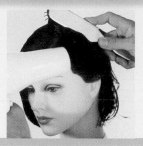
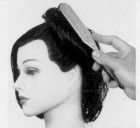

5. Direct air flow into the trough of this second wave. This is forming the alternating wave pattern. Dry thoroughly using this process. If desired you may continue into yet a third wave formation.

6. The finished style is asymmetric in nature. The waved lighter side of the style creates directional movement and control. This waving technique may be used on a variety of lengths.

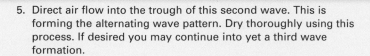
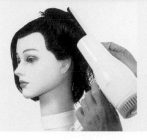
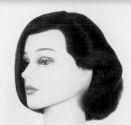

𝓛et's figure out this answer ourselves, using some commonsense logic:

Combined population of United States and Canada	300 million (approx.)
Percentage of population with heads	100
Percentage of heads with hair	80 (approx.)
Total heads of hair	240 million

Now if each of those heads uses, on average, just one eight-ounce bottle of shampoo per month, how many bottles of shampoo is that per year?

240 million x 12 months = 2.88 billion bottles of shampoo per year

Now, if each of those bottles of shampoo costs an average of $4, that's more than $10 billion a year spent in the United States and Canada–and that's just for shampoo! It doesn't even include conditioners, sprays, styling aids, scalp treatments, and so on, and so on, and so on. In truth, American and Canadian consumers spend more than $25 billion a year on hair care products.

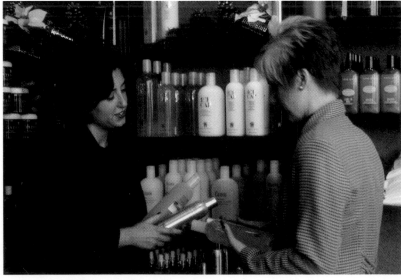

About 90 percent of that money—more than $20 billion—is spent in supermarkets, discount stores, and drugstores. (Is it any wonder that manufacturers of these products spend a couple of billion dollars a year on television advertising?) Yet the majority of the people who are buying these "over-the-counter" (not professional salon) brands do, at some time, receive salon services from a professional stylist.

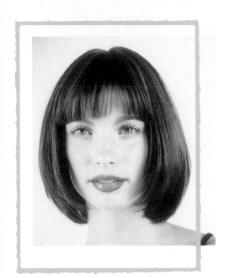

Curling Iron on Diagonal Back Blunt

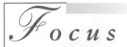

Overview

Curling irons are used to execute complete hairstyles or put finishing touches on others. Here, the basic blunt cut has not been totally altered. However, the curling iron technique shown here gives the hair added body and more control in the finished design. The hair can be left straight or transformed into an updo. The texture created from the curling iron procedure will add strength and holding ability to an updo style.

Focus

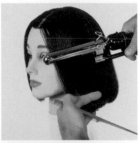

Silking the Hair—This is the process of sliding down the hair shaft lightly with the curling iron in an effort to lay down the cuticle of the hair and warm the hair to assist in rearranging the hydrogen bonds and accept curl more readily.

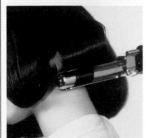

Bumping the Ends—This is a slight bend or "C" shaping performed with the curling iron to soften the ends of the hair.

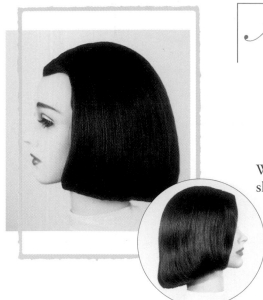

A pply
Curling Iron on Diagonal Back Blunt

With your clients, these technical steps will follow consultation, shampoo, and power or towel drying.

1. Take a small section of hair. Place the curling iron against the length of the hair. Adjust or subsection the hair panels as required according to hair density and amount of curl desired.

2. Slide the iron down the hair shaft to silk the hair rendering it more flexible and receptive to curling.

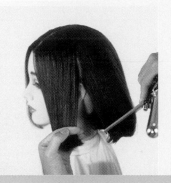
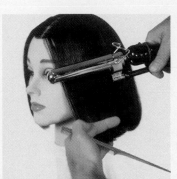

3. This iron has a revolving handle for ease in curling. Clamp the iron onto the hair strand three-quarters of the way down its length.

4. Close the iron and slide it to the ends. Roll at least three turns. Place your thumb and forefinger against the hair to check temperature. If it is too hot, release the hair.

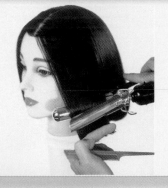
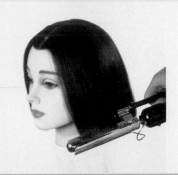

5. Subsection the hair as needed.

6. Thoroughly brush through with a bristle brush for the finished style. This technique will give strength to the finished style. The finished diagonal back blunt cut has a strongly defined line and volume at the weight line area created with the curling iron technique. Use this technique of bumping the ends on any blunt cut with the curling iron aligned with the ends of the hair.

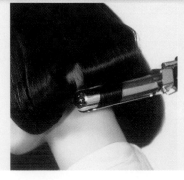
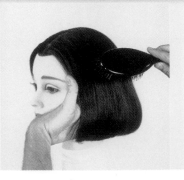

Apply this technique to different lengths, colors, and cuts for almost endless possibilities.

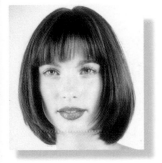

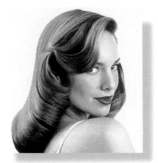

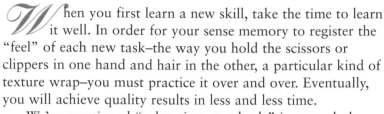

Time is Money
Part 1:

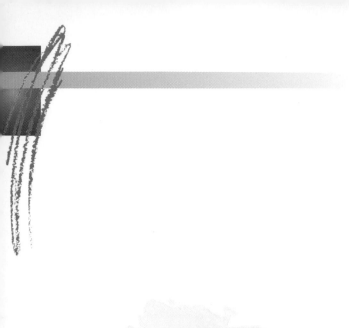

*W*hen you first learn a new skill, take the time to learn it well. In order for your sense memory to register the "feel" of each new task–the way you hold the scissors or clippers in one hand and hair in the other, a particular kind of texture wrap–you must practice it over and over. Eventually, you will achieve quality results in less and less time.

We've mentioned "salon time standards" in several places. The reason that time is so important in a salon is that time is what salons have to sell. And time is limited. The only way a salon–or a stylist who is paid on commission–can make more money is to provide more client services in the available time.

Example: You work in a salon that charges $20 for a shampoo, cut, and blow-dry. This service takes you 45 minutes, but you don't like to be rushed, and you like to take a break after each client, so you ask that your cut-and-blow-dry clients be booked an hour apart. If you begin at nine in the morning and end at five, with an hour for lunch, and every hour is booked with a shampoo-cut-blow-dry, you've done seven cuts and styles at $20 each. $20 x 7 = $140. If, for example, you receive a 50 percent commission (which is slightly above industry standards):

Your pay for the day	$70
Divided by 8 hours	$8.75 per hour
Multiplied by 5 days	$350 per week
Multiplied by 50 weeks	$17,500 per year

All of this assumes that clients never cancel and that you never have an empty slot. If just one slot doesn't book, your income is reduced to $60 per day. But you're still in the salon for eight hours, so your pay goes down to $7.50 per hour, $300 per week, and $15,000 per year.

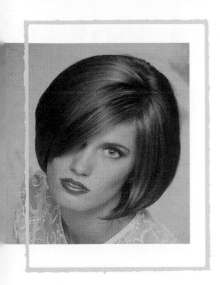

Back Combing

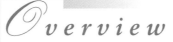

on horizontal blunt

Overview

To back comb, you comb the hair toward the scalp so that the shorter hair meshes to form a cushion or base for the top or covering hair. Back combing is the best way to create a hairstyle with full volume—as well as a method of control. While this style is modeled after the classic bouffant, the use of a texture comb and good holding spray will reinforce the hair's movement and add dimension for a contemporary look.

Focus

Feeding the Hair—Hold the hair firmly and feed it evenly into the comb while you push the hair lengths toward the base.

Blending Hair—Remember to work in small sections to ensure that the hair blends together.

Back Combing—Back combing on top of the strand causes closeness, while back combing underneath causes fullness.

Comb-out Brush—This brush has soft, flexible fine bristles.

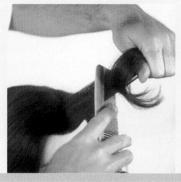

Apply
Back Combing on Horizontal Blunt

With your clients, these technical steps will follow consultation, shampoo, and power or towel drying.

1. Starting in the front section, hold the hair straight out and place your comb approximately midstrand.

2. Holding the hair firmly, slide your comb down to the base area. Remove the comb from the section and repeat. (Note that the left hand is feeding the lengths into the comb.)

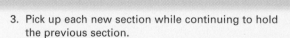

3. Pick up each new section while continuing to hold the previous section.

4. While you're holding both sections, lock in and connect them evenly.

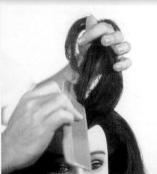
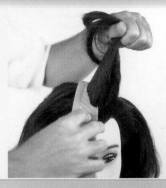

5. Continue to work through the fringe section, keeping it together and organized.

6. Begin back combing the side section, holding the hair close to the face. Curve the lengths down and around toward the face as back combing. Repeat this process on the other side.

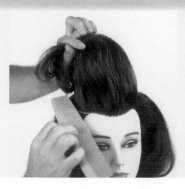
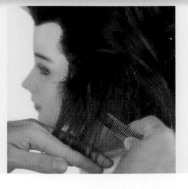

STUDENT COURSE BOOK

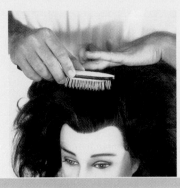
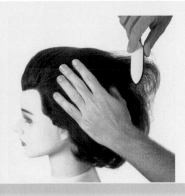

7., 8. Using a soft comb-out brush, begin to smooth the hair in the lines and direction that the back combing was completed. Work delicately along the top surface of the hair as not to remove the back combing.

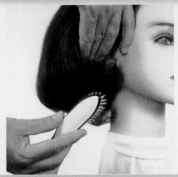
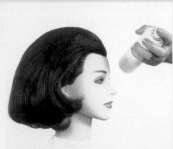

9. Continue smoothing the hair all the way around the head. Mold and place the directional movement and volume areas.

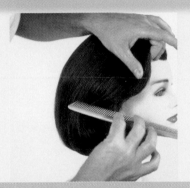
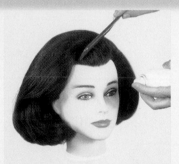

10. Once the structure of the style is complete, spray lightly with the direction of the hair.

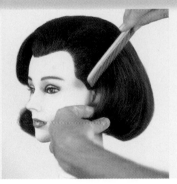
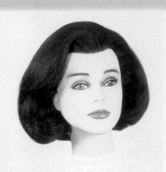

11. Use a large comb to trace over the surface, refining it. Place the comb at the end of the hair and use it to nudge in detail or movements. Create a wave movement by tracing a wave into place at the temple area.

12. Use a wide-toothed texture comb and spray to reinforce these movements, and to add dimension if desired.

13. Hold the hair in place while using a comb to stretch the movements for a more natural flow. Balance the shape.

14. The finished design may be adapted for more subtle volume or more accentuated volume. This style will have holding power throughout the day. This is truly a classic silhouette.

Explore

Apply this technique to different lengths, colors, and cuts for almost endless possibilities.

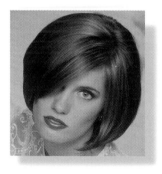

Time is Money
Part 2:

We've talked before about the importance of time standards. Remember the stylist who performed seven shampoo-cuts-blow-drys a day? Now let's look at the income of a stylist who works more quickly and who also sells chemical services to clients. This stylist's skills have improved to the point where she can complete the following services in the times given without rushing or giving clients the sense that they are on an "assembly line":

Times

Shampoo, cut, and blow-dry	30 minutes
One-process color, cut, and style	15 minutes application, 45 minutes processing, 30 minutes shampoo, cut, and style
Foils and perms, with cut and style	90 minutes

Prices

Shampoo, cut, and blow-dry:	$20
One-process color, cut, and style	$55
Foils and perms, with cut and style	$80 (average)

Now a productive day might look like this:

9:00	Client 1: One-process color application	$55
9:30	Client 2: Cut and style	$20
10:00	Client 1: Finish	—
10:30	Client 3: Perm, cut, and style	$80
12:00-12:30—Lunch		
12:30	Client 4: Foil, shampoo, cut, and style	$80
2:00	Client 5: One-process color application	$55
2:30	Client 6: Cut and style	$20
3:00	Client 5: Finish	—
3:30	Client 7: Perm, shampoo, cut, and style	$80
5:00	Off book	——
Total services		$330

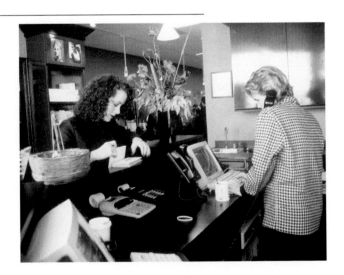

At a 50 percent commission, this stylist earned $195 in eight hours, or $34.38 per hour. That's $975 for a five-day week, which amounts to nearly $50,000 per year–more if you count tips from clients and commissions on retail products sold to clients.

Can you see how different days can bring different pay? You've seen two different stylists. Both have the same technical abilities. Both work 40 hours per week. Both service seven clients per day. One earns $15,000 per year; one earns more than $50,000. The difference is time and how efficiently each uses it.

Which stylist would you rather become?

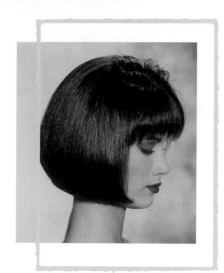

Blow-drying Graduated Blunt

Overview

This style begins with the graduated blunt cut that you completed in the haircutting part of the program. Styling this cut with an asymmetric look is very slimming to the face and answers the needs of the client who wants to move her hair off her face. Again, the simple movement of the brush and blow-dryer through the hair will create body and ornamental effects without diminishing the sculptural silhouette of the cut.

Focus

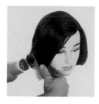

Concave Shape—This is a hollowed or indented movement in the finished form of the hair created with the brush and dryer.

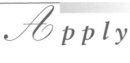

Apply

Blow-drying Graduated Blunt

With your clients, these technical steps will follow consultation, shampoo, and power or towel drying.

1. Apply a styling product of your choice, and work it through the hair. Use a side part as a design part.

2. Begin contouring in the nape area with the rubber based bristle brush. Directionally flow the hair outward from the center back on either side. The air flow follows the brush as it closely contours the hair against the head.

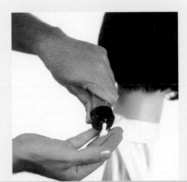
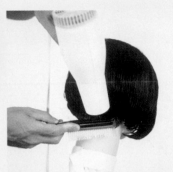

3. Above the occipital begin parting out along a diagonal forward. Insert the last two rows of the brush to lift and direct the hair as blow-drying. Continue upward and maintain the brush as drying along the diagonal forward.

4. Continue this process into the sides and up to the side part. Lift the hair out from the base area according to the amount of base lift desired. Turn the ends and dry to bevel the ends under.

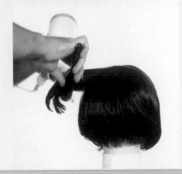
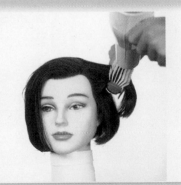

5. Repeat the process on the other side of the head. Concentrate on using precise blow-drying technique. Alternate the brush through the lengths and bevel the ends for a rounded weight line.

6. Finish blow-drying the front area, paying particular attention to the base area and mid shaft. The ends will be dried upward. Grasp the ends in the brush and turn upward to create a flipped effect.

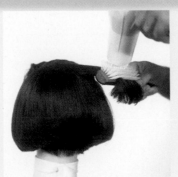
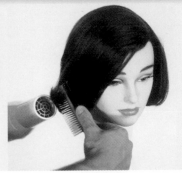

Reflect

Explore

Apply this technique to different lengths, colors, and cuts for almost endless possibilities.

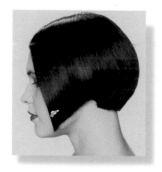 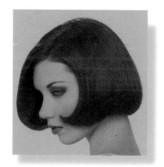 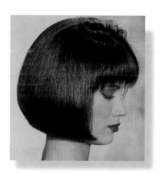

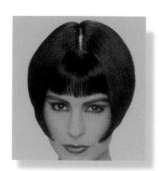

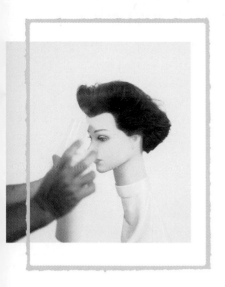

Blow-drying Low Graduation

Overview

This style begins with the low graduation mid-length cut you completed in the haircutting part of the program. The use of radial sections through the interior of the head makes the blow drying of graduated shapes fast, easy, and efficient. You'll use both the round and paddle brushes to get the most volume for this style.

Connect

Blow-drying with Holding Spray

Using a holding spray and blow-dryer on the hair at the same time allows the spray to reach all of the hair's surface internally, giving extra hold.

Focus

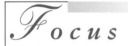

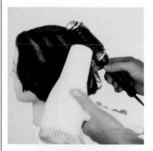

Directional Setting with Round Brush—This is the technique of rolling the hair through the interior around a round brush either vertically or diagonally and blow-drying the section. It gives the maximum amount of volume to the hair.

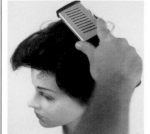

Paddle Airflow Brush—Slightly smaller than the larger paddle brush, this brush has air-flow vents that allow quicker drying suitable for all lengths of hair except with massive density.

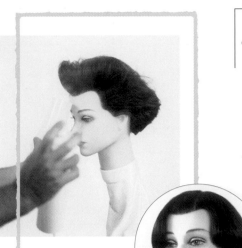

A p p l y

Blow-drying Low Graduation

With your clients, these technical steps will follow consultation, shampoo, and power or towel drying.

1. Apply a styling product of your choice, and work it through the hair. Use a round brush to part the hair into diagonal sections through the interior.

2. Work around the head using the dryer to follow the round brush positioned diagonally.

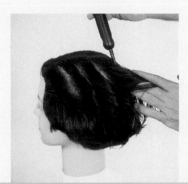

3. In the top area, direct lengths forward, then roll towards the base as blow drying. This will maximize volume given the over-directed base. Continue this technique toward the front hair line area. The front fringe section is rolled using the same technique to create a volume effect in this area.

4. Use a paddle airflow brush to stretch the shape and brush into place.

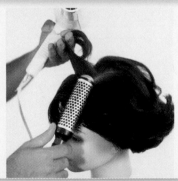
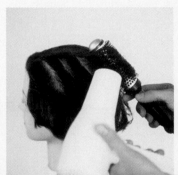

5. Use a hair spray and dryer technique to finish the design. Spray directionally up and into the front hairline lengths while following with the blow dryer. This will create enhanced directional hold, body, and lift. Again, brush through with the large paddle brush to loosen the lines of the style.

6. The finished style is very commercial and wearable for a large number of clientele. The technique may be adapted on a variety of other haircuts.

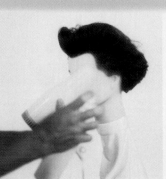
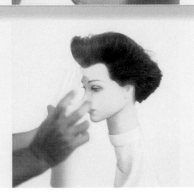
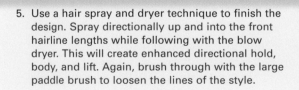

Reflect

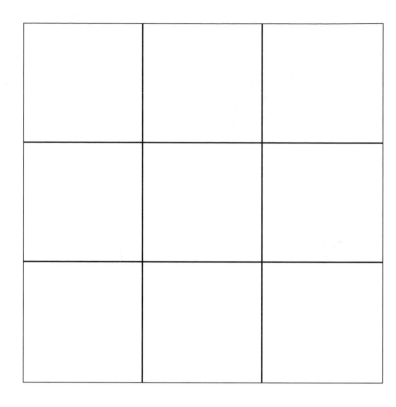

Explore

Apply this technique to different lengths, colors, and cuts for almost endless possibilities.

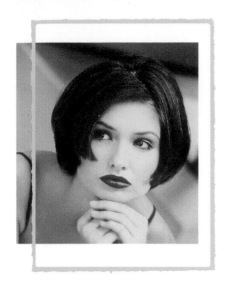

Blow-drying Blunt with Graduation

Overview

The blunt cut with a graduated front offers the client a classic style with a contemporary twist. It is a popular and versatile style that's also relatively easy for the client to maintain between appointments. The use of a good spray shine will give the hair a healthy glow—and gives you, the stylist an opportunity to retail the product to the client for home use.

Connect

Damp and Dry Hair

To create a straight shape, use small sections. Always lay damp onto dry hair, then stretch and smooth. This allows the hair to be dried quickly and evenly.

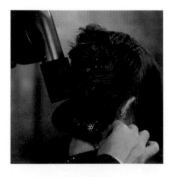

Focus

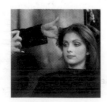

Spray Shine—The use of a shine enhancer in a spray container not only gives the hair a strong, healthy look, but enhances the natural fall of the cut as well.

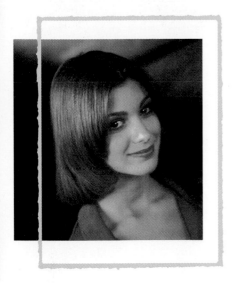

Apply
Blow-drying Blunt with Graduation

With your clients, these technical steps will follow consultation, shampoo, and power or towel drying.

1. Apply a combination of styling products of your choice and work the products through the hair. Layering products is a sophisticated way of getting the exact results that you want. This takes excellent product knowledge.

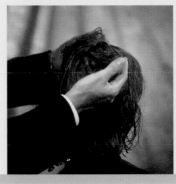

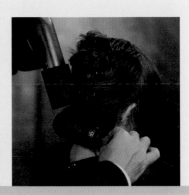

2. Start at the nape using a large round brush. Revolve the brush as directing the airflow. Work concisely and neatly.

3., 4. Continue through the back section. Focus on your neatness and your speed.

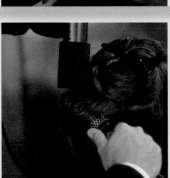

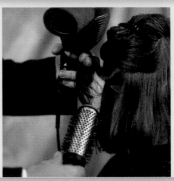

5. Hold the crown section up and away from the head for added volume. Direct the airflow from the base area outward to the ends. Note how easily the bristles of the round brush pick up and stretch these lengths. Direct into the center back.

6. Continue through the side section, holding the hair out from the head and following with the round brush to curl the ends.

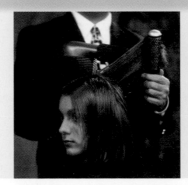

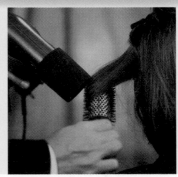

7., 8. Dry the fringe area by using a round brush toward the face.

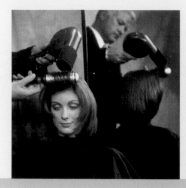 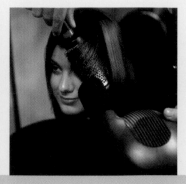

9. A spray shine is applied to accentuate a glossy surface finish.

10. Finish the design and detail the ends.

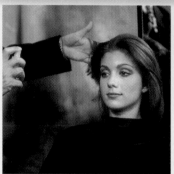 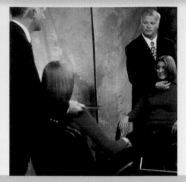

11. The finished style is sleek and smooth, suitable for all occasions.

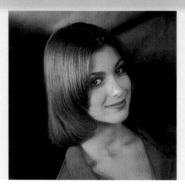

There is always room at the top.

Daniel Webster

R eflect

E xplore

Apply this technique to different lengths, colors, and cuts for almost endless possibilities.

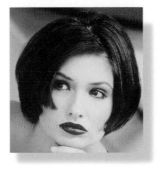

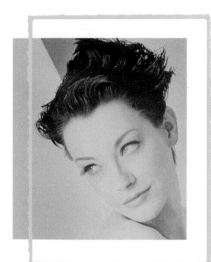

Blow-drying Graduated Horizontal

Overview

This style begins with the graduated, short-length horizontal cut you completed in the haircutting part of this program. As with the mid-length, graduated style, the keys to creating body and movement are the use of the round brush and your blow-drying technique. Because of the shorter hair length, you'll use a large-tooth comb and your fingers to stretch the hair in front; this adds an interesting contrast to the tapered back.

Connect

Finger Styling

The use of your fingers allows the natural movement of the hair to respond to your styling, and speeds up drying. This technique is best suited to hair that falls into style easily and has some natural volume and movement. It's an informal, natural look.

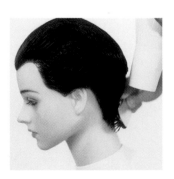

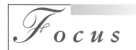

Natural Volume and Movement—Use fingers to create lift and design while styling.

Base Control Technique—Use a round brush to create the effect of a roller while blow-drying. Consider the position of the round brush to the base (the base control) according to the desired results.

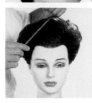

Texture Comb—This wide-tooth comb is used to create dimension or separation for a natural look.

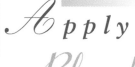

Apply

Blow-drying Graduated Horizontal

With your clients, these technical steps will follow consultation, shampoo, and power or towel drying.

1. Apply a styling product of your choice.

2. Work the product through the hair.

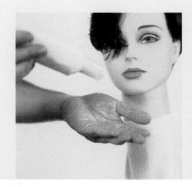

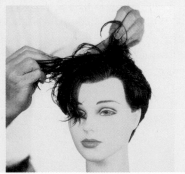

3. Begin to dry the hair in the nape area, using a brush to direct and shape the hair.

4. Using a round metal brush, roll sections of hair in the back of the crown and blow-dry. A one diameter base area (to the size of the brush) is rolled to position on base for perfect volume.

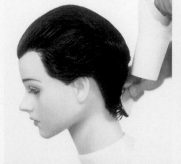 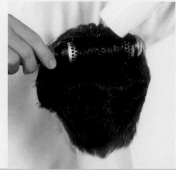

5. Move forward in the crown area, one section at a time, using a one diameter on-base technique. The hair is held 45 degrees (.785 rad) from the center of the base and rolled.

6. Secure the rolled hair with long clips at the scalp.

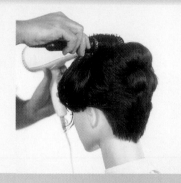 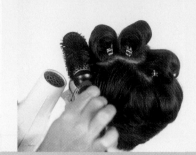

7. Continue to blow-dry rolled sections working toward the front hairline area. Clip each section as completed.

8. Remove the clips through the interior. Complete the side section by connecting the side hairline lengths with the front fringe area. Lightly spray as directing the airflow.

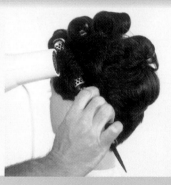 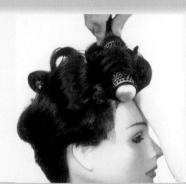

9., 10. Comb through the set with a texture comb to blend and shape the hair.

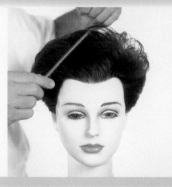 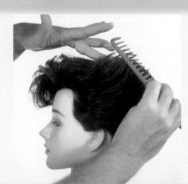

11. Use your fingers to place and style the ends. Continue to place the hair into the style lines. Lightly spray.

12. The finished style features lift and movement in the crown with a softly directed fringe.

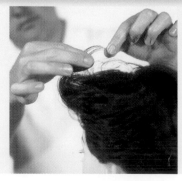 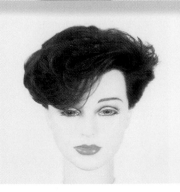

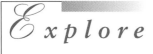

Reflect

Explore

Apply this technique to different lengths, colors, and cuts for almost endless possibilities.

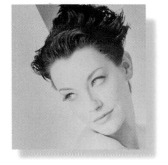

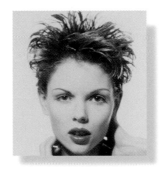

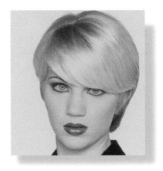

Think? Why think! We have computers to do that for us.

Jean Rostand

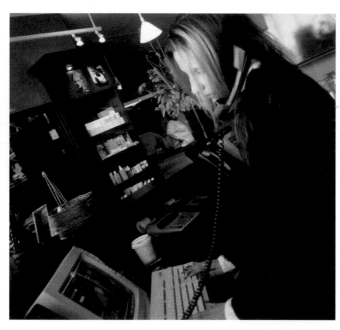

$\mathscr{M}$any of the tasks we've discussed already, such as appointment scheduling, client record keeping, and communicating with clients by mail—as well as others we haven't yet discussed, such as retail product inventory control—can be made simpler and more efficient through the use of a computer. Many salons today use computers for these tasks, and several companies have designed software systems specifically for the salon business.

Computers store and report information in a variety of ways to help salon managers monitor salon operations and then set goals for improving them. Computers generate reports that tell you:

◆ **The average length of time being spent for each client service.**

◆ **What percent of salon hours are productive hours, and what percent are considered "downtime."**

◆ **The average amount of money spent by each client on services and retail goods.**

◆ **The actual "cost" to the salon of each service and product it sells. This helps in making decisions about what prices to charge and what goals to set for more efficient and profitable operations.**

With the regular reports generated by the computer, the manager can set goals for improvement, and get regular progress reports. Don't be surprised if computers are in your salon future. If you're not familiar with how computers work, grab your first opportunity to take an introductory class. Nearly every school system offers adult education classes in computers. Most libraries have computers that the general public can use, also.

The Dispensary

Quality is never an accident.

Will A. Foster

Dis•pen•sa•ry: a place in a hospital, school, or camp from which medicines and first aid supplies are dispensed.

The salon dispensary is the room or area where the color solutions, relaxer and wave chemicals, rollers, brushes, combs, towels, capes, and a wide variety of other "tools of the trade" are stored. The name "dispensary" has its origins in the medical profession. (So do many of the traditions of today's hair salons. Did you know that, in an earlier part of this century, hairstyling students wore nurse uniforms and caps?)

The history and definition of the name "dispensary" should give you a clue about how important a place it is. For reasons of both efficiency and safety, rules and procedures must be carefully followed in the dispensary. Chemical spills must be cleaned up. Everyone in the salon should do their part to make sure the dispensary is properly stocked and the items in it handled properly and always cleaned thoroughly. You are learning about how infection and disease can be spread in a salon if such procedures are ignored. As a salon employee, you will be expected to help with stocking, arranging, and maintaining the dispensary.

When you see that a product is running low, follow the procedures you have been taught so that it can be reordered. Never put an empty bottle back, and always read the labels and instructions if you're not familiar with a product or ask someone who is. The health and safety of many trusting clients are in your hands. Take your responsibilities seriously.

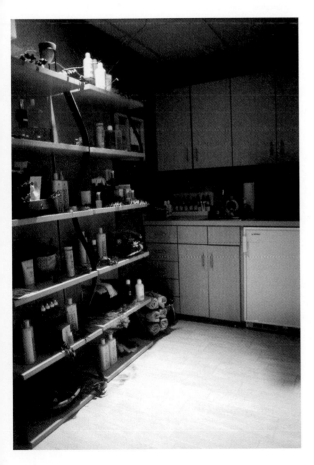

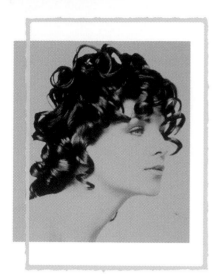

Curling Iron on Graduated Horizontal

Overview

This technique employs a curling-iron set with back brushing for a finished yet natural style that is suitable for all occasions or environments.

Focus

On-Base Curling Iron—The curling iron sits between its base partings.

Light Brushing—Run the brush gently through the hair so as not to brush out the curls.

Finger Separation—Accomplished by running your fingers through the hair. This technique gently separates the curls.

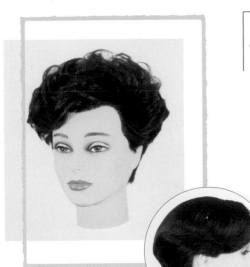

Apply

Curling Iron on Graduated Horizontal

With your clients, these technical steps will follow consultation, shampoo, and power or towel drying.

1. Place the iron at the base of the hair. Close the iron.

2. Slide it through to the ends of the hair.

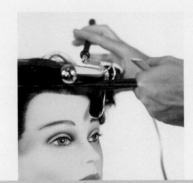
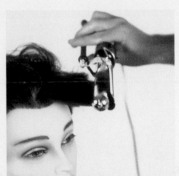

3. Roll it down to the base.

4. Place a hard rubber comb between the iron and scalp area. Continue to roll sections around the head. Note the base control used here. The hair is rolled using a 45 degree (.785 rad.) angle from the base to position the curl on base. Continue working with diagonal sections through the top.

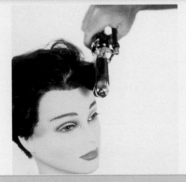
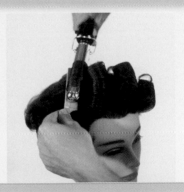

5., 6. Continue this procedure throughout the head. Use the comb to pick up and curl short perimeter lengths.

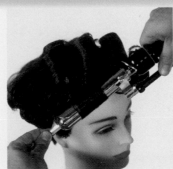
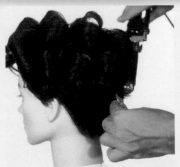

7., 8. Begin back brushing. The hair sections are held down and the back brushing is done along the top surface.

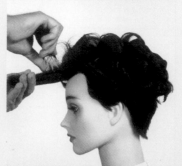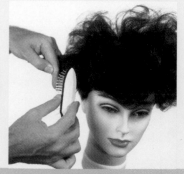

9. Use your fingers for texture and separation.

10. Lightly brush over the top surface of the hair.

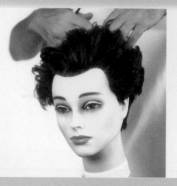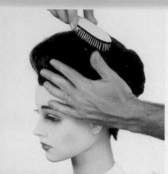

11. Push the airy volume into place. Separate the hair with a texture comb and/or your fingers.

12. Personalize the shape for the client. Check for proportion in the shape. Spray and balance the design.

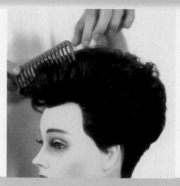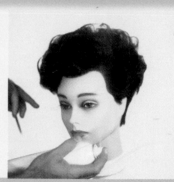

13. The finished style features expanded volume, movement and texture.

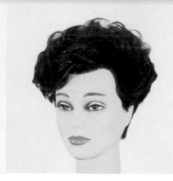

Apply this technique to different lengths, colors, and cuts for almost endless possibilities.

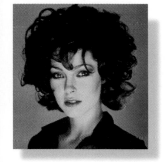

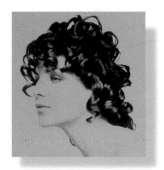

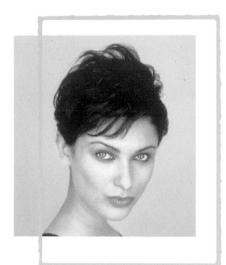

Blow-drying Layered Square Shape

Overview

The styling of shorter shapes is usually dictated by the way in which the hair was cut. Clients choose shorter shapes because they want ease of handling—so the finish should be easy care, too.

Connect

Styling Aids

Styling products make the hair more manageable during the drying process. They also give it the body it needs to hold the hairstyle. Your choice of styling aid will be determined by the client's hair type, the hairstyle, the features of a particular product, your personal preference, and the salon's policy. Remember to read the manufacturer's guidance notes.

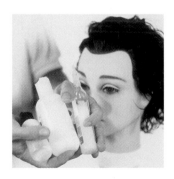

Focus

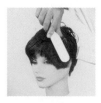

Short-Cut Styling—Many times a short cut just needs a light blend with the brush and dryer to achieve the desired lift and form.

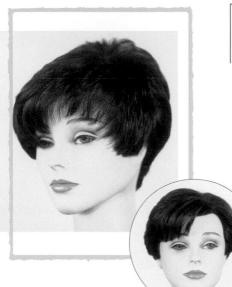

Apply
Blow-drying Layered Square Shape

With your clients, these technical steps will follow consultation, shampoo, and power or towel drying.

1. Distribute the hair into the style lines. Next, apply a styling product of your choice. Here a liquid gel is used for sleek control.

2. Work the product through the hair. A foam is applied to the crown area for more airy volume.

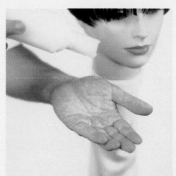
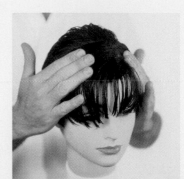

3. Begin to dry the front area. Direct the lengths and the air flow into the desired movement. The airflow is directed along the top surface. A vent brush facilitates even, thorough airflow.

4. Work around to the nape. Again the lengths are closely contoured.

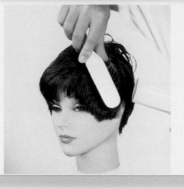
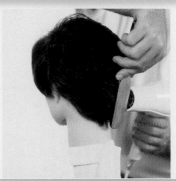

5. Switch to a round brush and begin to work the crown area, with the goal being to maximize volume in this area.

6. Continue through to the side section on either side connecting with the directional placement in the crown.

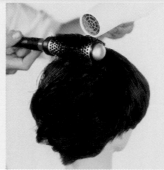
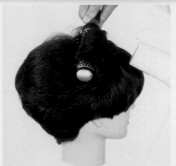

7. Comb the hair with a wide-toothed texture comb.

8. Detail the ends with your fingers, using a small amount of spray or pomade on the finger tips.

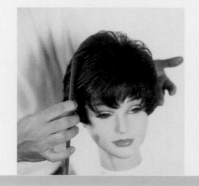
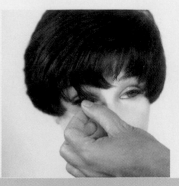

9. Spray to finish. Lift for volume in the crown—balance the shape while spraying.

10. Use your creative artistry to finish this design. Directional movement, volume, and enhanced texture are all features of this finished style.

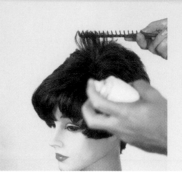
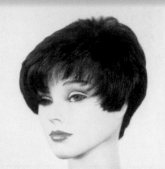

Getting an idea should be like sitting down on a pin; it should make you jump up and do something.

E. L. Simpson

Reflect

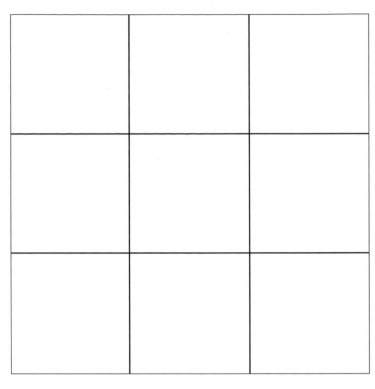

Explore

Apply this technique to different lengths, colors, and cuts for almost endless possibilities.

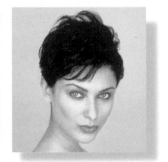

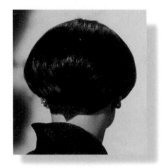

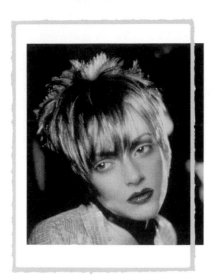

Thermal Styling on Tapered Layers

Overview

The use of proper technique on short hair is the key to a well-finished style. Know which areas you want to remain close and which you want to create volume in. This will tell you how to approach the style and what styling products to use in each area.

Connect

Blow-drying with a Brush

The movement of your brush back and forth in opposite directions creates a loose texture; it deflects the hot air, reduces its heat, and dries the hair nearest the scalp. It creates a style that has a more natural look, instead of a structured design with little movement.

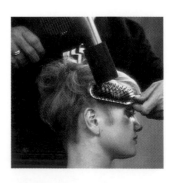

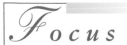

*F*ocus

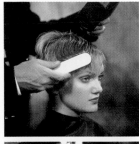

Curvature Shape—This describes the movement of your brush and dryer in a round, curved design.

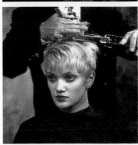

Directional Curls—Directional curls add strength to the design and give a more finished look. Use a curling iron to create them.

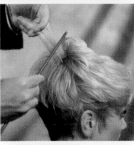

Texture Comb—Use a wide-toothed comb to create dimension or separation for a natural look.

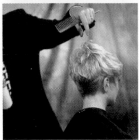

Combination Treatment—The use of one or more treatments or liquid styling products can customize the creation of texture, hold, and shine.

Dreams can be realized if you work hard.

Warren G. Jackson

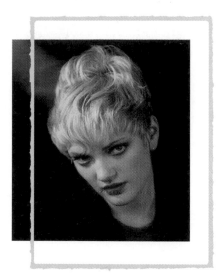

With your clients, these technical steps will follow consultation, shampoo, and power or towel drying.

1. Apply a styling product of your choice and work through the hair. Dry the nape area close to the head by following the brush with your dryer. Trace closely at the lower nape area to create a contoured silhouette.

2. Through the crest area insert the brush at the base and lift out to create fullness through this area.

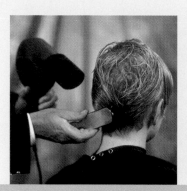
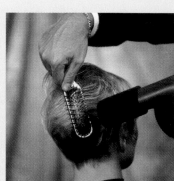

3. Lift the hair in the crown section, also following the brush with your dryer. Direct the air flow into the over directed base area to create maximum volume.

4. Begin to lift the top section directing the hair orward from the crown. Then turn the brush directionally sideways through the front fringe area.

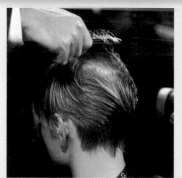
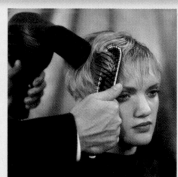

5. Mold the top section into a curving shape, following the brush with your dryer. Direct the air flow into the trough of the wave, then alternate direction into the next wave.

6. Roll the hair over your brush and begin lifting the side section. Continue until the head is complete.

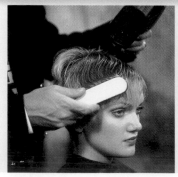
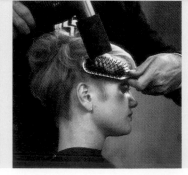

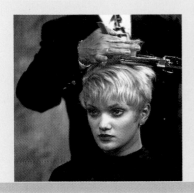
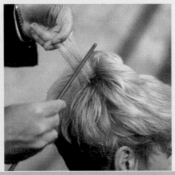

7. To add strength to the design, use a medium-size curling iron to make directional curls. Curls radiate out from the crown area.

8. Use a texture comb and your fingers to rake through the hair, separating and detailing the design.

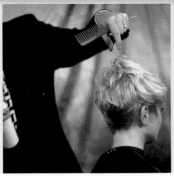
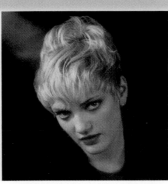

9. Spray to support the movement and volume as placing and detailing the lengths.

10. The finished style features a sculpted feeling that accentuates the short tapered haircut.

Twenty years from now you will be more disappointed by the things you didn't do than by the things you did do.

Mark Twain

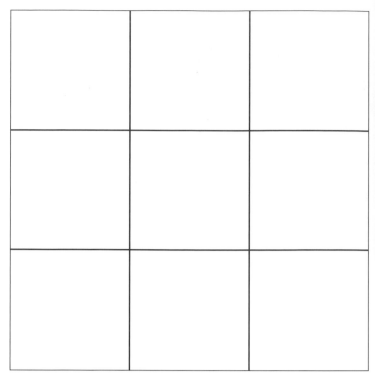

Apply this technique to different lengths, colors, and cuts for almost endless possibilities.

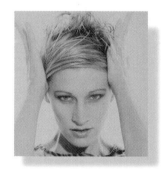
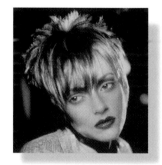
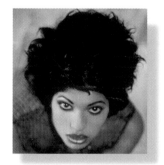

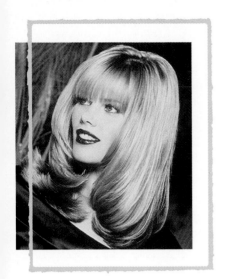

Hot Roller Comb Out on Perimeter Layers

Overview

This style begins with the perimeter layered cut you completed in the haircutting part of this program (see page 134). The use of hot rollers will create a style with body, strength, and hold. With these tools you can create a contemporary look that will hold—and still look soft.

Connect

Roller Diameter

The diameter of the rollers you use will dictate the degree of curl or wave achieved in the hair, as well as affecting the amount of base lift produced. Rollers that have small diameters will produce tight curls and maximum volume in the hair. Large-diameter rollers will produce a soft wave movement in hair—along with subtle base lift.

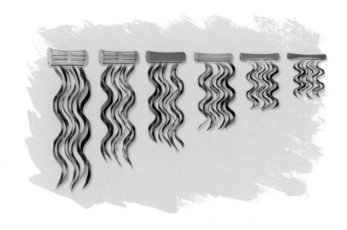

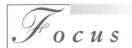

F o c u s

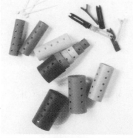

Hot Roller—This tool is available in a variety of sizes. The length and amount of the hair wrapped around the roller, the size of the roller, the base control and the direction of the roller all affect the finished hairstyle by creating lift, volume, and/or indentation.

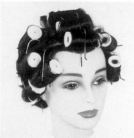

Directional Set—Place all of the rollers in the same direction to create a smoothness in the finished design.

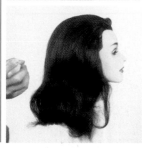

Scale Out the Design—This process involves defining or identifying the correct proportions for the shape and size of the design.

Nothing happens unless first a dream

Carl Sandburg

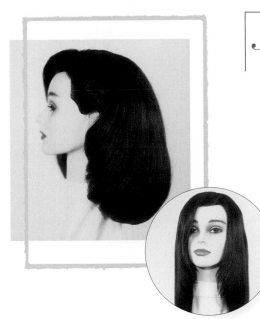

$\mathscr{A}$ pply
Hot Roller Comb Out on Perimeter Layers

With your clients, these technical steps will follow consultation, shampoo, and power or towel drying.

1.,2. It is important to scale out the design and roll directionally, making sure that all of the rollers are moving in the direction you want. In this case the rollers are set through the center top rolling back and toward the face through the sides.

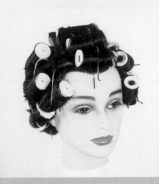
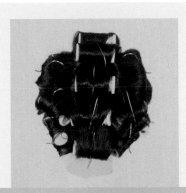

3.,4. Comb out and dry mold the set.

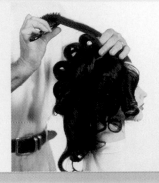
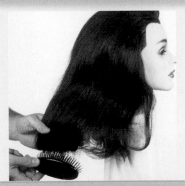

5. Apply a shine product and begin back brushing the hair.

6. Spray for added support.

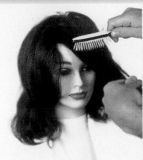
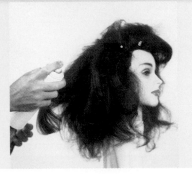

7.,8. Brush in structure and begin to detail. A light touch when combing, as well as a complete follow-through with your brush, can add to a perfect result.

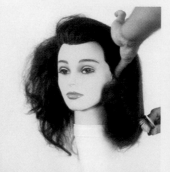 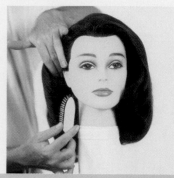

9. Finish with hair spray.

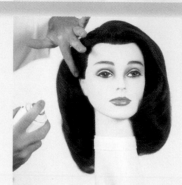

Transformation literally means going beyond your form.

Dr. Wayne Dyer

Reflect

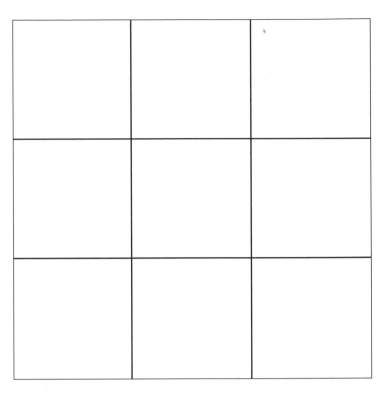

Explore

Apply this technique to different lengths, colors, and cuts for almost endless possibilities.

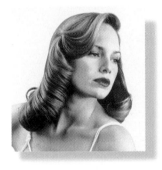

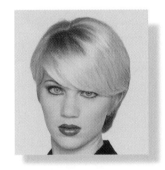

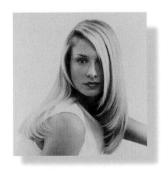

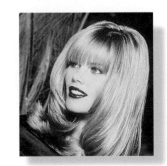

texture comb out of wet set/perimeter layers

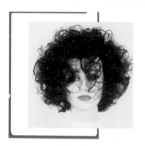

*W*hen the client requires exceptional hold you may want to consider a set set with traditional rollers. Vary the roller size accordingly to create the desired textural movement and expansion of the shape. This is an excellent way to introduce a client to temporary textural changes in her hair, perhaps inspiring a chemical waving process to be performed during the next visit.

1. Using a wet set you can create firm, resilient texture that provides maximum strength and volume.

2. Apply a styling product of your choice. Here a silicone shine product is used.

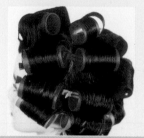
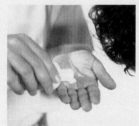

3. Use the fingers and a texture comb to gently break up the set and place.

4. Detail the ends as needed and adjust the volume. Lightly spray for hold.

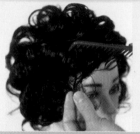
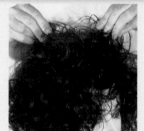

5. The finished style is full of defined curls, creating movement and lush texture. This strength is a result of the wet set.

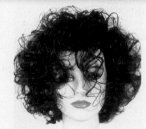

comb out of velcro
set/light layers

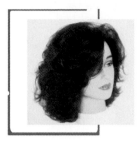

*T*his type of set is recommended for clients who need more body than a round brush and blow-dry styling can provide—but less than an electric curler or traditional set. Many clients want styles with a very full and bouncy look. Replacing the hair onto the Velcro rollers creates that desired fullness.

The Velcro-type roller will create a fuller look than brush and blow-dryer, but a softer and more natural look than the traditional roller set. Since these rollers grip the hair easily and tightly, be careful not to pull or entangle the hair in the process.

1. Apply a styling product of choice. Use a round brush to form curl formations throughout the entire head.

2. Replace the curl formation with Velcro rollers, apply one diameter on-base to engage the roller within the base area. When the head is complete, leave the rollers in place for a few minutes.

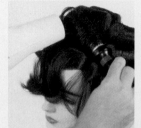
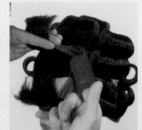

3. Brush and dry mold the set into the style lines.

4. Use a silicone shiner to massage through the hair lengths enhancing texture and shine.

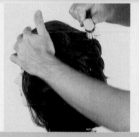
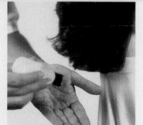

5. Detail and spray. Check for balance and harmony in the silhouette. Use a large toothed texture comb to do final detailing.

6. The finished style features a tousled, textured feeling, created with round brushing and Velcro roller setting combined.

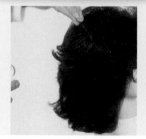
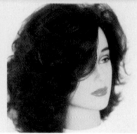

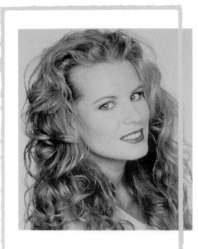

Blowdrying Curly Hair/ Heavy Layers

Overview

This technique for drying textured or overcurly hair will distort the curl as little as possible, giving the hair a clean and healthy look that's free from frizziness. You'll use both a vent brush and a blow-dryer, allowing you to lift the hair for quick drying and natural separation.

Connect

Blow-dryer Options

Don't overheat the hair; excessive heat can damage it, and can cause your client discomfort. Also, avoid holding the airflow against the hair in one place for too long, because this can overheat and damage the hair.

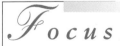

Focus

Low-Speed Drying—Using low-speed air from the dryer and a gentle touch will allow the curls of the hair to fall into place naturally. This technique is best used on layered or mid-length shapes or shorter.

Vent Brush—The vent brush has holes throughout its base to allow the warm air to penetrate to the hair in every position.

Apply
Blow-drying Curly Hair/ Heavy Layers

With your clients, these technical steps will follow consultation, shampoo, and power or towel drying.

1. Thoroughly towel dry the hair. Apply a styling product of your choice and work it through the hair.

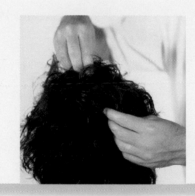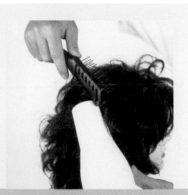

2. Use a vent brush to provide thorough, effective air flow onto the hair while creating volume.

3. Use small, gentle finger movements to separate the hair.

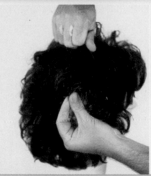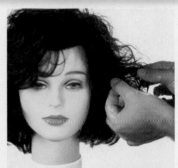

4. Finish the design by separating the textured hair with the tips of your fingers.

5. The finished style shows enhanced textural movement and volume.

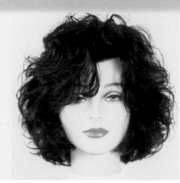

Apply this technique to different lengths, colors, and cuts for almost endless possibilities.

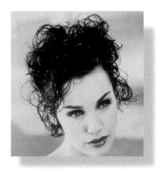

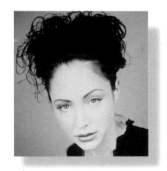

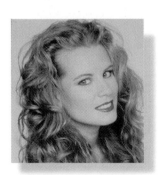

Is Retailing
Part 2:
Really Important?

*I*f most salon clients use shampoo, why don't they buy it in the salon? Simple. Salons and stylists have not placed the importance they should on making sure that their clients use professional products. Let's look at what would happen in salons if every salon client spent just $10 on hair care products to use at home. (Remember, that's $10 they're going to spend anyway, but on a product that might not be right for their hair.)

"Average" salon:

5 stylists x 30 clients each per week = 150 clients per week

150 clients x $10 each = $1,500 per week in retail sales

x 52 weeks = $78,000 per year

On average, salons pay about half of the retail price for the products they sell. So through retailing, a typical salon would add $39,000 a year to its profits without hiring one more person. At the same time, each of the five stylists, if paid 10 percent commission, would add about $1,560 per year to their income. All this just for making sure that clients–who, we know, have to buy hair care products somewhere–bought their products in the salon, where a professional stylist who knows what their hair needs can help them select the right products.

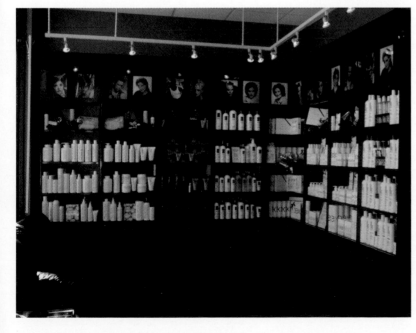

Then, instead of the current $2 billion a year that clients spend on hair care products at the salon, they'd be spending $15 billion a year, more than half of the total expenditure! (And we haven't even begun to discuss nail products or cosmetics.)

Is retailing important? It should be. And it will be if, one by one, stylists begin to understand just how important it is.

diffusing curly hair

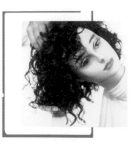

*A*diffuser is a blow-dryer attachment that spreads the flow of air over a greater area so that it does not come out the end of the dryer so fast. This dries the hair more evenly and slowly, and allows textured or naturally curly hair to maintain its wave pattern. The light layered shape is shown fully textured with shiny, luscious, spiral curl formations created with a diffuser technique of drying.

1., 2. Towel or power dry to remove excess moisture. Apply the styling product of choice. Tilting the head in a variety of directions, allow the hair to rest in the saucer of the diffuser. Gently lift and diffuse the hair. Press the diffuser up towards the scalp area. This will encourage curls to form.

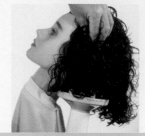 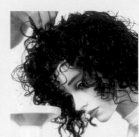

3. Have the client tilt her head from side to side and continue until the entire head is completely dry. It is the free fall of hair away from the head coupled with the diffusing action that creates the springy, resilient curls. Apply a light spray if desired as well as a silicone shiner to finish the style.

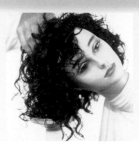

Always bear in mind that your own resolution to succeed is more important than any other one thing.

Abraham Lincoln

Salon Hygiene:
Safety and Comfort

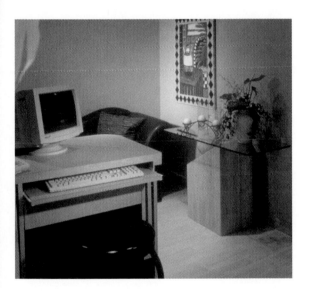

The word *hygiene* means "clean" and "healthful." You might not think of this word when you think of a salon, but it is important for everyone working in a salon to pay attention to the "health" of the salon environment.

Chemicals used for both hair and nail services give off gases. If smoking is permitted anywhere inside a salon building, even if it is limited to the break room or reception area, the gases in secondhand smoke can combine in sometimes dangerous ways with the gases in the chemicals being used.

Clients and employees wear a variety of perfumes and cosmetics, and certain combinations at certain times can lead to allergic reactions of both skin and sinuses–even in people who've never experienced allergic reactions before. An air bubble in a container can cause the chemical inside to spray in all directions when first opened, so wearing safety glasses and gloves is a wise move when you're preparing and applying chemicals.

Even the noise level of a salon–the roar of dryers, volume of the stereo system, ringing of the phone, and loud laughter of clients and stylists who've become good friends–can contribute to creating a stressful environment. Is a stressful environment appropriate for a business that specializes in personal service and attention? No, we don't think so, either.

These issues are important to you, as a stylist, as well. If you spend your day inside a space where chemicals are being used and proper ventilation isn't, you could become susceptible to a range of illnesses and immune system difficulties, including certain types of cancer.

As one stylist in a salon, you can do your part by observing all safety procedures when handling chemicals. Be aware of the salon atmosphere, as well. Too often, we grow accustomed to certain smells, noises, and other sensory assaults, and we forget that other people aren't.

If you suspect that chemical fumes are not being properly ventilated, let the salon manager know. If the music playing seems to annoy the clients, ask the salon manager or receptionist to change it. If clients frown and wince when you apply chemicals, that's a sure sign they are uncomfortable. Pay attention to product ingredients and chemical combinations, and learn what works best for you and your clients. It will be your responsibility as a licensed professional to understand and observe proper salon hygiene.

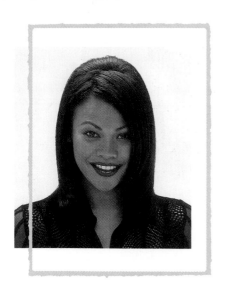

Press and Curl on Heavy Layers

Overview

A press and curl is a temporary thermal straightening technique used for very curly or kinky hair; the hair will revert to its natural state when shampooed. It may also be affected by perspiration, humidity, or other elements. No chemicals are used in this service—a growing number of clients do not want chemicals in their hair. If they are on medication, pregnant, or have extremely dry scalps, clients will want a press and curl because it is chemical-free.

Connect

Blow-drying Dry Hair

Use the blow-dryer to soften textured hair in preparation for pressing. Imagine a sheet of wax or a piece of clay; if you handled this for a while, it would become softer and more impressionable. In the same way, the heat from a blow-dryer will relax the hair somewhat, making it more receptive to the higher heat used in pressing.

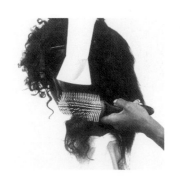

Silking Hair

Done by exposing the hair to heat briefly and without much pressure, the purpose of silking hair is to smooth it in preparation for curling. Think of pulling a ribbon over a hot lightbulb. The heat softens the hair, making it more impressionable to the curling iron.

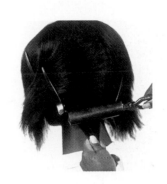

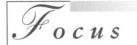

Focus

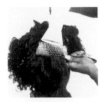

Drying Hair for the Press and Curl—Start this procedure with dry hair. Blow-drying the hair when it is dry will make it softer and easier to press.

Electric Pressing Comb versus Thermal Comb—Pressing combs' main difference is in their heat source—directly from electricity or from heat stored in them from a stove or electric heater. Electric combs have a cord which limits movement, and takes 15 minutes to heat. Thermal combs have no cords and can get exceedingly hot.

Silking Hair—Place the barrel of a closed curling iron on top of the section of hair you're getting ready to curl. Slide it down the hair shaft. Now open the curling iron and do not close it again until you get to the end of the section of hair. Closing it could cause hair breakage.

Breakage—Damage to the hair can cause it to split and break off. In this case, breakage can be caused by improper use of the curling iron. Be sure to keep the iron slightly open as you slide it down the hair shaft to avoid damage to the hair.

Protecting the Scalp—Always place a hard rubber (heat resistant) comb between the scalp and the section being ironed.

Perimeter—The outer line of a hairstyle is its perimeter.

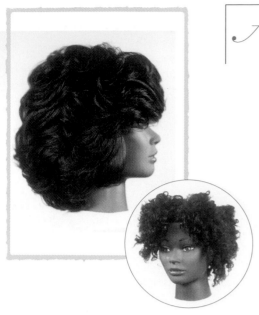

Apply
Press and Curl on Heavy Layers

With your clients, these technical steps will follow consultation, shampoo, and power or towel drying.

1. Shampooing the hair before a press and curl is not recommended when working on a mannequin. Working with dry hair allows you greater manageability.

2. Divide the head into four quadrants. Work your way up through the first section of hair using a blow-dryer with nozzle, and a hard rubber brush to heat and straighten the hair. Work section by section then stretch through the top surface.

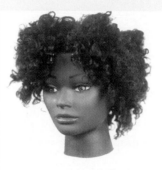
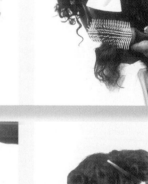

3. Continue this technique through all sections of the head to prepare for the pressing.

4. Divide the hair into four quadrants. Divide each section into 1 1/2" (3.75 cm) horizontal sections. Both an electric pressing comb and a thermal comb should be tested before being placed on the hair. Holding the hair firmly in one hand and your pressing comb in the other, direct the teeth of the pressing comb into the hair as close to the scalp as possible. Comb outward to the ends. Turn the back of the pressing comb to press the section.

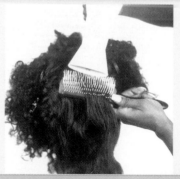

5. Press the comb through the hair, rotating it to bring the barrel against the lengths. The teeth guide the hair only, the barrel does the straightening. As you finish each rotation, the teeth of the comb should be pointing toward you.

6. Hold the hair as you move down the shaft until you've pressed the very end of the hair. Keep the hair taut to facilitate straightening.

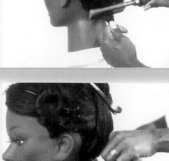
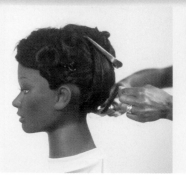

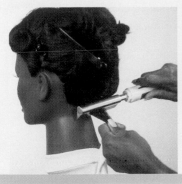
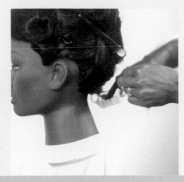

7. You would use the same technique with an electric pressing comb.

8. Note how the pressing comb is turned while working down the length of the hair.

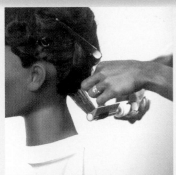
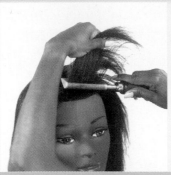

9. While the technique of pressing with an electric comb is the same as with a thermal comb, you will have to go over the hair two to three times more.

10. When you've finished the interior, press the hair along the perimeter. Hold the hair with a gentle but firm tension as you pull the comb through the hair.

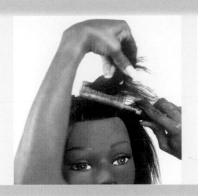
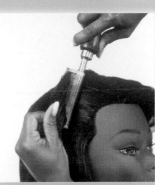

11. No sectioning is needed when you press the hair along the perimeter.

12. Holding the hair firmly, continue pressing the outer perimeter hairline.

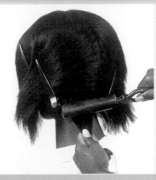
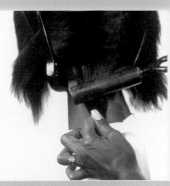

13. Divide the hair into four sections starting at the nape. Test the heat of the iron by placing it on a white paper towel. Take up one of these 1 1/2" (3.75 cm) sections and test your curling iron by placing it on top of the section. Slide the iron down the hair shaft while firmly holding the hair—this is called silking the hair. Remember to always leave the curling iron slightly open until you get to the end of the hair.

14. Hold the hair and slightly open curling iron. Firmly slide the curling iron down the hair.

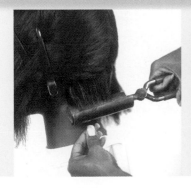
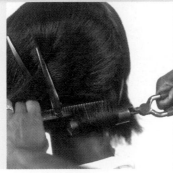

15. When you get to the ends of the hair, close the curling iron and work the ends of the hair into the middle of the curl.

16. Placing a hard rubber comb under the curling iron is imperative if you are going to roll the curling iron to the scalp.

17. Hold the curling iron in the hair until you can no longer see the ends of the hair. Slide the iron out of the curl.

18. Slide the curling iron until you reach the end of the hair.

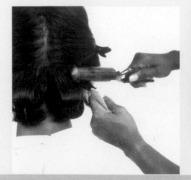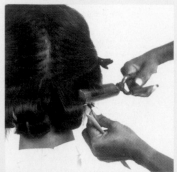

19. Use a hard rubber comb to protect the scalp.

20. Place the styling comb between the scalp and curling iron to protect the scalp. Work upward toward the crown.

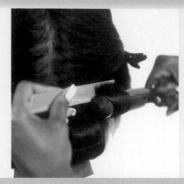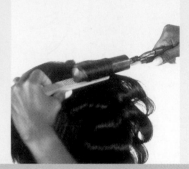

21. Moving to the side, continue curling the hair.

22. When you are not rolling the curling iron toward the scalp, be sure to direct it away from the client's scalp with your hand. Place your fingers between the client's face and the curling iron.

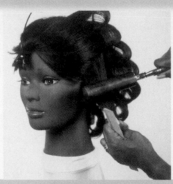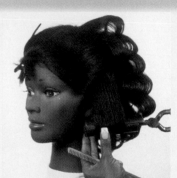

23. Complete the curling technique by moving up the section of hair into the interior.

24. The press and curl is complete and ready to be styled. Notice the smooth lines of the curls.

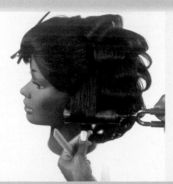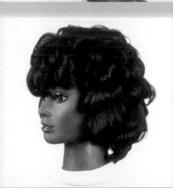

25. Using a rake-type of styling comb, comb the hair toward the back of the head.

26. As the rake styling comb moves toward the back center of the head, smooth your hand over the hair in the same direction.

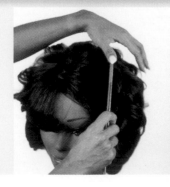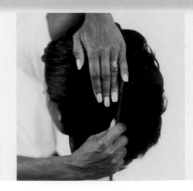

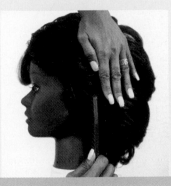
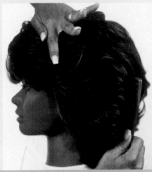

27. As you reach the center back of the head, stop and, applying pressure, push the hair toward the front.

28. Pushing the hair toward the front will create a layered look.

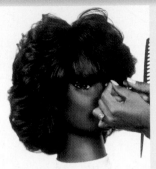
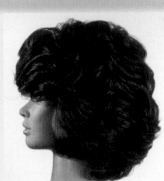

29. Repeat on other side, pulling out pieces of hair to softly frame the face. Detail the surface for the desired textural movement.

30. The styled press and curl creates a softened shape with textural and directional movement and dimension.

Cherish your visions and your dreams as they are the children of your soul; the blue-prints of your ultimate achievements.

Napoleon Hill

Reflect

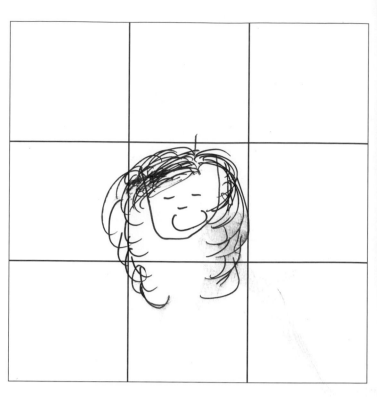

Explore

Apply this technique to different lengths, colors, and cuts for almost endless possibilities.

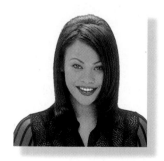

The Appointment
Schedule

You've read already about the importance of time to a salon business, and to a stylist's earnings. (We'll return to the topic later, too.) Here's a list of salon services, and the amount of stylist's time that the average mid-price, full-service salon schedules for each:

Men's or child's haircut (no shampoo)	20 minutes
Shampoo, cut, and blow-dry	30 minutes
Style finish (hot rollers, curling iron)	30 minutes
Chemical wave set (short hair)	30 minutes
Chemical wave set (long hair)	45 minutes to 1 hour
Chemical wave set neutralizing, rinsing	15 minutes
Single-process color application	15 minutes
Foil application	30 minutes to 1 hour
Manicure	30 minutes
Complete set of applied nails	60 minutes
Nail fill	45 minutes

Managing your time so that you stay on schedule is important to your income; and it is also important to your clients. Many of today's clients are "on the run" with work and home responsibilities. If they make an appointment for 5 P.M., they expect to be in the chair at 5. And they don't expect an appointment that usually takes an hour to last any longer than that.

Getting off schedule with one client can throw you off schedule for the rest of the day, and you simply don't need that kind of stress. Consider, too, that if you work in a salon with a large staff, one that includes specialists, a client who's having more than one service done might be scheduled with more than one employee. In this salon, one employee's falling behind can really mess things up!

No matter where you work, each day before you leave the salon, check the appointment book for the next day. If you have an appointment as soon as the salon opens, be there at least 15 minutes beforehand. When the client arrives, your station should be set up, and you should be ready to go.

Don't dawdle between clients, take unnecessary breaks, or spend too much time at lunch. Put in a good, busy, eight-hour day, and you'll have plenty of time to rest when it's over. You'll be so energized from doing good work and making good money for it, however, that you probably won't need to rest—and you'll have plenty of money to use for play!

Success is nothing more than a few simple disciplines, practiced every day.

Jim Rohn

There are several facts about each client that are important to know and record on a card or salon computer system. Some facts are important for the salon, some for the stylist. Good record keeping always benefits the client because it helps the salon and stylist meet her needs, and remember from visit to visit the important details that make every salon visit special for every client. Listed below are some of the items you'll want to make note of. (You can begin right now with the clients you service in school; it's never too early to get in the habit of keeping good records.)

General Information ▼

Client's Name and Address:	For mailing thank-you cards, reminders, and special promotion notices.
Client's Home and Work Phone Numbers:	For confirming appointments; or to call the client if a stylist is ill, giving her the option of rescheduling with another stylist that same day or at another time.
Birth date:	For sending birthday greetings, a nice customer service touch.

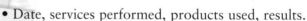

Service Information ▼

- Date, services performed, products used, results.
- Notes about client likes and dislikes learned during consultation.
- Client service plan.
- Samples of hair after a color service, to check color retention on her next visit.
- Home hair care products recommended, retail products purchased.

Good record keeping helps build rapport between client and stylist. It connects one visit to the next, creating a continuum of customer service and personal care. It shows your client that she matters to you. It reminds you what salon retail products your client uses so that you can make sure she doesn't leave without them—which makes her life easier and your paycheck fatter.

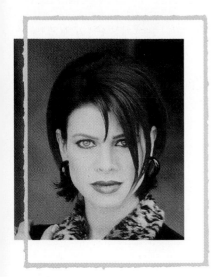

Blow-drying Full Layers

Overview

Here's another example of styling the hair to conform to the contours of its shape. The finished style highlights the shape of the cut, and the drying technique you use accentuates the layering above the ears and through the top of the head.

Connect

Blow-drying with a Comb

Work with your dryer and comb to keep the shape of the cut intact with minimal volume. Use your comb to draw the hair into place and mold it into a shape that still allows for movement in the finished style.

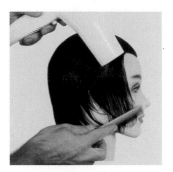

Focus

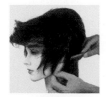

Detailing—Detailing with your comb and fingers will maintain the angular shape of the cut.

Apply
Blow-drying Full Layers

With your clients, these technical steps will follow consultation, shampoo, and power or towel drying.

1. Apply a styling product of your choice and work it through the hair. Holding the hair very close around the perimeter shape with a comb, dry the hair, following the comb with the dryer. This will keep this area very closely contoured.

2. Move to the fringe area next. Using a rubber-based blow-drying brush, overdirect the hair to create volume and fullness. Note how flat the base area is held as turning the ends back and toward the side.

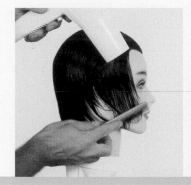
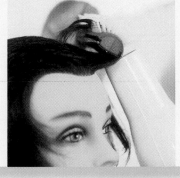

3. Continue into the crown area.

4. Comb through the nape area if it needs lift.

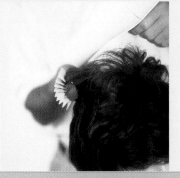
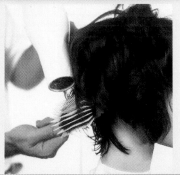

5. Blend and connect the side sections with the front.

6. Use a texture comb to separate and detail the lengths. Back comb the crown area, then detail, using your comb and fingers.

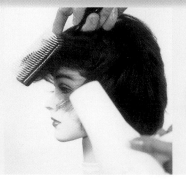
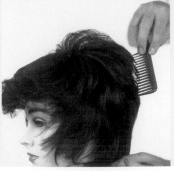

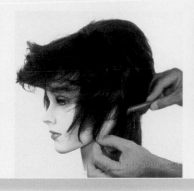
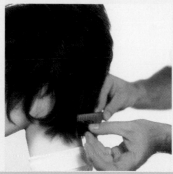

7. Continue detailing. This is where your artistry is expressed.

8. Detail the edges. Spray for the desired hold.

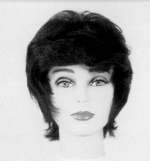

9. The finished style shows closely contoured layers through the exterior with an emphasis on directional volume through the fringe and crown areas.

The difference between the impossible and the possible lies in a person's determination.

Tommy Lasorda

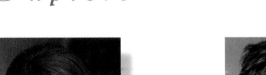

Reflect

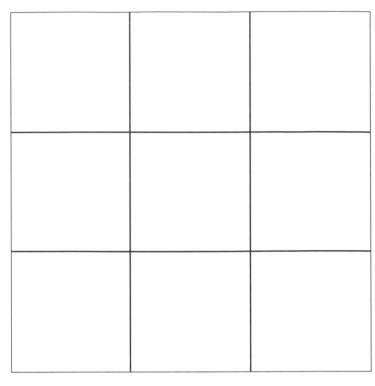

Explore

Apply this technique to different lengths, colors, and cuts for almost endless possibilities.

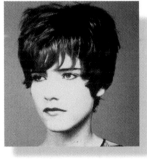

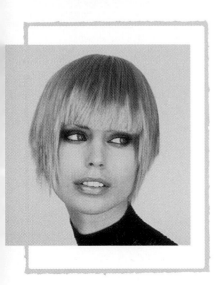

Blowdrying High Graduation

Overview

This style begins with the high graduation cut you completed in the haircutting part of this program (see page 172). As with many of the shorter styles in this program, you should use tools in the drying process to conform to the shape of the cut. The key to finishing this style is moving the brush through the hair as you direct heat from the dryer onto it.

Focus

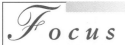

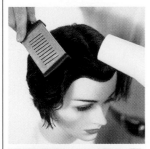

C-Section—This is the movement of your brush in a wave pattern that resembles a letter C. The movement can be small or large—large enough to contour to a given area of the head.

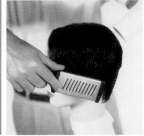

Metal Vent Brush—This brush is designed to allow maximum drying efficiency and heat transfer.

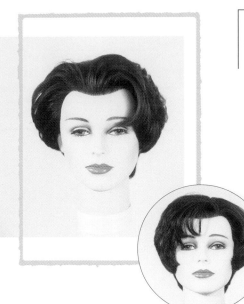

Apply
Blow-drying High Graduation

With your clients, these technical steps will follow consultation, shampoo, and power or towel drying.

In this design, the highly graduated haircut has been styled for a back swept flow away from the face.

1. Apply a styling product of your choice and work it through the hair. Comb and direct the hair into the style lines in preparation for blow-drying.

2. Use a metal vent air brush to wave a C-section while following the brush with your dryer. Insert the brush into the hair and form a curved movement. Direct the air flow into the movement. Repeat on the opposite side.

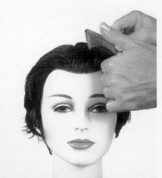
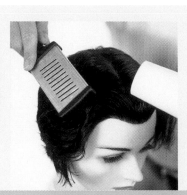

3. Follow through to the ends of the hair. The brush is used to mold movement. Follow the brush with the blow-dryer tracing in a curvature movement.

4. Use a round brush to lift and bend the hair around the face in a directional manner. Use this technique throughout the sides. Brush the hair in back to contour and blend to surrounding lengths. Use a spray, texture creme, or silicone shiner for the desired finish.

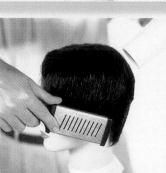
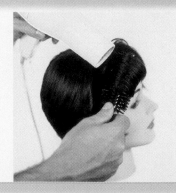

5. The finished style enhances the graduated movement through the back and the layers that frame the face.

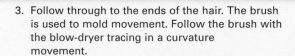

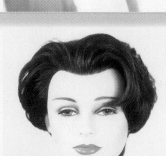

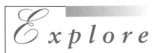

Apply this technique to different lengths, colors, and textures for almost endless possibilities.

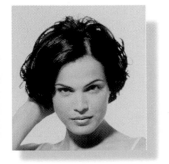

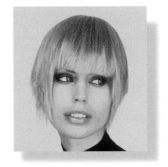

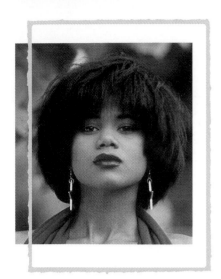

Wrapping Layered Graduation

Overview

Wrapping is a technique for keeping straightened hair smooth. The hair design can be left as is, close to the head, or combed out. You can also create wrapped styles with extra volume by using rollers that are wrapped in a single direction at the top. This traditional wrap technique will create a style that lasts as long as a week. It's perfect for active clients—it makes hair more manageable, and gives it added movement. This can be done on wet or dry hair.

Connect

Wrapping

The wrapping technique uses the same principle employed in rolling hair. When you roll hair, you wrap a section of hair around a roller to give it the roller's shape; the smaller the roller, the tighter the curl. The same thing happens when you wrap hair around a head. The hair takes on the shape of the head, which works like a huge roller to keep the hair smooth.

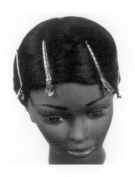

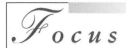

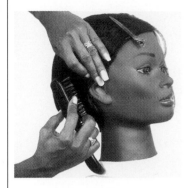

Position for Wrapping—Hold one hand at the top of the head; with a pivot motion, wrap the hair on the outer perimeter of the head. Do not brush or push the hair to the back; the correct way is to always brush the hair clockwise around the head. Try to think of the head as a roller; your job is to smooth the hair around the head.

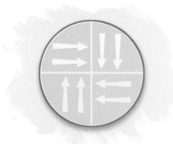

Comb the hair in a clockwise direction around the head. Follow the comb with your hand, smoothing down the hair and keeping it tight to the head.

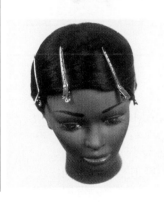

Use of Clips—Clips are used to hold the hair in place while you are wrapping it. Once all the hair has been wrapped and a neck strip has been stretched around the head, the clips will be removed. If the hair is wet, a light gel can be used instead of clips to hold the hair in place while you wrap it.

The highest reward for a person's toil is not what they get for it but what they become by it.

John Ruskin

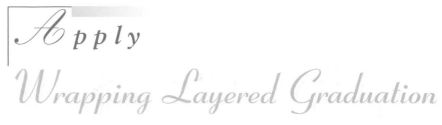

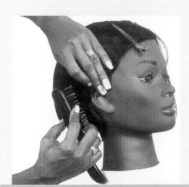

Apply

Wrapping Layered Graduation

With your clients, these technical steps will follow consultation, shampoo, and power or towel drying. The finished style is created through the use of a wrapping technique. This creates a smooth, glossy texture.

1. Brush the hair around the outer perimeter of the head.

2. Holding the hair in place with long clips, continue brushing around the outer perimeter of the head until you reach your starting point.

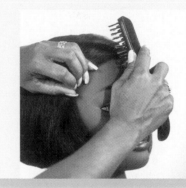

3. As your hands move, your body should also move in sync around your client's head.

4. Make sure you keep the hair low, so that it remains on the outer perimeter of the head.

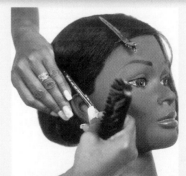
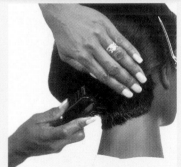

5. At this stage in the wrapping process, you can see how the hair smoothly follows the contour of the head.

6. Continue bringing the hair around the head, holding your hand securely (a pivotal movement is used).

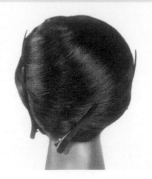
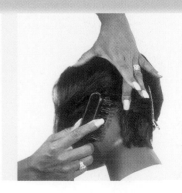

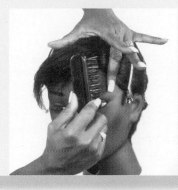

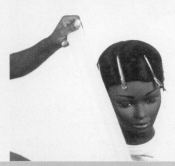

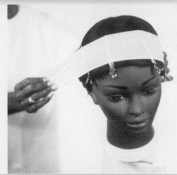

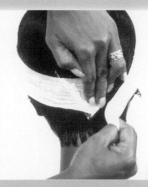

7. As you brush, continue placing long clips. Brush up and around toward the top front of the head clipping as you go.

8. Taking a neck strip, stretch it around the entire head.

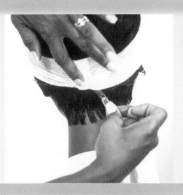

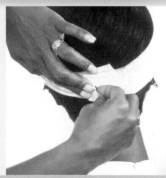

9. Place the neck strip over the clips.

10. Stretch the neck strip so that it overlaps at the ends.

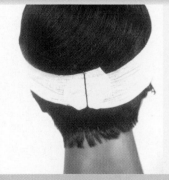

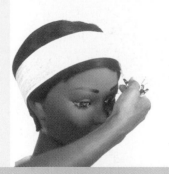

11. Holding the neck strip in place, start removing the clips. Remove the back clip first since you will need this area free for securing the ends of the neck strip.

12. Secure the wrapped strip with a bobby pin.

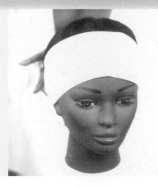

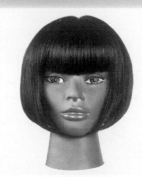

13., 14. Start removing the rest of the clips from the head.

15. If you have been working on a dry head, you will need to leave the hair wrapped for about 15 minutes. If the hair was wet, you will need to place the client under a dryer for 45 minutes to one hour, depending on the hair length, until the hair is completely dry. The longer you leave the hair wrapped, the smoother it will be.

16. Unwrap the hair and brush the straightened hair into the desired style. Shown here is one possible comb out of the wrapped hair.

*R*eflect

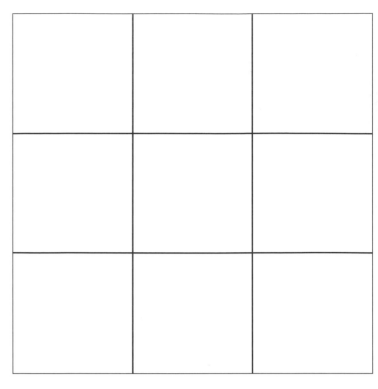

*E*xplore

Apply this technique to different lengths, colors, and textures for almost endless possibilities.

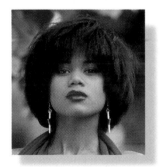 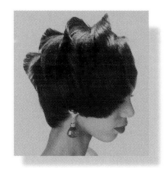

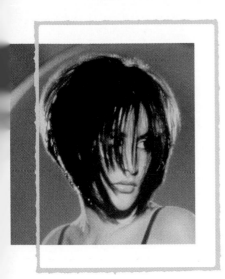

Blow-drying Layered Razor Cut

Overview

Razor cutting provides a wide range of opportunity for you to express your artistic and professional talent. And it gives you another way to achieve the ultimate objective: to design a hairstyle that enhances your client's appearance. The key here is the minimal manipulation of the hair. If you blow-dry the hair while moving it in place with your fingers, you'll create a style that truly highlights the detailed texture within the razor cut.

Focus

Small Rubber-Base Paddle Brush—This vent brush is used for added fullness. It allows for quick drying given the maximum air flow through the brush.

Placing Textured Hair—Use the fingers to arrange hair when finishing. The hair is massaged between the fingers to dry quickly while building in volume and texture.

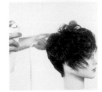

Personalize the Design—Place hair in the style based on the characteristics of individual clients and the desired expression.

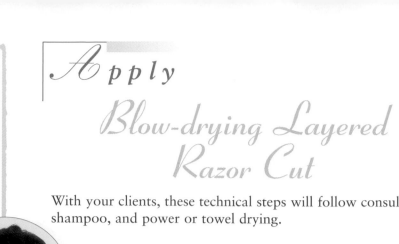

Apply
Blow-drying Layered Razor Cut

With your clients, these technical steps will follow consultation, shampoo, and power or towel drying.

1. Apply a styling product of your choice and work it through the hair. Use your fingers and a dryer to gently nudge the textured hair into place. Use your fingertips to separate the textured ends. Notice the massaging action used to add texture and body as drying.

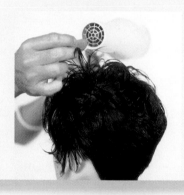
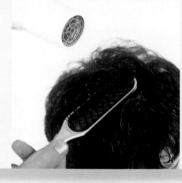

2. Use a small rubber-based paddle brush to add fullness. In this style the lengths are turned up and forward toward the face.

3. Use a brush around the face to add strength and direction. The brush will add polish to the lengths. Alternate the brush with the fingers to accentuate texture.

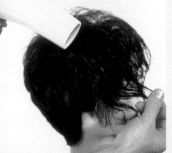
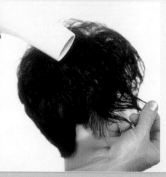
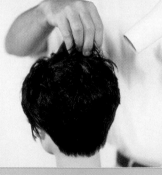

4. Use your fingertips to soften and personalize the design.

5. Finish with a combination of spray and blow-dryer for added volume, separation, and texture.

6. The finished style is light and airy with soft fringe-like lengths around the face.

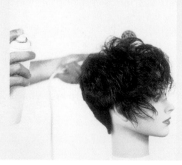
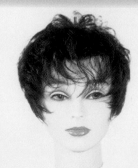

Explore

Apply this technique to different lengths, colors, and textures for almost endless possibilities.

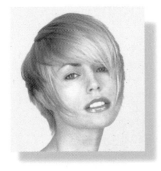
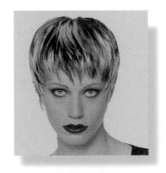
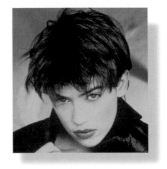

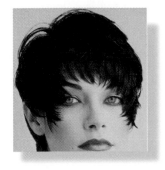
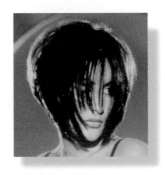

blow-drying uniform layers

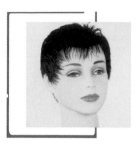

*T*his is a perfect example of a haircut's ability to stand alone with a minimum of finishing. This style is extremely contemporary and flattering to the face, yet it requires very little maintenance. While the cut features a heavily layered or textured effect, styling gel will maintain its structure but soften the overall look. The control of this style depends on the type of styling product selected.

1. Apply a styling gel to the hair and work it through. This creates a wet and very textured look.

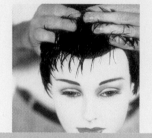 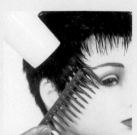

2. Use a texture comb to detail the edges. Use a dryer to set the shape in place. Contour the comb closely as drying. Use cool air as drying this area around the face.

3. The finished style frames the face with a fringe-like effect that contrasts with the extra short gelled layers.

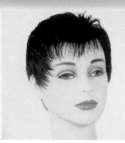

The starting point of all achievement is desire.

Napoleon Hill

Reception
Area

Success is in the details.

A P Erkkila

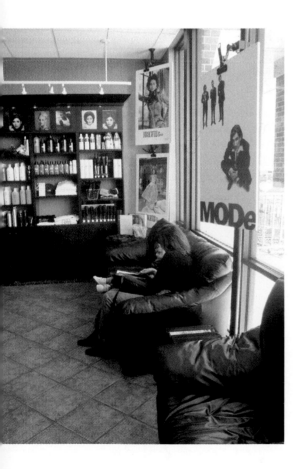

*L*et's take a look at two salon reception areas:

1. Salon Slop-PÈ ▼

A new client enters a crowded, messy reception area. The decor is nice enough, but there are magazines scattered about and dirty Styrofoam coffee cups left sitting on tables. There's a person behind the desk who might be a receptionist, but she's talking on the phone and doesn't even make eye contact. Someone else–it looks like a stylist–is back there checking the appointment book, and still another stylist-type person in a lab coat is chatting with a client who is paying for a service. No one pays any attention to the new customer for two, three minutes. Finally, the receptionist hangs up the phone, writes in the book for a minute or two, and then offhandedly says to the newcomer, "Oh hi, can I help you?"

2. Salon Superb ▼

Same new client. Same decor. But the reception area is neat and tidy, music is softly playing, and this time, when the client walks in, the three employees notice that someone new is present. The receptionist on the phone smiles at the newcomer and makes eye contact; the stylist who's checking the book immediately comes out from behind the desk and says, "Hi, I'm Tom, one of the stylists here at Salon Su-Perb. Our receptionist, Gail, is on the phone, so may I help you?"

The client replies, "I'm Jillian Anderson I have a two o'clock haircut, but I'm not sure who the stylist is." Just then the receptionist hangs up the phone and Tom says to her, "Gail, I'd like you to meet a new client, Jillian Anderson. She has a two o'clock appointment."

Gail steps out from behind the desk immediately, smiles, and extends her hand to clasp Jillian's. "Thank you, Tom. I'm sorry, I was unable to greet you as soon as you came in. Yes, our senior stylist, Andrew, is looking forward to meeting you. He will be ready in about five minutes. May I hang up your coat and bring you coffee, tea, or a soft drink?"

If you were a client, which salon would give you a better first impression?

Texture Services

A New Approach

Texture is best described as the visual and tactile quality of a surface. We are surrounded by textures in our environment. When it comes to hair, each individual hair strand has a texture that affects its look and feel—fine, medium (normal), or coarse. And the hair as a whole has texture, or movement. Does it look radiantly straight, smooth, and sleek? Or does it have shiny, sensuous curls that make for dynamic movement and volume? As a texture service specialist, you will be able to give your clients the hair texture they want.

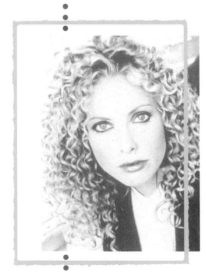

Bricklay set

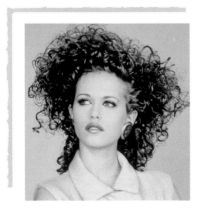

Curvature set

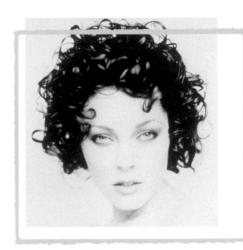

V" formation set

This service category has seen and continues to see dramatic changes as we enter the 21st century. For one thing, styles have changed. Instead of bouffant hairstyles, clients now request easy-care, easy-wear haircuts. Texture services allow you to offer each client a variety of expressions to customize her haircut. These services can be the foundation for styling versatility!

Today's culture, too, has changed. Today's client seeks instant gratification from her salon visit. Hair manageability is one of the most frequent requests that she'll have. A texture service can play a large role in helping each client manage her style on her own between salon visits.

And finally, technology has changed. There are two basic types of texture services—waves, or the introduction of movement or wave into the hair; and relaxers (sometimes called retexturizers) which remove wave or curl from the hair in varying degrees. And the incredible advances in technology in the chemical systems used for both types today have made the texture service very desirable for the client—while also quite lucrative for you, the cosmetologist!

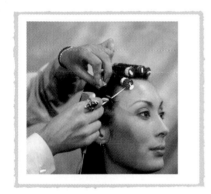

Texture service

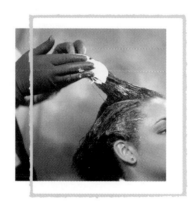

Relaxer service

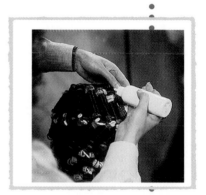

Follow manufacturer's instructions.

Manufacturers of professional waving and relaxer systems continue to research and develop state-of-the-art formulas. You will be exposed to these formulas while you are in school as well as when you enter into the salon world. Manufacturers provide excellent product education in the form of seminars and printed material. You will be instructed in school to "always follow the manufacturer's directions." This is an excellent maxim to follow, given the tremendous amount of research and experience that it takes to bring a product to the professional marketplace.

Marketing the texture service involves thorough knowledge in three areas: terminology, technology, and tools.

Terminology

Communication has never been as important in the salon as it is today. Your communication with each client before, during, and after the service-consultation is an ongoing process throughout the entire service. This is especially important when it comes to the texture service, which many clients still think of as a "permanent." Permanent is a term not often used in the salon world today—particularly not when you're consulting with the client. The most progressive salons do not use this word at all—to great effect! The word perm conjures up for many clients an image of a very undesirable experience she may have had in the past, or perhaps the perm that her mother used to get. It does not conjure up a pretty picture. So if you propose a "perm," your client may very well say to you, "Oh, no thank you, I had a horrible experience with a perm years ago, and I said I would never get one again."

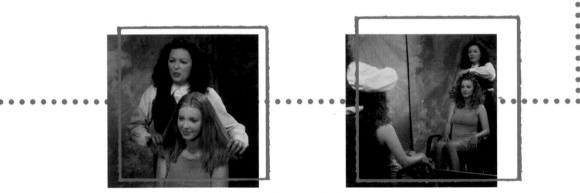

Service consultation

So how do you talk to your client about the wonderful benefits of today's texture services? Well, start with asking her what types of problems or frustrations she has with her hair. Then you can tell her in non-threatening, non-technical, and result-oriented words how you're going to "provide the solution" to her problems. Use beauty or fashion-oriented words that she can easily accept: "directional movement," "style support," "more volume." (If you were to ask 100 women what they wanted more of in their hair, probably 99 of them would answer, "more volume"!) Help her visualize what her hair could look like, then tell her she can have this—through a waving process. Explain that the process uses revolutionary formulas that will maintain her hair's healthy condition, and you are well on your way to creating a texture service for your client.

Study the texture design menu here. Many salons have successfully used this type of approach to promote their texture service category. Naturally, you would add your own or your salon's prices to this menu.

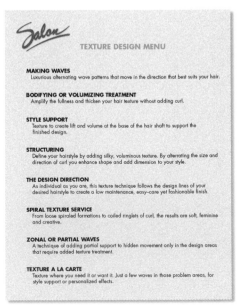

Texture Design Menu

TECHNOLOGY AND TOOLS

Now that your client has agreed to a texture service, you must deliver it! Below are some concepts fundamental to this category.

Setting

Setting the hair is a very non-threatening term for the client. It refers to arranging your tools into the pattern for waving. You can set using either a rolling or a spiraling technique.

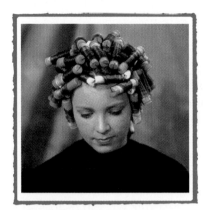
Setting the hair

The Rolling and Spiraling Techniques

The rolling technique involves rolling the hair onto a tool from its ends to its base—just as you would roll a scroll, with each turn overlapping the turn before. Rolling creates a strong undulation and enhanced dimension in the hair.

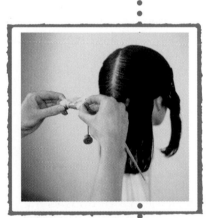
Rolling technique

The spiraling technique involves spiraling the hair around the tool from its ends to its base. Unlike the rolling technique, the hair does not overlap; the spiral formation moves along the length of the tool. If you used tools of the same diameter to roll and to spiral, the spiraled tool would create less length reduction in the hair.

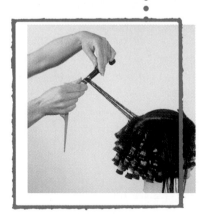
Spiraling technique

Textural Movement, Directional Movement, and Volume

These are the three primary textural effects that you'll strive to create for your clients. They are interrelated, and each a part of the decision process. As you consult with your client, you'll together determine the amount, direction, and dimension of movement in her hair.

Textural Movement

Textural movement is how "active" the hair is. It is determined by the size and diameter of the tools you use to set the hair; small tools will create high-energy motion, while larger tools will create smoother, softer wave patterns in the hair.

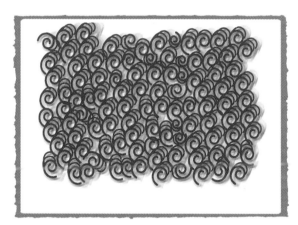

Small tools create high-energy motion.

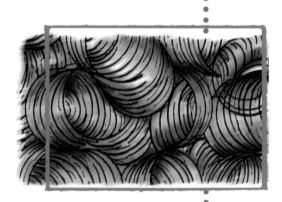

Large tools create soft wave patterns.

Directional Movement

Once you and your client have chosen the amount of movement to create, you'll decide the direction of movement. Will the client want to wear her hair all back off her face, or forward onto her face? Will she want the movement to contour around the curve of her head, or perhaps to move in alternating waves throughout the head or an area of it? The pattern or arrangement into which you set the hair will determine its flow of movement.

Remember that your client expects to "love" her new texture on the day she receives it; she doesn't want to wait until it "relaxes a little bit." Setting her hair directionally and chemically waving it to move into the style lines will give her this.

Direction can refer to how the tool is positioned on the head—horizontally, vertically, or diagonally. And it can refer to how a complete head of hair is set within a directional pattern—bricklay, straight, curvature, alternating waves, and so on. (Refer to Chapter 11 in Milady's *Standard Textbook of Cosmetology* for the basic block rolling method.)

The hair will take on different texture qualities when rolled horizontally, vertically, or diagonally. Consider this when planning your setting pattern. The base area will move in the direction that you roll the tool; the fall of the wave or curl will also undulate according to how you roll.

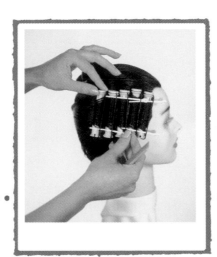

Vertical direction

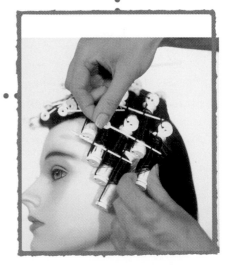

Diagonal direction

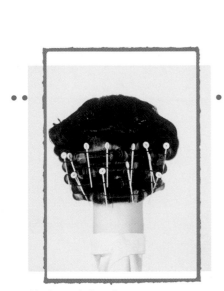

Horizontal direction

The Patterns

Bricklay

The bricklay pattern simulates the actual technique of bricklaying. You offset base partings from each other from row to row, to prevent any obvious splits in the finish. The flow of hair is very blended and harmonious. Different bricklay patterns use different starting points (front hairline, occipital area, and crown, for instance). Naturally, this starting point affects the directional flow of the hair. The bricklay pattern accommodates either rolling or spiraling the hair.

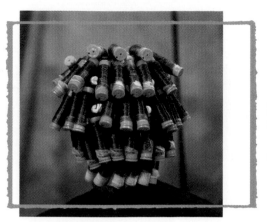

Bricklay pattern

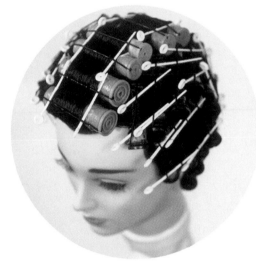

Contour pattern

Contour

In the contour pattern, straight and curvature directional movement combine. You roll panels in a direction back away from the front hairline, contouring to the curves of the head. You can adapt the rolling direction within individual panels in many different ways; study the variations here.

Curvature

In curvature setting, movement curves within sectioned-out panels or molded shapings. Partings and bases radiate throughout the panels to make the desired turns around the curvature of the head. This requires you to create trapezoid-shaped bases through these curvature areas.

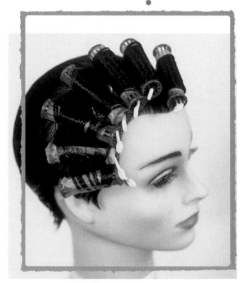

Curvature pattern

Straight

In straight setting, you set all tools within a panel to move in the same direction, and position them on equal size bases (each base should be the length and width of the tool). Study the example here. Hair may be set straight forward, straight back, straight down, and so on.

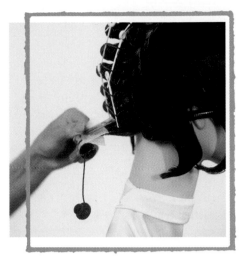

Straight pattern

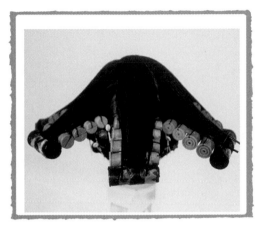

Angular stack pattern

Angular Stack

In the angular stack pattern, hair is progressively positioned away from the head on stacking sticks; this creates texture along the ends of the shape only. Also called a pyramid set, the stack will angle according to the shape created. Generally, you part the hair into panels. Take bases straight through the panels as you work from the perimeter area of the panel to the top. The nape area is bricklayed to provide extra support and texture.

"V" Herringbone

The "V" herringbone or alternating wave formation resembles the herringbone pattern popular in woolen fabrics. In this pattern, you set tools within adjacent panels to move either towards each other or in opposite directions from each other—creating an alternating wave pattern. Measure out the panels according to the length of the tool you're using and set the tools within the panels diagonally. Study the pattern here.

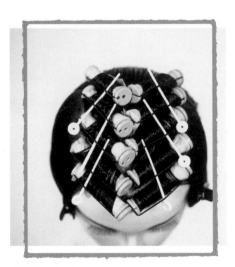

"V" herringbone pattern

Volume

You can create volume in your client's style in two ways: by creating base lift (this depends on which base control you use), and by creating textural movement in the hair. The more textural movement in the hair, the more expansion of the shape is possible.

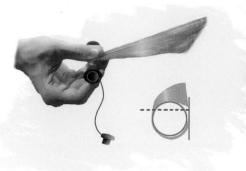

Base Controls

This term refers to how you position the texture tool in relation to the base area. The base controls most often used are the one-diameter, on-base and half-off-base controls; it is also possible to use a one-diameter off-base control if you wish to greatly diminish base volume. Over-and underdirected base controls are also possibilities. These produce dramatically different results at the base areas. Study the examples here (and see Chapter 11 in Milady's *Standard Textbook of Cosmetology* for more information).

One diameter base control

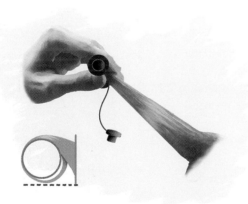

On-base control

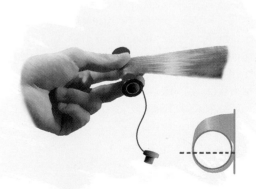

Half off-base control

Volume and Indentation

Volume setting expands the shape for fullness. Lift the base and stem using your desired base control, and turn the tool under.

Indentation rolling creates hollowness and space in the shape. Keep the base area flat, while turning the stem and tool upward.

Whether you use curvature or straight directional movements, combining volume and indentation creates contrast and interest in the style. Indentation is especially effective when used around the perimeter of the shape to create a very natural hairline movement.

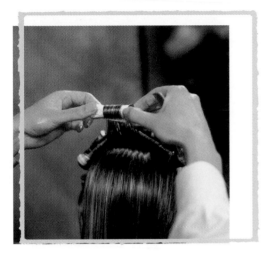

Volume setting

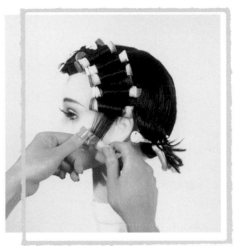

Indentation rolling

Volume in the Cut versus the Styled Shape

When you perform a texture service to accentuate volume in your client's style, decide with her whether she will wear her hair dried or diffused naturally, or use blow-drying and curling iron techniques. This will determine the tool size you use. The smaller the tool, of course, the greater the expansion and volume of the style. This volume may be controlled or diminished in finishing the hair, if desired. And softer, minimal movement in the hair, such as that created in a body or style support wave, may have its volume accentuated through thermal styling, wet setting, or other styling techniques.

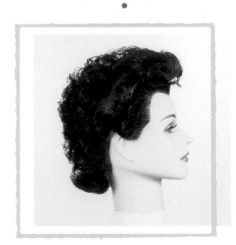

Indentation in nape

Tool Selection

As mentioned, the texture you create in the hair depends on the tool diameter you choose. Another factor in tool selection is the length of the hair. For blunt, graduated, and layered shapes, consider the length arrangement and structure of the haircut.

Once you've selected the setting pattern you'll use, you need to decide the arrangement pattern of the tool sizes within the set. Study the examples here.

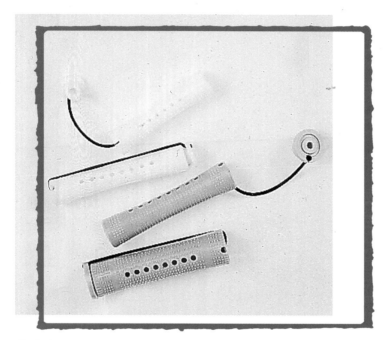

Tool sizes

Using the same-sized tool throughout the head will create the same-size texture.

Alternating the tool sizes and/or directions will introduce a rhythm of harmonious yet different textures into the style. This can provide visual interest, especially when the style is dried naturally or diffused.

Using a progression in tool sizes, particularly one that relates to the length progression in the cut, will create a desirable flow of textural movement.

Consider that on haircuts that feature a weight buildup (such as blunt and graduated cuts), you may wish to use a smaller tool on the underneath lengths, then progress or change to a larger-size tool on the longer lengths.

Specialty Techniques

In addition to the primary setting techniques—the roll and spiral—consider the following specialty techniques.

Double Tool

In this technique, two tools are positioned along a single section of hair. It's most often used on midlength or longer hair where two texture patterns are desired. Stack or piggyback the tools or use the insertion technique.

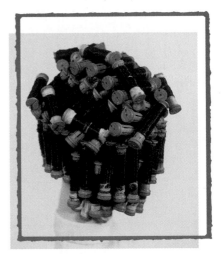

Double tool technique

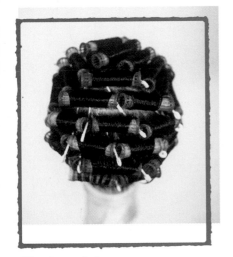

Weaving technique

Weaving

In weaving, zigzag partings divide base areas. You can perform the weave either on or off the scalp. Roll the hair in opposite directions within a single base area; measure out this area to the size of the two tools combined. This technique is used for very effective blending between tools that move in opposing directions, so as not to create a split. It's also used to create a transition from rolled areas into the natural, untreated hair that is left unrolled.

Twisting

Twisting the hair before you spiral it will enhance volume in the finished texture. Use this technique on longer lengths of hair that you're spiraling onto conventional texture tools. It is also an excellent technique for harder-to-wave hair types. Use a nonalkaline waving formula on this set to avoid excessive swelling of the hair.

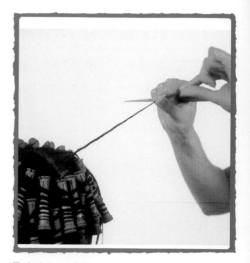

Twisting technique

Nothing is as real as a dream. The world can change around you, but your dream will not. Responsibilities need not erase it. Duties need not obscure it. Because the dream is within you, no one can take it away.

Tom Clancy

Optimizing and Closing Your Texture Service

The bottom line is to satisfy your client the first time around. Review Chapter 11 in Milady's *Standard Textbook of Cosmetology.* Do not skip any of these steps, particularly thorough hair saturation with waving and neutralizing lotions, meticulous timing, rinsing, or towel blotting procedures. Diligence in these areas will truly pay dividends in having a satisfied client!

And don't forget the essential step of teaching your client how to properly care for her new texture. She should know how to use liquid styling formulas to finish her hair at home, and she should take home the formulas that will keep the magic of her new hair texture and style living on after she's left the salon.

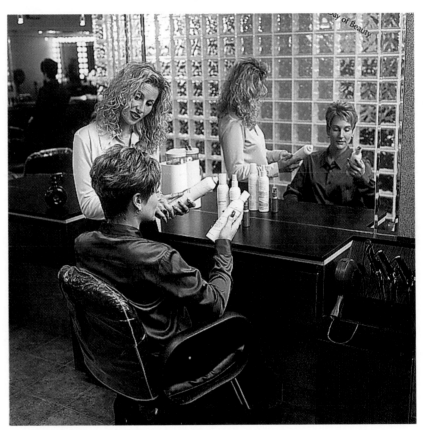

Communicate home care to the client.

Mary Beth Janssen

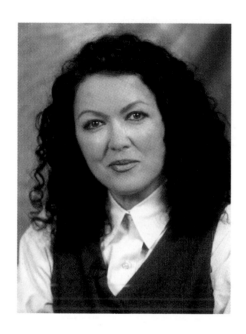

Throughout her 1,500-hour training in cosmetology, Mary Beth Janssen aspired toward working in a top salon, and that's exactly where she got her first job, as a full-time assistant. The salon was staffed by eight successful stylists and owned by a top competition stylist. Mary Beth spent six months shampooing clients, sweeping up hair, applying color solutions, processing permanent waves, and observing before she was given a chair of her own.

"I gave the best shampoo in the greater Chicago area," said Mary Beth with a smile, adding, "but I didn't have enough experience cutting hair." So the salon owner took Mary Beth under her wing and taught her how to cut hair until she was proficient. After a year in the salon, Mary Beth was encouraged to enroll in an advanced 1,000-hour teacher's training course.

After graduating from teacher's training, Mary Beth taught beauty school for nine months, and then her technical, as well as people skills, and the people she met in the industry began to open doors for her. She was sent to the Netherlands to teach haircutting to Dutch educators. From there she spent several years traveling all over the world as an educator for a well-known international cosmetology education company before being named that company's International Artistic Director, a post she held from 1981–1993.

As the Creative and Education Director for a major product manufacturer from 1993-96, Mary Beth helped develop and market a line of shampoo, conditioner, and liquid styling products, which included overseeing product development, package design, and advertising and publicity campaigns to introduce the products. In late 1996 she formed her own company, The Janssen Source, Inc., which provides creative and educational services to major manufacturers and publishers in the beauty industry. Mary Beth is a widely sought speaker in the areas of beauty and wellness integration. She is the technical editor for this course as well as the author of the technical segments on texturizing.

Over the years, Mary Beth developed a private clientele of celebrities and also designed hair and makeup for TV, feature films, and magazine layouts.

Mary Beth is more than technically talented. She also has a keen aptitude for business and a gift for reaching people. She speaks of her career as a "journey" that, as she gained more awareness of who she was and what skills she could offer, resulted in one door after another opening up for her. She urges all other beginning stylists to respect their intuition, to listen to both their heads and their hearts, for she says, "If you are doing what you love to do and communicating with people, doors will open for you, too."

"There is a tremendous shift in the way people are looking at wellness today," she added. "And our industry is at the heart of it. The professionals who work in hair salons and day spas providing services to clients are truly caregivers in every sense of the word."

Mary Beth believes that caregivers have to care for themselves, too. She teaches beauty professionals how to achieve wellness and wholeness, telling her students that, "If you can maintain lightness of being, your joyfulness and energy with your last client of the day will be just as sublime as with your first client in the morning."

To achieve this, Mary Beth says, "Nurture and strengthen your body with rest, meditation, nutritious food, pure water, and exercise. And feed your mind by continuing to seek knowledge and wisdom in your craft, as well as engaging in a widely diverse range of "topics" or hobbies. Seek out the people who's energy will be the best for you, and work with them and through them to achieve your goals. Then, when you have attained success, reach out and help others."

Floyd Kenyatta

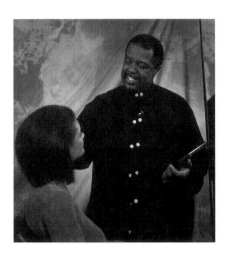

Floyd Kenyatta, who with Charlene Carroll authored the groundbreaking black hair education in this course, is president of Floyd Kenyatta Enterprises, founder of the U.S.A. Black Hair Olympics Team, and chairman of the U.S. Council of Black Salon Owners. As Global Ambassador for John Paul Mitchell Systems, he travels around the world to advance the art and science of black hair design. His business interests include marketing and distribution of the Kenora haircolor product line, which he created. He is the exclusive U.S., Canadian, and Caribbean importer of Sabi salon furnishings and equipment of Italy, and the exclusive U.S. importer of the high quality line of GIS flat irons.

As a young man, Floyd left his boyhood home in North Carolina for the bright lights of New York City, where he landed a job as a busboy at the Playboy Club. So how did he go from busboy to renowned hair designer and millionaire businessman?

"A co-worker of mine told me her husband was making a lot of money as a hairdresser. Several members of my family were barbers and beauticians, and I got to thinking it would be a great way to create my own work environment, be an entrepreneur, and spend my work hours around beautiful women."

With that goal, Floyd enrolled at Wilford Academy in Manhattan, one of only two black students among 1,200. He credits a teacher and mentor he met there, Anthony Colletti, with inspiring him to excel. "Here was the man who had developed many of the techniques being used in the salon industry, and who had written one of the major textbooks, the very textbook I was studying; and he was right next to me, teaching me." Years later, that same teacher would induct Floyd Kenyatta into the Wilford Academy Hall of Fame.

But before fame came a lot of hard work, first as a shampoo assistant in an "uptown, upscale" black salon in New York City where, says Floyd, wealthy clients would send helicopters to fetch the owner so that he could style their hair for weddings and other special events. Watching this man work, says Floyd, gave him the confidence to open his own business. So he headed "back home" and learned the hard way that "what works in New York City doesn't necessarily work in Maryland or North Carolina. You have to understand your territory and your environment, know your market and know your audience, and then tailor your skills accordingly."

Floyd opened his first salon only two years after graduating from cosmetology school, and he said he made a common mistake: "I did everything based on emotions—how it looked, how it felt—and I didn't understand the numbers side of my business." He soon learned that, as he said, "The secret to success is understanding your numbers."

He obviously understands them now, or he wouldn't be driving to business appointments in a Rolls Royce or motoring around the Chesapeake on weekends on his 32–foot yacht. Given his notable business success and international reputation for excellence and innovation in black hair design, what one last pearl of wisdom would Floyd Kenyatta give to industry newcomers to help them be as successful as he has been?

"In order to sell anything to anyone, you first have to get that person's attention."

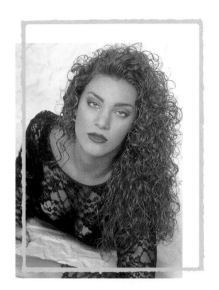

Bricklay

roll and spiral technique

Overview

The bricklay pattern is a classic technique for arranging or setting the tools in position for waving. It creates a smooth flow of movement because base partings are offset from row to row.

In this design, we transform the shoulder length horizontal blunt cut to create luxurious wave patterns, movement, and dimension. Many clients desire this type of texture result.

The Rolling and Spiraling Techniques

These two techniques are fundamental for creating a wide variety of textural effects. The techniques remain the same whether the pattern of application is within directional, curvature, or straight movements.

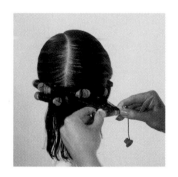

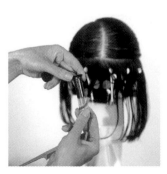

Connect

The Bricklay Pattern

The bricklay method comes from the world of architecture and translates easily to the patterns in which you arrange tools for waving patterns.

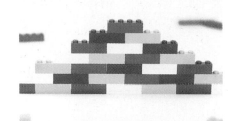

* ✳ Aesthetic in nature—no splits between rows providing fluidity/ flow of movement

* ✳ Functional in its use—inherent strength and support of movement within the structure

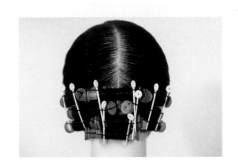

The width and length of base sections may be adjusted for the techniques of rolling or spiraling.

Difference Between Rolling and Spiraling

The rolling technique involves rotating the tool to wrap the hair evenly around it. Think of rolling a diploma or scroll. Spread the hair evenly along the tool and roll smoothly toward the base. This creates a strong undulation.

The spiral technique involves winding a strand of hair along a tool from one end to the other. Think of winding a ribbon around a dowel. This creates natural-looking elongated texture.

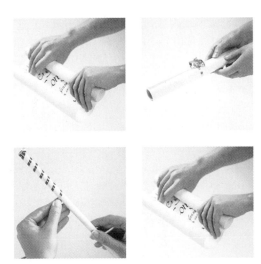

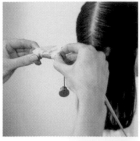

Rolled—Rolling technique creates an undulating back and forth movement that creates strong support and volume. Notice the horizontal positioning of the tool.

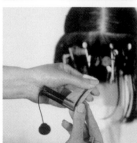

Spiraled—The elongated texture formation of a spiraled length of hair will create a highly natural look. This technique will create less length reduction. Note the vertical positioning of the tool.

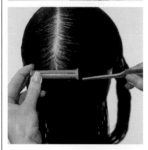

Use of Different Tool Lengths/Diameters—Adjust the length of the tool according to the area of the head and length being worked on. The tool diameter in this design is smaller in the nape for extra support on shorter lengths and larger through the longer interior lengths.

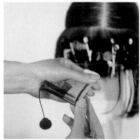

Hair Distribution and Tool Position for Spiraling Technique—Hold the spiraled lengths diagonally out from the center base area to create a base control that is half off–base.

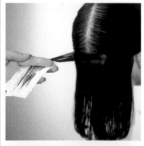

End Paper Technique for Spiral—To facilitate smooth spiraling of lengths, turn the end paper lengthwise and fold in half over the ends of the hair. (See Milady's *Standard Textbook of Cosmetology* for other end paper methods to be used.)

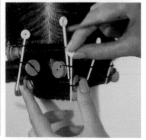

Proper Method of Using Picks—Picks are long, plastic strips that slide beneath the bands to ease pressure on the hair where the band is fastened. It's important to turn the band toward the outward top of the tool before inserting the pick. Using picks properly will ensure smooth, resilient, uncompromised lengths of textured hair.

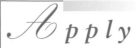

Apply
Bricklay
roll and spiral technique

After your consultation, drape the client, shampoo, and cut the hair according to the directions for the Horizontal Blunt Cut.

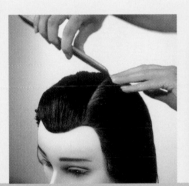

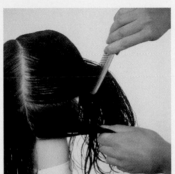

1. Begin the procedure of setting by sectioning the hair off through the natural side part, curving towards the center crown.

2. Start at the center crown and part down the center back vertically. Part horizontally from the occipital area to the center back of the ear on both sides to subdivide the nape area.

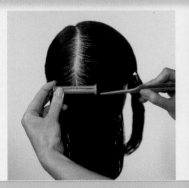

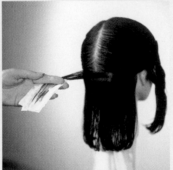

3. Begin at the top center area of the nape section by placing the rod and parting out to the length and width of the rod (a one-diameter base size).

4. Comb the hair straight out from the base parting. Place two end papers over the ends in preparation for rolling the hair smoothly. This is a double end paper method.

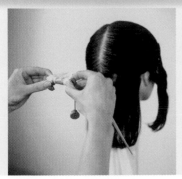

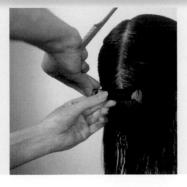

5. Position the rod at the ends and begin to roll the hair smoothly toward the base area, maintaining the hair position straight out from the base as rolling.

6. Secure the band and cap across the rod when reaching the base area.

7. Continue to roll the hair lengths on either side of this center rod. Use the length of rod and amount of rods needed to complete this row.

8. Offset the rod positioning in the next row from the center top rod. This will ensure no hair splits between rows. Adjust rod length as needed to adapt for your client's head size, hair line, etc.

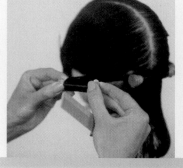 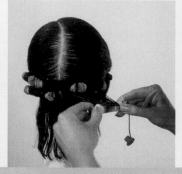

9. Complete the bricklay rolling technique in the nape area. Position picks through the bands. Turn the band toward the top of the rod before inserting the pick.

10. The completed nape area indicates a bricklay pattern with horizontally rolled rods.

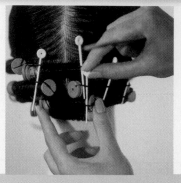 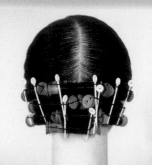

11. Part out 1"(2.5 cm) wide subsections, for spiraling the hair onto rods vertically from center back to the front hairline. The 1"(2.5 cm) width can vary depending on the amount of base lift desired.

12. Part out base sections that are approximately the width of the rod. Comb the lengths diagonally outward from the base area in preparation for spiraling the hair.

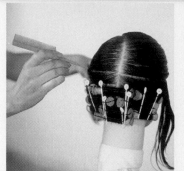 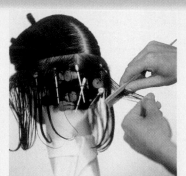

13. Fold the end paper lengthwise over the ends.

14. Place the end of the rod at the ends of the hair and roll at least 1 1/2 revolutions to secure the ends. Note how the end where the rod will be secured is toward the bottom.

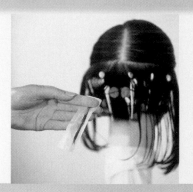 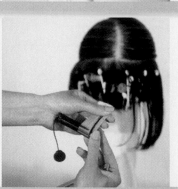

15. With the ends secure, spiral the hair onto the rod. Secure the rod at the bottom when reaching the base area.

16. Continue to use this method of spiraling lengths onto the rod working toward the side front hairline area. Maintain consistent hair sections as spiraling.

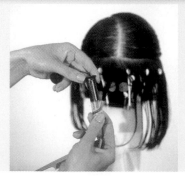 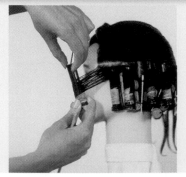

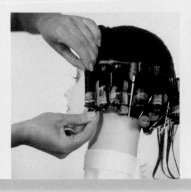
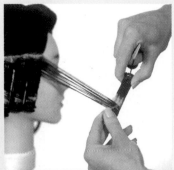

17. Secure the rod at the bottom. Proceed to the other side of this section.

18. Follow the same procedure of spiraling along the length of the rod, maintaining a slight diagonal position.

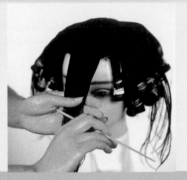
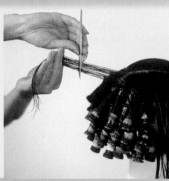

19. Continue to divide the hair as you work upward into the 1" (2.5 cm) subsections.

20. Working around the curvature of the head, be aware of the distribution from the curve of the head. Hold the hair diagonally outward before spiraling.

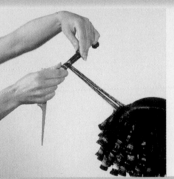
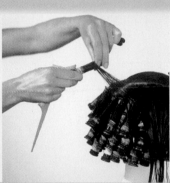

21. Secure the ends of the hair (1 1/2 to 2 revolutions) at one end of the rod, and then proceed to spiral lengths along the rod.

22. Maintain a slight diagonal on the rod as spiraling toward the base before fastening to secure.

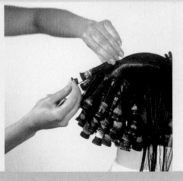
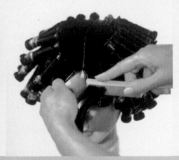

23. Fasten to secure.

24. Continue to subdivide as you work upward.

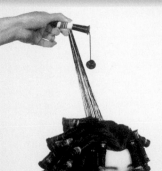
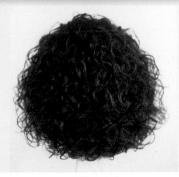

25. Note how the rod is positioned to allow for fastening along its bottom. Notice how each row of rods overlaps the previous sections.

26. Consider the possibilities! This technique may be adapted to create a wide variety of style effects. The finished texture result creates dimension and adds dynamic movement to the blunt shape.

Explore

Apply this technique to different lengths, colors, and cuts for almost endless possibilities.

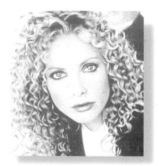

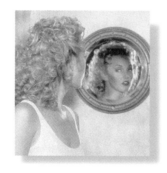

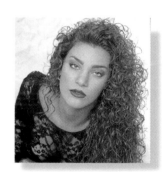

bricklay-roll and spiral technique I

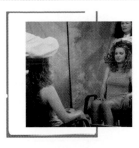

*I*n this finished texture, a full head of sensuous ringlets creates a highly kinetic effect, truly beauty in motion. The interesting mix of textural qualities in this style creates a very natural look that many clients will want.

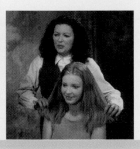 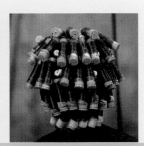

1. This client's thick, dense, long hair has never been treated chemically. For the desired style, we will spiral the hair lengths to create full explosive volume and texture with lots of movement.

2. In the finished wave set, note the alternation between two different rod diameters, and their positioning. The white rod's diameter is smaller than the larger rod's diameter. This smaller rod is rolled horizontally throughout to alternate with panels of spiraled rods positioned vertically to add texture, strength, and definition.

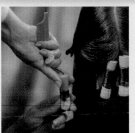 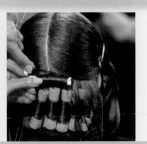

3. Spiral hair throughout the first panel in the same direction, then release the next section to be rolled, measuring this section to the diameter of the smaller rod. Beginning at the center back, distribute the hair straight out from the base area and roll horizontally from the ends to the base.

4. Fasten the rod at the base area and roll the remainder of this section horizontally. Extend the next 2" (5 cm) panel into the side area. All rods in this panel are spiraled and overlay the rods underneath, requiring these rods to be lifted when applying lotion to the lower rods.

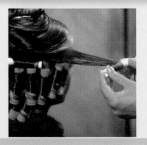 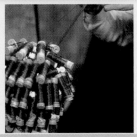

5. Continue this alternation of horizontally rolled rods with spiraled rods positioned vertically within the panels.

6. Take sections across the top of the head and distribute the hair up and out from the base area. Adjust the rod sizes and positions as you approach the front hairline to fit the needs of the client. In the front hairline area, roll the smaller rods orward to create more movement around the front hairline, framing the face.

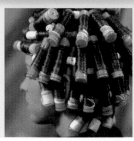 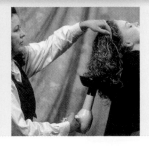

7. The completed wave set shows the alternation of rod sizes and positions. Note how the alternation in the top area of the head moves across the top, not around the curve as you did around the exterior area.

8. Apply a firm-hold conditioning foam and, using a diffuser attachment, have the client drop her head back so that the hair falls freely. Gently cup the hair up into the diffuser attachment and gently massage, lift, and separate the hair as needed, but do not scrunch it.

Consultation

Y ou've been told over and over that, to be successful, a stylist needs "good communication skills." But what exactly does that mean?

To answer, let's look at the literal (dictionary) meaning of the word:

com-muni-cation

_____

_____

_____

_____

_____

_____

There are two important Latin root words here: *com* (which means "with") and *muni* (which means "people").

So communication means, in its most basic sense; "with people."

Whenever you interact with a client, a coworker, a supervisor, or an employee, you are "with people." You are, in effect, always communicating. Communication is the basis of all relationships. How well you communicate will determine your success as a stylist, a colleague, a supervisor, or an employee.

Good communication is necessary for a successful consultation, and a successful consultation is the start of a good client relationship.

Good communication is as stimulating as black coffee, and just as hard to sleep after.

Anne Morrow Lindbergh

bricklay-roll and spiral technique II

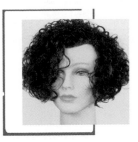

*T*he spiral and roll bricklay technique that was done on the longer blunt cut is used here on shorter lengths to create a natural springy ringlet formation. In this next style, the textural result was created on a variation of the graduated blunt cut at jaw length.

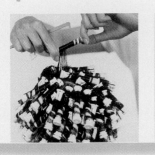

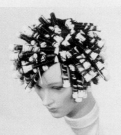

1. Use the same technique that was outlined earlier to progress upward through the set. Maintain consistency of hair distribution and rod positions as you progress through the wave set.

2. Adjust for the natural part, if required. Here, use picks to support the rods away from the forehead to clear this area for client comfort.

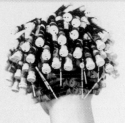

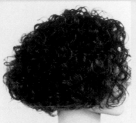

3. Adjust the rod size, length, and setting pattern as required for the desired result.

4. The spiral technique can be highly effective on shorter lengths, particularly blunt and graduated forms—it creates a natural ringlet effect.

Consultation
Step 1:
Connection

*N*othing is more important to the relationship between stylist and client than what happens in the first few minutes of each visit—whether from a new client or one who's returning for the tenth time. If you don't "connect" on both a personal and a professional level from the beginning, your job will be much more difficult than if you do.

It is not as easy as it sounds. Imagine you're in the salon on a busy day. Ten employees are hurrying about as 20 clients are in various stages of service, and still more wait in the lobby. You have just finished an intense two hours with a new client who has required a lot of attention and emotional energy from you. Now, out of the corner of your eye, you see your next client sitting there in the waiting room with a hopeful smile on her face (because she's hoping that you will work your same magic for her).

What do you do? Do you whisper to the receptionist to cover for you for a few more minutes while you sneak away for a soda break and a chance to get your wits back about you? Or do you take a deep breath, walk up to the next client, smile and in your warmest, most sincere voice, "Hello, you must be Angela Barrie. I'm Jack Daws, and I'm so pleased to meet you. Welcome to The Salon."

If you're destined to be a top performer, you'll know which one is correct.

Greeting
The Client

It's not the hours you put in, but what you put into the hours that counts.

E. James Rohn

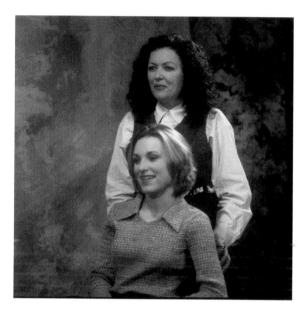

The connection between stylist and client begins in the first few seconds, during the greeting. Remember that earlier we said, "You never get a second chance to make a first impression." The way you greet your client, and your client's response to you, will set the tone for the entire service visit. Make a good impression during the greeting, and everything after that will go much more smoothly.

Let's review a few key phrases that give you clues to a successful greeting:

◆ **Smile**
◆ **Eye contact**
◆ **Speak slowly and clearly**
◆ **Sincere voice**
◆ **Reach out to shake hands**

And there's one more—"Take a deep breath." Going from client to client can be compared with changing partners when dancing. You have to get used to the different style of each one. Like dancers, some clients move more quickly than others; some are more likely to touch than others, some are more confident and outgoing, while others have a hard time coming out of their shells to express themselves.

The most skillful stylists are like good dancers. They know how to adjust to each new client just like dancers adjust to each new partner, making their partner look good in the process. You may be a naturally "bubbly" person or you may be quiet, but when you meet your opposite in a client, it's your responsibility more than it is the client's to adjust your style so that the relationship can work. If you come on too strong with a shy client and make her uncomfortable, don't blame the poor communication that results on her. After all, you're the one making a living at this. It's your job to pick up on the clues that each client gives off, and to adjust your approach each time. Here's another way to look at all this: It's as if you're adjusting the volume on the stereo. For some clients, you can "turn up" your personality full blast. For others, it better be just a murmur.

By the time you get through this program, you'll have a lot more information and skills to use to help you communicate with clients. Pay attention. That's what it's all about.

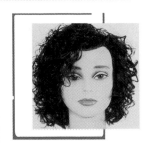

*T*he spiral technique is used here on the light layered haircut to create enhanced volume throughout its shape. This shows the versatility of the spiral technique—which can be adapted to all lengths of hair. In this wave set, you'll use soft bender rods to spiral the hair lengths. These rods come in a variety of diameters and lengths. Adjust according to the length of hair and the results you're looking for. Here, a progression of diameters is used—smaller throughout the nape area, progressing to midsize throughout the crest area, and large throughout the top.

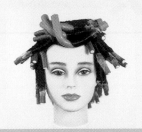
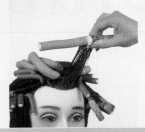

1. Take partings throughout each section on a diagonal to create a directional influence in that section. Directions alternate within each row.

2. Comb the hair lengths on a diagonal from the base area. Secure the ends of the hair at one end of the tool by revolving or rolling the ends 1 1/2 to 2 turns around the rod.

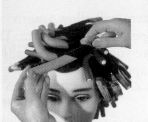
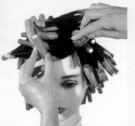

3. Begin spiraling the remaining lengths of hair toward the base area.

4. Secure the tool at the base area by turning its end in the opposite direction from how you spiraled the hair.

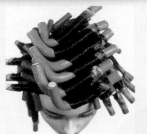
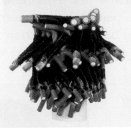

5., 6. In the finished wave set, you can see the progression of the rod diameter sizes—smaller at the nape area, to mid-size around the crest, to larger at the top area of the head. Directions alternate from one spiraled panel to the next.

Whatever you do, do it with all your heart and soul.

Bernard Baruch

And consider the A-line skirt or dress. On the human anatomy, this line is not only waist defining, but also kind to larger-hipped forms, given the outward flow, movement, and expansion of the lower hemline area. The ultimate expansion of the A-line shape is achieved by adding a crinoline underneath the skirt. This same expansion effect can be achieved with the angular stack set.

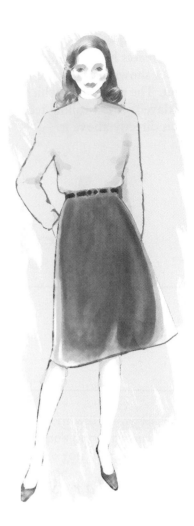

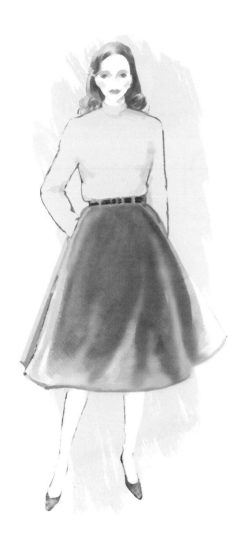

Expansion Possibilities

The expansion of the shape depends directly on the cut shape itself, and on how you stack the texture rods along the edge of that cut shape.

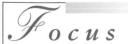
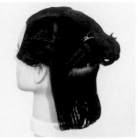

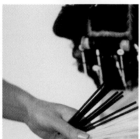

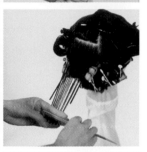

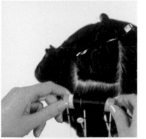

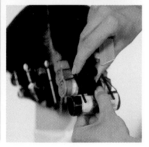

Sectioning Pattern—This is an important first step when you set the angular stack pattern. For this style, subdivide the nape area from the remainder of the head. Section off the remainder of the head into panels that reflect the width of the rod you're using. Panels radiate around the top curved area of the head, working off a side part.

Stacking Sticks—A variety of stacking sticks are available to angle the rods along the ends of the hair.

Positioning the Stacking Sticks—After you roll the second rod within a panel, drop it slightly away from the base—over and on top of the first rod (which you rolled all the way to the base). Gauge and adjust the angle of the sticks according to the length extended out and down from the crown area toward the area to be stacked. This will give you a good estimate of the angle you'll need to allow you to roll the top lengths within a panel at least 1½ turns around the rod. This is the minimal amount of rolling required to engage and wave the hair; any less and the rod would not hold in place.

Rolling/Stacking Procedure—Once you've positioned the stacking sticks, work through the rest of the panel, sectioning it out, combing the mesh of hair through and underneath the sticks, rolling the rod up to the two sticks positioned, and directing the band over the top of the sticks to fasten on the other side. Continue to the top of the section.

Progression of Rod Sizes—In this set, rod sizes progress according to the cut shape. The top lengths have only the softest bend on the ends of the hair—creating the most natural-looking result possible. Yet, because you use smaller rods underneath, you also create the support system that allows the shape to be expanded.

Motivation is like food for the brain. You cannot get enough in one sitting.

Peter Davies

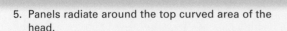

Apply

Angular Stack

After your consultation, drape the client, shampoo, and cut the hair according to the directions for the Diagonal Forward Blunt Cut.

1. In the finished wave set, the panels are rolled to stack at an angle away from the head. Determine this angle by reaching the top length out to the stacked area and rolling it 1½ to 2 turns, to create a bend on the ends.

2. Bricklay the nape area first with a roll technique. Within the individual panels, the rod sizes will progress from medium to extra large.

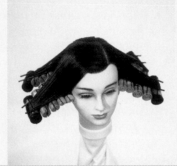
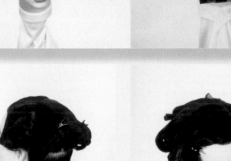

3., 4. To create this wave set, work from the side part and section off the panels you're going to stack; they should be the width of your rod. You can measure panel widths along the bottom area, where the stack will begin. Adjust throughout the interior area according to the curve and size of your client's head. Section off the nape area from the top of the ear on each side; this will be rolled in a bricklay pattern.

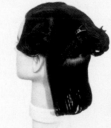
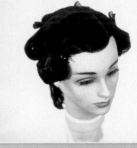

5. Panels radiate around the top curved area of the head.

6. Roll the nape area holding the hair straight out from the base area, to create halfoff-base rod positioning. Adapt medium and long rods to fit into this area. When you complete the nape area, position picks to secure the rods and prevent band marks on the hair.

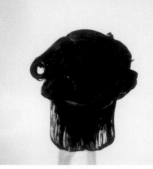
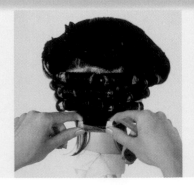

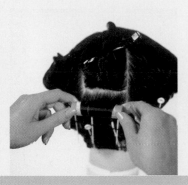

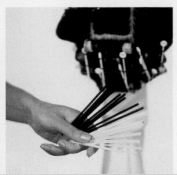

7. Begin the angular stack in the back panels. Roll a large rod from the ends to the base area, along the bottom of the panel. Use a one-diameter base size and roll with hair directed straight out from the base area, so that your rod is positioned halfoff-base.

8. You can use plastic or wooden stacking sticks to angle the rods out and away from the head.

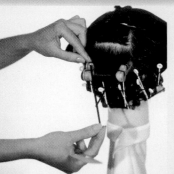

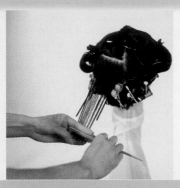

9. Before setting a panel, direct lengths from the top of the panel down toward the stack areas to gauge the angle for the stack. Roll a second rod into position, dropping it over and below the first rod you rolled. Position the sticks underneath and through the bands at the outer areas of the rod on each side.

10. Continue to work upward through the panel. Comb and distribute the hair smoothly through the positioning sticks.

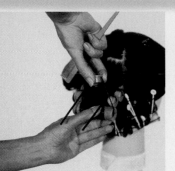

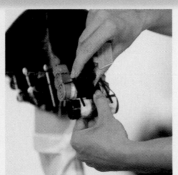

11. Position double end papers. Place a large rod (note the progression in rod size) and roll it up to rest underneath the sticks. Grasp the band and cap and stretch over the top of the sticks to secure the rod to the sticks at the predetermined angle.

12. Continue rolling strands until all lengths are stacked at an angle along the perimeter area of the cut lengths. You'll use the largest rod here to complete the progression of the texture movement.

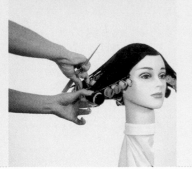

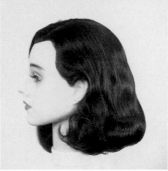

13. Use this same technique throughout all of the divided panels. During the processing and neutralizing procedure, take the client back to the shampoo bowl and using a gentle pressure, rinse and blot. Realign the angled stacks as needed in between these parts of the service.

14. The finished texture provides tremendous versatility for the client who likes a smooth design, yet wants control around her perimeter weight line.

Reflect

Explore

Apply this technique to different lengths, colors, and cuts for almost endless possibilities.

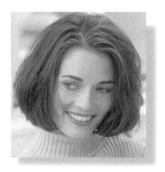

Establishing
Rapport

Give the world the best that you have, and the best will come back to you.

Madeline Bridges

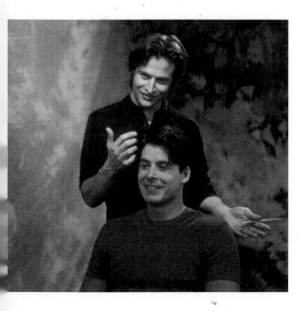

Rapport is defined as "a relationship of mutual respect and comfort." Think about someone with whom you have good rapport. What makes that relationship so good, so comfortable? Do you share all the same opinions and ideas and tastes? That's an easy way to find rapport, but it's not a common one. More likely, your best relationships are good because you are different but able to deal with each other's differences with mutual respect and affection, so it really doesn't matter that you don't agree on everything. You're in rapport, so you can disagree without being disagreeable.

So how do you get to that point with each client? And how do you adjust to each client's personality without completely losing yours in the process? You needn't hide what makes you special—just find that common thread between you and each client on which you can build rapport.

With some clients, the rapport begins before you even meet. It's based on your reputation. If you have been requested by a client because you have built a great reputation, she has already begun forming some opinions about you, and they're probably pretty positive. On the other hand, even if you're just starting out in your first job, you can put each and every client at ease and start to build rapport by being a genuine, caring, nice person.

Remember the clues we gave you for making a connection? Smile, make eye contact, be warm and sincere, reach out and shake hands. Let's not forget the most important: With each client, take a deep breath, and take the time to get to know her on a personal level and to discover how to make your relationship with her one of mutual respect and comfort—a relationship of rapport.

After all, the more clients you can make comfortable with you, the more clients you will have—and keep, for a long, long time.

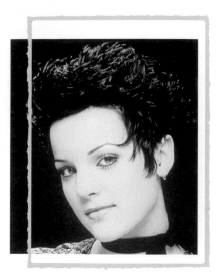

Contour Set

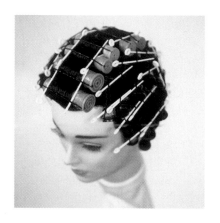

Overview

This classic texture set waves the hair into a formation that provides the client with great versatility. Whether diffused, for soft natural movement that accentuates the dimension of the style, or blow-dried smooth, for voluminous style support, this set pattern is an important one to add to your repertoire of skills.

This set pattern encircles the curved contour of the head. Within panels, roll the hair directionally. These panels surround a central panel, which you part out from the front forehead area to the center nape. Then divide the remaining profile (side) areas to reflect the directional movement that you're looking for in this area, along with other considerations, such as the size of the client's head. Your rods progress in size from larger in the interior, where the longest lengths are, to medium size around the perimeter, where more support is desired. You have many options in rod size; you can see some on the next page.

This set pattern is versatile enough to be used on virtually any cut shape—blunt, graduated, or layered. Here, it accentuates the shape of the diagonal back blunt cut.

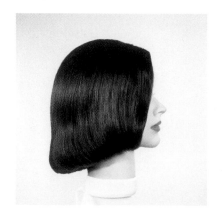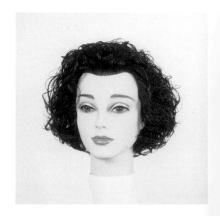

C onnect

Circling the Head

You may have heard the expression circling the globe. The world is round, of course, and even if you choose to travel around it using the straightest route possible, your route will still be curved. Or you may choose the scenic route, meandering from one spot to the next, not necessarily in a straight line.

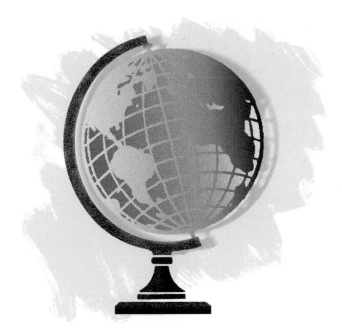

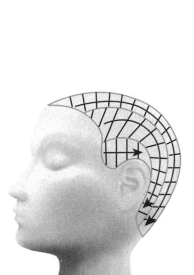

Choosing the "route" you'll take around the curved shape of the head with setting panels is much the same. It is essential that you develop a sensitivity to the shape of the head and its many planes and curves. In this basic directional set, a center panel travels in a straight line from the front forehead area to the center nape, moving around the curve of the head. The texture created by this pattern will flow backward off the face as well as sideways, to blend into the side or profile areas.

Other options to consider in the top front fringe area include: weaving a two-diameter base area—roll one woven strand forward, the other backward; or perhaps setting the hair directionally sideways off a side or center part (if you wish, you can also weave the area along this part). You'll set the profile areas to contour to the curve of the head from the front hairline area to the nape, providing a sweeping, curved movement back off the face that harmonizes with the top area.

In the style here, the area directly above the ear is directed back away from the face, and set vertically. You have other options in setting this area, too. They include: setting the hair in a forward direction; or perhaps diagonally up and back. In all instances, be guided by your client's hair length, shape, and chosen style.

Taking the Curves

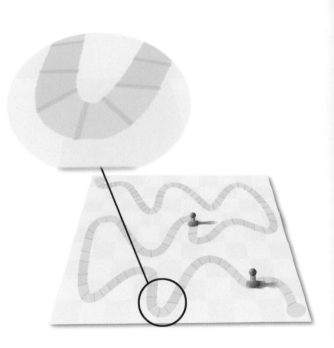

As you take and make the curves of the head with your parting patterns, it might help you to consider these examples of curvature shapes and movement.

Imagine that you're traveling the straightaways on your favorite board game. All of a sudden you need to take a curve—so you pivot along the inside, tight part of the curve. Your movement on the outside of the curve must be more expansive and wider if you're going to make the turn. Or consider the curved center section of a sectional sofa. It's narrow on its sitting edge, but widely expanded at its back edge, to "make the curve" from one straightaway to the next.

The same idea applies as you're setting the hair. You'll take base partings within a curving panel that are narrow at one end, in order to make the curve; the outside area of the base parting will remain wider. In other words, these partings and base sections radiate out from the inside of the curved area.

Through this area, make sure that you're setting relative to the lower parting. Don't set the rod in an overdirected position; this would distort the curvature flow, or movement, that you're seeking to create.

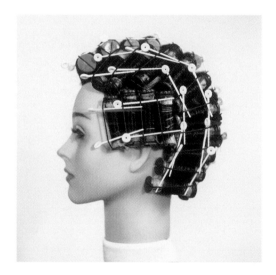

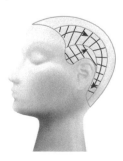

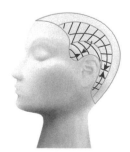

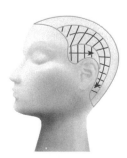

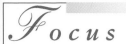

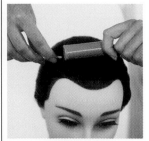

Sectioning the Hair—Distribute all hair off the front hairline. Section out panels that curve to fit the shape of the head. The central panel travels from the center forehead area to the center nape area and is as wide as the rod you're using. Divide the profile areas into two panels—one that curves from the temple area to the outside nape area, the other positioned directly above the ear.

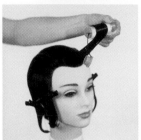

Parting, Rolling, and Rod Positions—Take straight horizontal partings throughout the central panel to create rectangular bases. In the outside of the profile area, take base partings that first angle, then radiate, around the curve. At this point, take partings horizontally to the nape. The partings throughout the area above the ear are taken vertically.

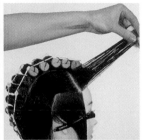

Base Controls—In the interior and front hairline area, you want to position the rod directly on base for optimal lift and volume there. Hold the hair 45 degrees (.785 rad) above the center of the base area for rolling this base control. Around the exterior or perimeter area roll straight out from the center of the base. Your rod should be positioned half off-base, which slightly diminishes the base lift and volume.

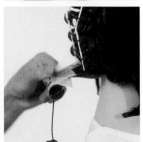

Rod Sizes—Use a progression of rod sizes to match the progression of lengths in the cut. This will create a very natural end result. In the underneath and perimeter areas, use smaller rods (for support and expansion of shape); set the longer interior lengths on larger rods for a looser, more languid wave pattern.

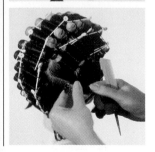

Base Lift—Blunt shapes generally require more base lift in the interior area. Fine hair with less integrity around the front hairline will require less tension on the base.

Apply

Contour Set

After your consultation, drape the client, shampoo, and cut the hair according to the directions for the Diagonal Back Blunt cut.

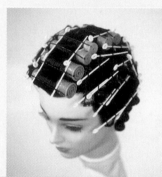

1. Here's the finished wave set. The texture tools curve to fit the shape of the head as they move away from the face. A central panel that is the width of the longest rod extends from the center forehead area to the center nape. On each side of the head, the partings curve from the temple area to the outside nape area.

2. Prepare to set this pattern by directing all lengths back away from the face. Comb and distribute the hair smoothly.

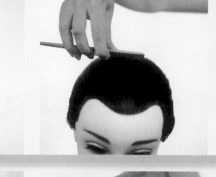

3. Beginning at the front hairline area, part out a panel as wide as the rod you've chosen. Position the rod at the center top area to provide a guide for parting off the panel on each side. Take the parting along one side from the forehead area to the crown.

4. Part out the other side of the panel to the crown. Separate the hair gently on each side of the part; try to maintain the original backward hair distribution.

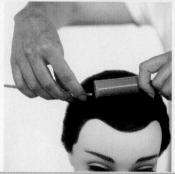
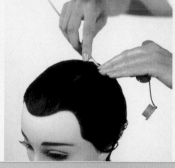

5. Continue this procedure throughout the back area of the head. Position the rod centrally, then part from the crown to the nape.

6. Part out along the other side of the rod length to complete the central back panel.

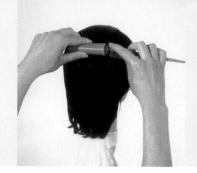
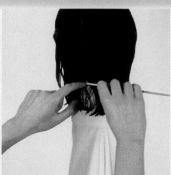

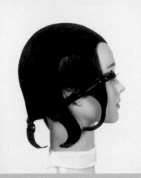
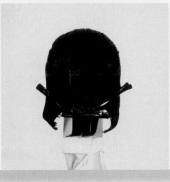

7., 8. Use this same technique for sectioning out panels on each side. Place rods at an angle at the temple area to measure panel width, because the desired direction moves down and back through this area. Keep in mind that this set is being done on a mannequin head, however; every client you work on will have differences in head shape, head size, hairlines, and growth patterns.

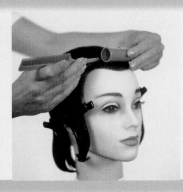
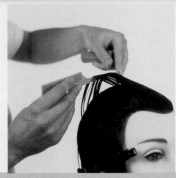

9. Use the rod to measure and section out the base area to a one–diameter base size. You'll use extra-large-diameter rods through the center top to match the longer lengths of hair there. Progress to large-diameter rods around the exterior of the shape, which has shorter lengths.

10. After parting across with the tail end of your comb, lift the tail end up and back through the hair as shown. Try not to disturb the surrounding hair.

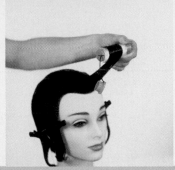
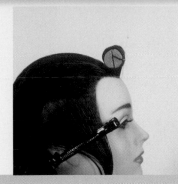

11. Comb the hair smoothly 45 degrees (.785 rad) above the center of the base. Apply double end papers to the ends of the hair. Roll the lengths from the ends to base area.

12. The rod will position itself on its base area given the angle of rolling. This technique is used to create strong base lift, hence volume, through the top area.

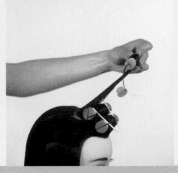
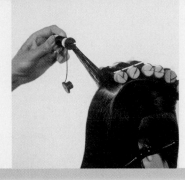

13. You can insert picks while you work through the set. After the set is complete, the picks will support the rods while keeping the band away from the hair. Continue to roll lengths through the top area using the same rolling angle.

14. At the lower crown area, you'll make a change in both rod size and base control. Comb the hair straight out from the center of the base area in preparation for rolling. The rod will position itself half off-base, which will slightly diminish the amount of base lift.

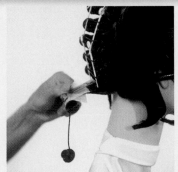
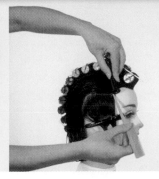

15. Comb the hair straight out from the base and continue to roll lengths straight toward the center nape.

16. Use the rod to measure and diagonally part out the base area. Roll the rod so that it positions itself at a diagonal.

17. After parting, lift the tail end of your comb up and back through the hair. Try not to disturb the surrounding hair in the panel.

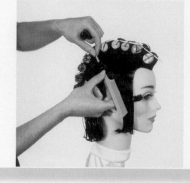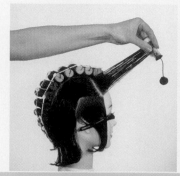

18. Comb the hair 45 degrees (.785 rad) diagonally above the center of the base area. Using this technique in the side areas around the front hairline gives extra base support and lift.

19. Roll the rod to the base area and fasten. Assess the hairline strength, density, and growth patterns on your client to determine the most appropriate base control. Fine hair with less integrity around the front hairline, for instance, will require less tension; you might also want to use a halfoff-base control.

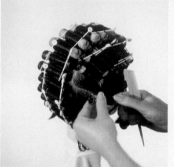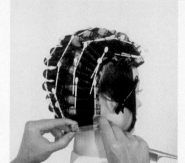

20. As you round the curve of the head toward the back area, change your base control: Hold the hair straight out for rolling and positioning the rod half-off-base. Note the diagonal rod positioning.

21. As you turn toward the nape area, your base sections will be slightly wider along the outside edge of the panel; this will allow you to turn from the diagonal back position to a downward direction. On the mannequin, taking one or two base sections around this curve should be enough.

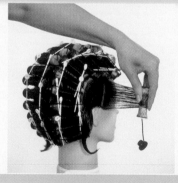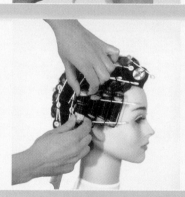

22. Continue to roll lengths through to the nape area. Use shorter rods in this panel to adapt to its width.

23. At the area above the ears, section vertically beginning at the front hairline area. Direct lengths diagonally downward from the center of the base area, then roll to position the rod on base.

24. Roll all rods vertically and in a backward direction through this area for the client who prefers to wear her hair off her face.

25., 26. Here's the finished wave set again, seen from two different views. Observe the rod size and positioning from the top interior area toward the exterior. Note the directional movement within the panel areas—the hair goes back and off the face in a movement that echoes the curve of the head.

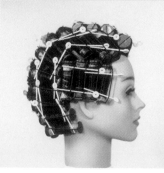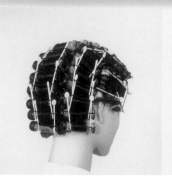

358

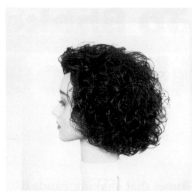
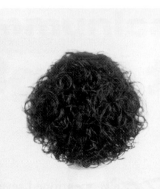

27., 28. The textural expression of movement and dimension in this design enhances the cut shape beautifully! And this texture is versatile enough to allow for a wide variety of style changes.

Reflect

Explore

Apply this technique to different lengths, colors, and cuts for almost endless possibilities.

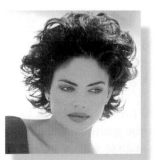
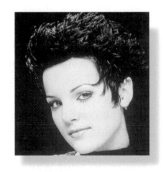
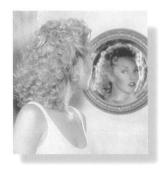

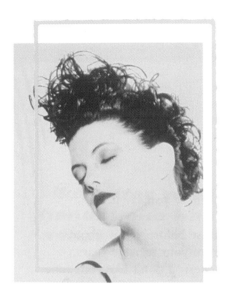

Bricklay

—roll technique

Overview

We've explored the concept of bricklay setting in the first technical—refer to page 332. In this style we explore using the bricklay setting technique to set the entire head (whereas up until this point only the nape area has been set with this technique).

This setting pattern will be one of your most often used in the salon. The flow of movement in this finished result is very natural and easily maintained by your client. Hair flows with no discernible splits between rows. The variables possible with this setting pattern will be explored at the end of this chapter.

Given that we're working on a mid-length graduated shape, this setting pattern will expand and enhance voluminous movement and dimension. The tool diameters used here will create a firm, resilient curl pattern.

Connect

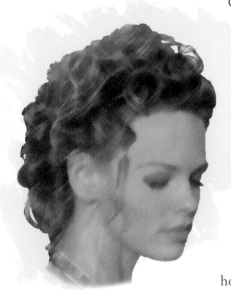

Clients today desire "instant gratification" with their hairstyle. This includes the results of their texture service—they would like to comb through or run their fingers through their hair and have it fall into place effortlessly. Setting and waving the hair into a direction that will work with their desired finished style is today's approach instead of setting hair into block sets (or "railroad track" sets) that take extra work to style.

The backswept direction off the face is a popular setting direction to be used as many women desire the qualities that it provides. It opens up and keeps hair from falling in the face. It moves hair back and up against the natural fall of gravity, creating desirable volume. The setting pattern for this set involves beginning at the front forehead area with the first tool placed—this will serve as the starting point for all subsequent partings through the top and sides to parallel each other—a shift takes place at the crown area to make the turn into the back area. At the crown horizontal partings are taken that continue down to the nape.

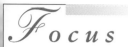

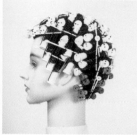

Full Head Bricklay Set using Rolling Method—The bricklay setting method will be used throughout the entire head to sweep the hair back off the face toward the nape. The base controls for this set are as follows: A one diameter on base tool position is initially used, changing to a one diameter half off-base control toward the perimeter of the style.

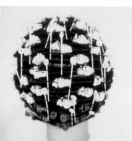

Setting Pattern—The rows for setting are adjusted according to the area of the head—on the top and sides, rows are set that parallel each other until the crown—making for diagonal positioning at the side areas. At the crown area rows are set with a horizontal positioning (also paralleling each other) through to the nape area.

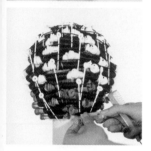

Tool Size—Tool size is medium until reaching the shorter nape lengths at which point a smaller tool diameter size is used.

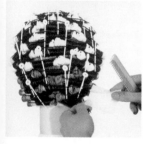

End Paper Technique—The bookend wrap method is used in the nape area where lengths are shorter as a double end wrap would be excessive for this length of hair.

> *It matters not what road we take but rather what we become on the journey.*
>
> *Michael Angier*

Apply *Bricklay*
—roll technique

After your consultation, drape the client, shampoo, and cut the hair according to the directions for the Low Graduation cut.

1. Begin the set at the front hairline area by parting out a base area that's the length and width of the longer rod you're using. Comb and distribute the hair 45 degrees (.785 rad) above the center of the base area. Apply a double end paper wrap. Roll from the ends to the base to position the rod on its base area.

2. In the row directly behind your first rod, take base partings that allow for two midlength rods to be offset from the center of the first rod.

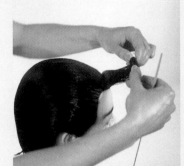
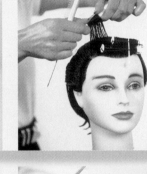

3. Insert picks underneath the bands to alleviate pressure on the hair.

4. Before you set the next row, study the area to be set. Adjust the rod length as needed to accommodate this area. Now begin the next row by positioning a rod at the center of the spot where the two rods met in the previous row.

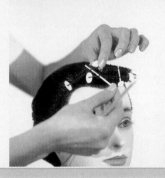
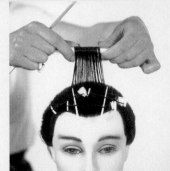

5. The pattern you see here is the one you'll use throughout the entire set.

6. Continue to part out rows that radiate around the curve of the head, extending around and down toward the side hairline area. Maintain precise parting out, distribution, and rolling of hair strands to create the bricklay pattern. Secure the rods and insert picks—either as you go or when you're finished.

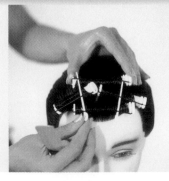
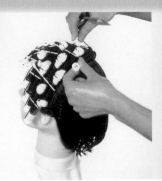

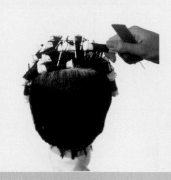

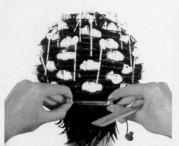

7. At the crown area of the set, stop curving rows around the front hairline. Instead, take rows that work around the back of the head in a horizontal fashion. Continue with the bricklay pattern. As you work from row to row, adjust the length of rod to fit into the area you're working on.

8. When you reach the occipital area, change to a smaller rod to create more curl definition, and support. When lengths become quite short, change your end paper technique. Fold single end paper in half to control and smooth the ends—this is called a bookend wrap.

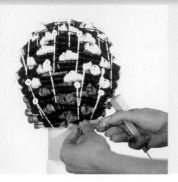

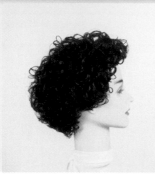

9. Complete the bricklay wave set in the nape area. As you move toward the perimeter area, progress to a one-diameter base size with the rod positioned half off-base.

10. The highly active texture and support in this design fully expands the shape, providing a tremendous amount of volume. The backsweep of hair from the face is highly prized by clients who want to make a textural statement but still easily maintain their styles.

Explore

Apply this technique to different lengths, colors, and cuts for almost endless possibilities.

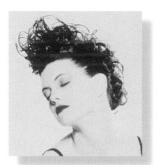

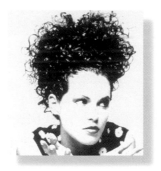

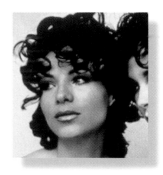

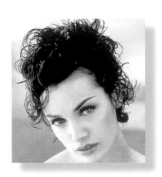

Verbal Communication
Part 2:
Content

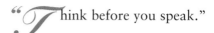

"Think before you speak."

As for the content of your communication, the actual words you say, remember: Salon clients are not your friends, even when they are your friends. In other words, when you're behind the chair, act as professionally as possible. Be polite and show good manners. The way you talk should not in any way make a client—even if she is someone you've known a long time—think you are anything but skilled, confident, and professional. Following are a few tips for talking the talk of a professional stylist:

◆ **Use correct grammar, such as "I have seen" or "I saw," "I have been" or "I was," "I have done" or "I did," not, "I seen, I been" and "I done." Also: "He/she/it doesn't" rather than "He/she/it don't." And: "I don't have any" instead of "I ain't got no." While we're on the subject of "ain't," forget you ever heard that word. If you weren't paying attention when grammar was being taught in school, get some help from someone you know who knows the rules, or pick up a book on the subject, and read it.**

◆ **Avoid slang and lose the "you knows," the "ums," and the "likes"—as in, "I'm like, you know, 'How could you do that, girl, when, like, we had those plans for um, like, forever;" Translation: "I let my friend know I was disappointed that she canceled our plans."**

◆ **Do not curse or use phrases that could offend a client. "That sucks!" might be written into every television sitcom script in America, but it's a poor choice of words for a professional stylist. Try "How unfair!" instead.**

Polite, grammatically correct speech is the sign of a skilled professional. Save your more colorful lingo for your personal time.

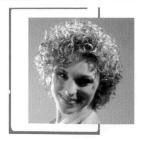

his highly textured style provides the ultimate volume and definition of the cut shape. Alternating texture diameters give a very natural curl. This type of texture can be diffused naturally or air formed with a round brush; you can also dry the texture in naturally, then use thermal styling tools, such as hot rollers or curling irons, to create a smoother finished effect. Before waving the hair, we'll perform a porosity and elasticity test to gauge its condition. The waving system used will be specifically selected for this hair type—a fine texture, a normal density and color treated.

1. In the finished wave set, two different diameter rods alternate in a directional movement swept back off the face. To add to the naturalness and flow of movement, each base part is weaved or zigzagged throughout the set. (See page 363.) Begin setting at the front forehead area by zigzagging the tail end of your comb along the scalp area to part out the first base area.

2. Note the base parting.

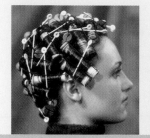
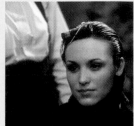

3. Roll this first section on the larger rod to position on base. The bricklay pattern will begin from this rod position.

4. Continue to roll row after row with the bricklay pattern. Zigzag the base partings and alternate rod diameter from row to row. At the crown, begin rolling half off-base. Note the zigzag base parting.

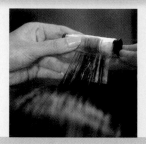
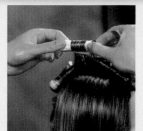

5. Continue rolling directionally toward the nape area. At the perimeter hairline area, roll the larger rod upward in an indentation technique.

6. The rods are directionally rolled back off the face and rolled diagonally at the sides, shifting direction at the crown to begin rolling horizontally downward. Apply the appropriate liquid styling tool, in this case a liquid gel, and diffuse hair for a natural finish.

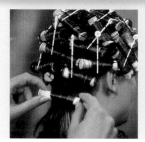
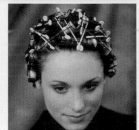

bricklay-roll technique II

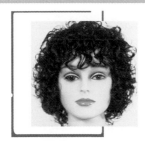

*I*n this design, the bricklay set will add texture to the classic heavy layered shape. The symmetry of the cut shape is quite conducive to this low-maintenance, easy-care, easy-wear style. All the hair around the front hairline is directed toward the face. The lengths framing the face give a softness to the facial features. Texture flows directionally from the crown area, providing voluminous movement and dimension.

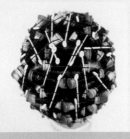 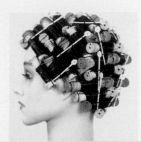

1., 2. In the finished wave set, all rods radiate from the naturalgrowth direction in the crown area. Direct all rods in the front area of the set forward in a bricklay pattern; all rods through the back area of the head flow from the crown downward in a bricklay pattern. Distribute the hair into front and back sections by parting out from the central crown area to behind the top of the ear on each side of the head. In the center crown area, which is directed forward, part out a base area to the length and width of the larger rod you'll be using for this set.

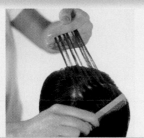 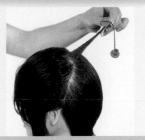

3. Divide the first sections using a weaving technique. (See page 363.) Move the tail end of the comb to alternate between strands of hair. Comb one of the woven portions toward the back area; you'll roll it, along with the back area of the head, later. The other woven portion will be rolled forward.

4. Distribute this strand of hair 45 degrees (.785 rad) above the center of the base, and roll it to the base, to create a one-diameter on-base rod position. This will provide lift in this area.

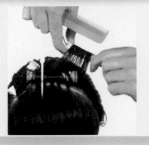 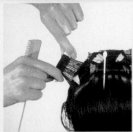

5. Begin to alternate rod sizes in the next row; adjust your rod lengths as needed to fit within the rows. Roll all rods in the front area forward, toward the face. In the third row, return to the central area to begin rolling from this area outward.

6. Work toward the outer side of the row on either side of the centrally positioned rod. Continue to alternate between the two rod sizes from row to row.

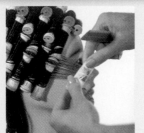 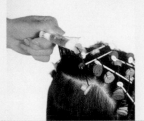

7. Complete the bricklay set in the front area by working to the front hairline. Adjust rod sizes and lengths to allow for the hairline lengths around the face. When the front area is complete, move to the crown area.

8. Part out a base area to the length and width of the smaller of your two rods. Distribute the hair 45 degrees (.785 rad) above the center of the base area for rolling. This will create a one-diameter on-base rod position, maximizing the volume in this area. Roll lengths back and down from the crown area.

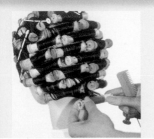 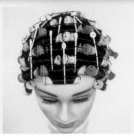

9. Alternate rod sizes from row to row through the back area. Finish the bricklay setting technique at the nape area.

10. In another view of the finished bricklay set, note how all rods directionally flow from the crown area outward toward the perimeter hairline area. Use picks to lift the bands away from the rods.

partial bricklay I

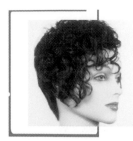

*T*his textural effect is well suited to shorter layered lengths of hair. In this style, the texture moves toward the face through the crest area while the directional movement is alternated through the interior lengths.

1. Here's the finished wave set. To start the set, section out the interior from the recession area and curve around to the crown on both sides. The panel directly below this should be the same length as your longer rod. Begin setting at the center back of this panel.

2. To alleviate any splits, weave the first base section you take. (See page 363.) Weave with the tail of your comb through this hair strand. Comb the upper part of the weave into the hair on the opposite side panel.

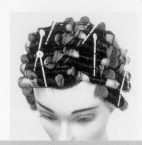
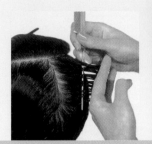

3. Roll this first rod to the base and fasten. Roll all rods throughout this panel to the half-off-base position. Continue through the section.

4. Roll one-diameter bases toward the front hairline area. Repeat this technique on the other side.

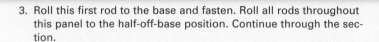
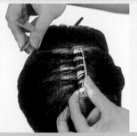
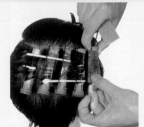

5. At the top, begin setting in the crown area by rolling your smaller-diameter rod forward, alternating with the next row being rolled with the larger-diameter rod in a backward direction. This will be the process used throughout the interior; smaller tool rolled forward, larger tool rolled back. At the front hairline, set the rod with a spiral technique. The hair is spiraled or elongated along the length of the rod to create a ringlet effect on the longer fringe lengths. Insert picks as needed.

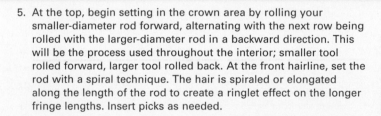
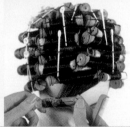
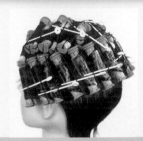
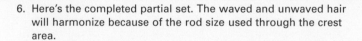

6. Here's the completed partial set. The waved and unwaved hair will harmonize because of the rod size used through the crest area.

7. Introducing texture into this short layered shape gives many options to the client—from air forming the hair into a smoother, sleeker look to diffusing into a natural textured finish.

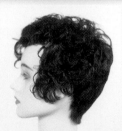

"Reading" the Messages
Clients Project

The most important thing in communication is to hear what isn't being said.

Peter Drucker

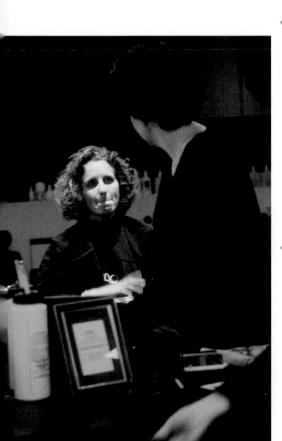

Once you become aware of the messages you project, you'll be able to learn something about clients from listening and observing. With practice, you'll "know" things about clients in the first few minutes of your greeting. For example:

◆ Voice, Volume and Speed

People who talk fast may be "hyper," or they may simply be nervous because they are in a new situation. And just like speed, volume also increases with excitement and nervousness. A loud voice can be the trait of a "Notice me—I'm important" kind of person. In either case, this person needs attention to put her at ease.

◆ Body Language

You can learn a lot from watching a person stand or walk. Arms across the chest signal a defensive or withdrawn position, as if the person is saying, "I don't agree" or, perhaps, "I'm not sure of myself." Someone who holds herself "tightly" in when she sits or walks is not comfortable or self-confident. Similarly, hands raised to cover the mouth while talking signals low self-esteem or insecurity. As you may guess, someone who does the opposite—who strides into a room, swings her arms, gestures and talks rapidly and loudly—is saying, "I'm entitled to take up extra space."

◆ Appearance

The first thing you might notice a person wearing is a smile. Nearly all people will smile at you if you smile at them—but are they also smiling with their eyes?

As a stylist who will be helping people create their personal images, you should pay careful attention to how each client dresses, the fashions she chooses, the colors, the amount of jewelry. Before you suggest a hairstyle for someone, you need to know how she perceives herself and what she believes is the image she portrays. Don't see your clients simply as "heads of hair" that you can design according to your whim. Look at the whole person, even inside the person, to determine how her hair and makeup can best reflect who she is and match her image at work and at play.

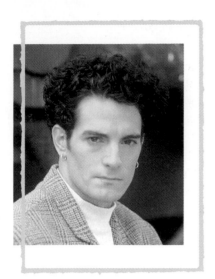

Curvature/Bricklay Combination

Overview

This design introduces you to several new concepts—along with some that you've already experienced. The set itself is a quick and easy way to introduce texture and body using an interesting tool—a vented roller that is secured with a pick. Curvature movement around the face, with a rolled bricklay pattern through the rest of the set down to the occipital area, creates a carefree, versatile texture. A variety of style changes is possible—the hair can be dried naturally, blow-dried with a round brush, molded, or wet set.

Connect

Partial Setting

Partial setting—in which you don't necessarily roll or set the entire head—is often used in waving the hair. This can apply to placing texture only in spot areas, such as the crown or the top of the head, to provide lift, volume, and support; or it can apply to setting tools only at the side front hairline, to directionally move hair off the face. Here the entire set is rolled— except for the nape area, which is left in its natural texture. This type of effect requires that the cut's shape be maintained to look its best.

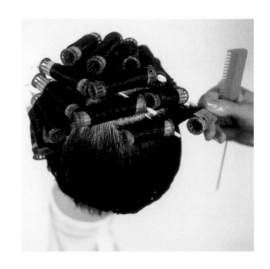

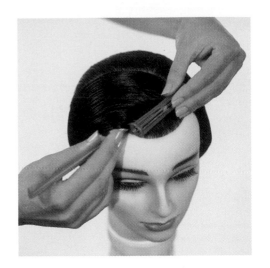

Curvature Movement

Refer to page 320 where we explored the concept of curvature movements for the first time. In this texture set, the curvature is around the front area, off a side part. Everyone's hairline in this area will be different, but essentially, you decide on the amount of curvature you want, then take base partings radiating around the hairline area. This will create tapered base shapes—narrower along the front hairline, and wider toward the back edge of the shape. This allows you to make the turn around the front hairline area.

Weaving Technique

To weave means "to form by interlacing threads, yarns, or strips of material." When you weave cloth, you form a fabric or texture. Weaving as related to hair involves zigzagging with the tail end of your comb along a section of hair, so that you divide the base area into two separate sections to be rolled. In this set, you'll use weaving to blend the area that you are rolling and the perimeter hairline, which you're leaving unwaved. You'll roll the upper base area. As a variation of the weaving technique, use two distinctly different tool diameters to create a very natural effect—place them in opposing directions to create "clash," hence volume, at the base area.

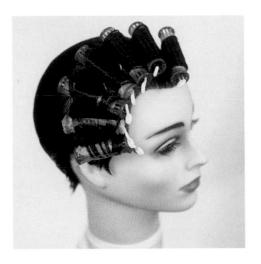

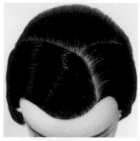

Sectioning/Setting Pattern—Section out curvature panels around the front hairline. Bricklay the top and center back with a rolling technique.

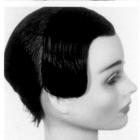

Parting Pattern—Use radial parts at the front to make the turn around the hairline area.

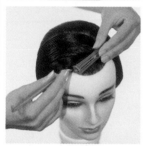

Tapered Base Shapes Through Curvature Movements—Your base shapes should be tapered around the front hairline area to facilitate the curving movement. Along the hairline area where the inside of the turn is taking place, the base width should fit the tool; the outside edge of the base will widen slightly. Roll the rod to sit relative to the lower base parting.

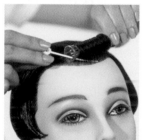

Vented Roller—The tool of choice in this set is a vented roller that is secured with a pick. This pick allows for great freedom as you set curvature movements. The roller is vented to allow thorough rinsing of solutions from the hair.

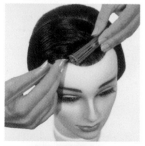

Base Control—Use a one-diameter, on-base roller control throughout the interior; use a one-diameter half-off-base roller control from the crest area downward (this will subtly diminish the base volume).

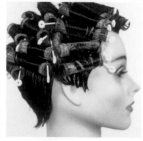

Weaving Technique—The weaving technique used around the perimeter allows the waved texture to blend into the shorter unwaved lengths.

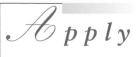

Apply

Curvature/Bricklay Combination

After your consultation, drape the client, shampoo, and cut the hair according to the directions for the Horizontal Graduation cut.

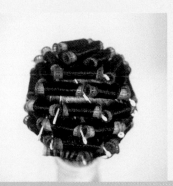

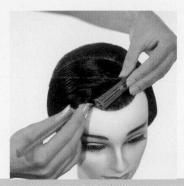

1. To create the finished wave set, set the lengths in a bricklay pattern from the top apex area of the head toward the occipital area, until hair becomes too short to roll on a large-diameter rod.

2. Begin at the top front hairline, placing the rod as a measurement for a one-diameter base size. Part out through the molded panel. Lift up and around so as not to disturb the remainder of the molded section. The base will be approximately 1 diameter in width at the front hairline area, then expand at the outer back edge of the panel.

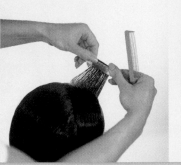

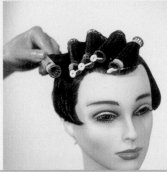

3. Holding the hair at a 45 degree (.785 rad) angle above the center of the base area, roll to position the rod on the base.

4. As you continue, take base sections whose outside area is slightly wider than the inside area. As you start to travel over the curved crest area of the head, take the hair sections straight out from the base. This will create a slightly diminished base volume as you move toward the shorter perimeter lengths.

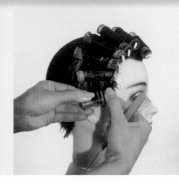

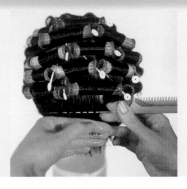

5. At the area above the ear weave the section as shown. Roll the top of the woven section to rest on base. Try to keep a large, open wave pattern here, to harmonize with unwaved perimeter lengths. If the length here does not roll onto the rod you've been using, do the weave on the section just above it. Repeat this on the other side.

6. Bricklay through the crown and back area. When you reach the shorter perimeter lengths, again use the weave technique to roll the last row of rods.

7. Roll the rods in this last row along the top of the woven section. Pick to secure.

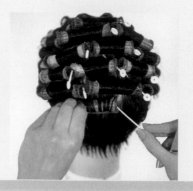

8. Again, the finished wave set.

9. In the finished style, note how the texture accentuates the shape while giving directional support and control to the hair lengths, for ease of styling.

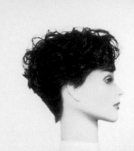

Focus on the power within you and let it guide you.

Louise Hay

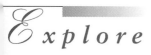

Reflect

Explore

Apply this technique to different lengths, colors, and cuts for almost endless possibilities.

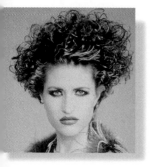

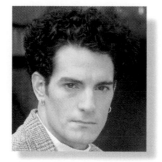

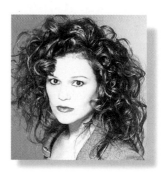

partial bricklay II

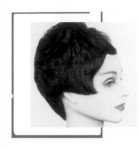

A very commercial and desirable approach to texture for many clients could be called "texture a la carte." This is the positioning of texture in only those areas where the client needs or wants support, lift, and movement. In this short layered shape, for instance, texture was introduced into the crown area only. We've elected to use a bricklay pattern within a diamond shape that reflects and complements the lines of the haircut.

Begin the procedure by studying the natural growth patterns through the crown area and determining the most appropriate beginning and ending areas for your set. Then distribute the hair around the curved region of the head from a pivotal area at the top of the crown, where the movement is to begin.

1. Create a zigzag base part in preparation for rolling.

2. You'll use very large diameter rods in this set to blend smoothly into the surrounding unwaved lengths of hair. Roll the first rod within the diamond shape. Continue to part out and roll rods from row to row using the bricklay pattern.

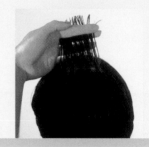
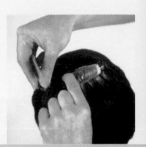

3. Continue the bricklay setting pattern within a diamond shape. The set diminishes at the upper occipital area.

4. Note the finished wave set through the entire crown area within a diamond shape. All base partings have been zigzagged. The set area is surrounded with cotton to protect the surrounding hair (unwaved) from the waving solution. You can apply a conditioning cream to the hair just outlining the set area before you place the cotton, to provide extra protection.

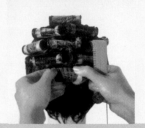
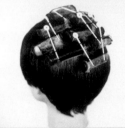

5. This finished style is a perfect example of texture a la carte—the partial crown volume balances the style, adapting to the client's face and head shape. It's a very contemporary approach to waving the hair, and it allows you to discuss texture with clients who would not consider a full wave set.

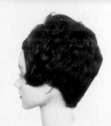

Asking the Right
Questions

"There is no new knowledge. There is only correct questioning."

Socrates, ancient Greek philosopher

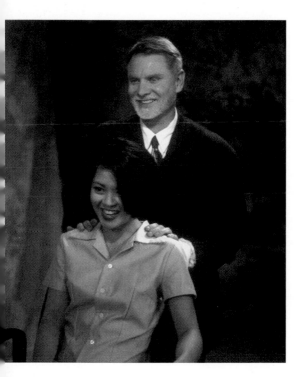

To get the information you need to help a client make style decisions, not only should you ask the right questions, but you must also ask them in the right way. When you are looking for facts, ask closed-ended questions. These are questions that have only one answer. When you want to understand a person's perceptions, ideas, and feelings, however, ask open-ended questions. Following are examples of both types of questions.

Closed-Ended Questions

1. Where do you work? What is your job title?
2. What activities do you participate in, such as swimming or other exercise workouts, that can affect the condition of your hair?
3. What time of day do you shampoo? How many days per week?
4. How much time do you have before work to style your hair?
5. Do you use a blow-dryer? Curling iron? Electric rollers?
6. What cleansing, conditioning, and styling products do you presently use? Do you like how they work?
7. Does your home use city water or well water? Is there a filter on your home water system?
8. Are you taking vitamins or any medications?

Open-Ended Questions

1. Tell me what you like about how you are wearing your hair now.
2. What would you change about your hair if you could?
3. Describe a hairstyle or length you've worn in the past that you really liked.
4. Tell me about past salon experiences that you either liked or didn't like.
5. Describe your home hair care regimen and styling routine.
6. Thinking about your position at work, what qualities do you need to project? How can your hair, makeup, and fashion help you project the right image?

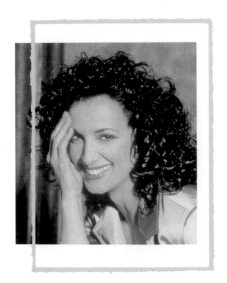

Spiral
with Circle
Tool

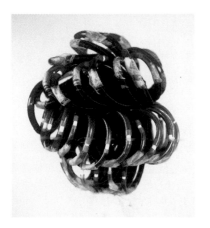

Overview

You first read about spiraling technique on page 318; you might want to review that section. In this design you'll build on your spiraling technique by using an elongated tool for extra-long lengths of hair. This allows you to work quickly and efficiently. The texture service will be done on the very long blunt shape combined with subtle long layers around the front area of the cut.

The circle tool is ideally suited to create a resilient, springy spiral texture in long lengths of hair. This long layered shape has been set with an alternation of tools that progress in size from panel to panel. This allows more movement on the underneath lengths of hair, then progresses to a lesser, yet still firm, amount of texture through the top of the design.

Connect

Spiraling Extra-Long Lengths of Hair

Adding texture to extra-long lengths of hair often requires special techniques and tools. These can reduce your spiraling time while creating an equality and resiliency of the spiral formation. And depending on the hair length, a conventional waving tool simply may not work. The circle tool's extra length, however, allows you to create resilient, firm spirals from the base to the ends—without minimizing length reduction. This is because the hair is spread over a longer length of tool.

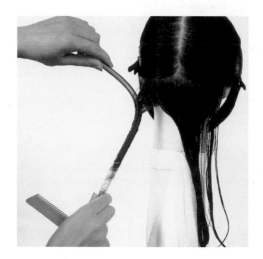

Alternation and Progression

In the world of art, alternation and progression are the patterns you use to arrange the elements within a design, a painting, a sculpture, perhaps woven fabrics, etc. Alternation is the sequential repetition of two or more elements in the design; this creates a rhythm or pattern. When you're setting tools, alternation means intermixing tool diameter sizes and/or directions to create a very desirable and natural look.

Progression is gradual change from one area to the next within a work of art. Gradual change, of course, implies movement—from light to dark, from large to small or small to large, from fast to slow, and so on. This set uses both alternation and progression.

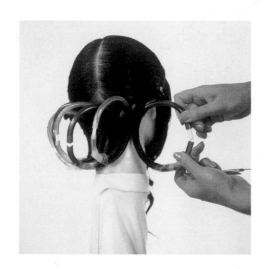

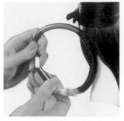

The Circle Rod—Choose the circle rod for extra-long lengths of hair. It minimizes length reduction of the hair, while still creating resilient, firm spirals.

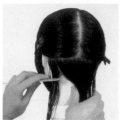

Sectioning/Parting Pattern—The depth of the panels or sections in this set is approximately 2 1/2" (6.125 cm). Take partings through the panels vertically and in a bricklay pattern. Alternate the direction of spiraled movement from panel to panel.

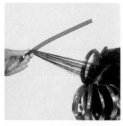

Base Controls for Setting—Within each panel you will want to consider the base control desired, whether one-diameter-on base, or half off-base, or even a hanging stem. The decision to have the tool sit within a base area versus hanging from it will determine the depth of the panel. Depending on the base control desired, the width of the panel will be parted out accordingly.

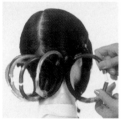

Direction of Setting—If you're spiraling the hair toward the right to create volume, begin spiraling on the left side of the panel. If you're spiraling the hair toward the left, begin spiraling your rods on the right side of the panel.

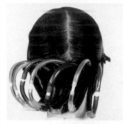

Alternation/Progression of Rod Size—Alternate rod sizes within each panel, as well as from the exterior to the interior.

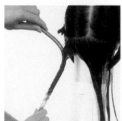

Spiraling Method—Angle each rod slightly toward the base area for consistent, even tension.

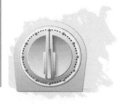

Optimizer Steps—You already know that you should follow certain steps in optimizing the waving of every head of hair. Still, you must be extra careful about these procedures when you're waving extra-long lengths of hair—particularly when it comes to saturating, timing, rinsing, towel blotting, and so on.

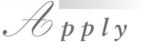

Apply Bricklay

After your consultation, drape the client, shampoo, and cut the hair according to the directions for the Horizontal Blunt cut. Notice that layers have been added on the side.

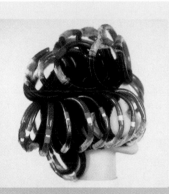

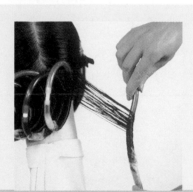

1. Here's the finished set. Bricklay the elongated, vertical base sections within each panel.

2. Begin setting in the nape area. Section out a panel approximately 2½" (6.125 cm) deep from ear to ear. Part out vertical base sections that are the same diameter as the rod you're using. To spiral, secure the ends of the hair, by applying a single end paper folded lengthwise, then rolling 1½ to 2 times to engage the ends of the rod. With the ends secured, begin to spiral along the length of the rod, working toward the base area.

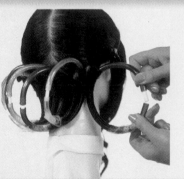

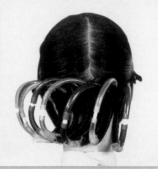

3. Maintain an even tension from the ends to the base area. Secure the rod by fastening the ends together. This will be the process used throughout the head.

4. Here's the completed nape panel.

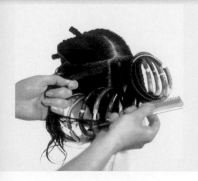

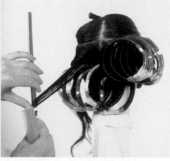

5. Section out the second panel above the first. Begin setting at the side opposite from where the first panel began, and move in the direction opposite the
direction you established in the first panel.

6. Secure the ends of the hair by rolling them along one end of the rod 1½ to 2 times, then spiral along the length of the rod. Maintain an even tension from the ends to the base area.

7. Secure the rod by fastening the ends together. Continue to work around the head.

8. Move to the panel encircling the crest of the head, and continue the same technique—but add yet another larger rod size into the mix. It alternates with the larger of the two rods from your second panel.

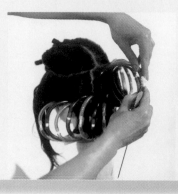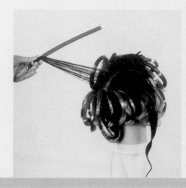

9. Within this panel, work toward the opposite side, using the direction opposite to the previous panel. Secure the ends and spiral toward the base using even tension. Note the angle for spiraling the hair.

10. Fasten the rod and work around toward the opposite side.

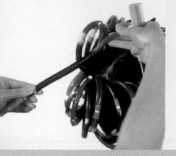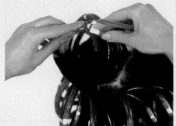

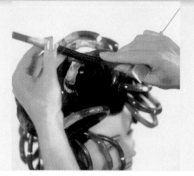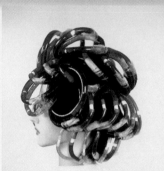

11. In the very top area of the head, begin spiraling lengths from the crown area forward. Note the angle of the rod: again, this ensures smooth tension on the hair.

12. Another look at the finished set shows the progression of rod sizes in an alternating pattern from the nape area to the top of the head. The rod directions are also alternated from one panel to the next. These techniques create a natural texture that mixes textural movement and direction.

Success is an inside job.

Ralph M. Ford

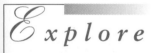
*E*xplore

Apply this technique to different lengths, colors, and cuts for almost endless possibilities.

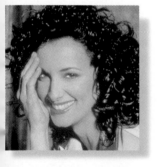

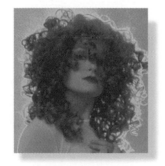

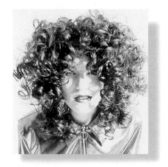

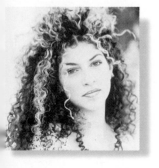

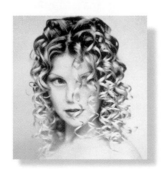

> **The opposite of talking isn't listening. The opposite of talking is waiting.**
>
> *Fran Lebowitz*

The key to successful communication is knowing what to say, knowing how and when to say it, and—just as important—knowing when to say nothing and listen.

Listen with your whole self. Don't just sit quietly and wait for the other person to be done talking so that you can take your turn. Don't "fake attention" by nodding your head and making eye contact, while mentally you're planning what you'll do over the weekend. If there's a pause in the conversation, ask leading, open-ended questions to help the speaker continue to tell you more about herself.

As you ask your correct questions in the correct way, be careful to listen actively to both the content of the client's answers and the hidden messages she's sending through the feeling part of her communication. Pay close attention to her voice, body language, hand movements, and other clues to help you understand what motivates her and how you can help this person achieve the image he or she wants. Don't make the mistake of paying attention only to the blanks you're filling out in the client questionnaire. As you ask each question, and as the client answers, look at her, and restate her answer to make sure you understand. This restatement is so important that we'll return to it very soon!

During the consultation, use style selectors, magazines, and anything else that is available to help clients communicate their thoughts and desires. They probably don't talk your technical language, so avoid "tech talk." Be careful not to interrupt. Don't assume you know what the client is going to say; don't finish her sentences for her; and watch for clues that she's uncomfortable. As an example, although alpha hydroxy acids (AHA) have been used for some time now, some clients will hear the word acid and get worried. If you see a frown, or a flicker of concern, be sure you explain to her satisfaction. Your response might be, "I don't know if you're familiar with alpha hydroxy acid. It's an ingredient that is extracted from various fruits and helps remove dead skin cells, tighten pores, and smooth away wrinkles."

twist spiral

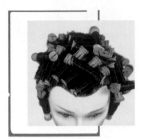

*O*n longer lengths of hair, you can spiral or roll with conventional wave tools—but you can't use conventional techniques because you would run out of rod space as you spiraled. Following, you'll see two techniques for using traditional rods to add texture to extra long lengths of hair.

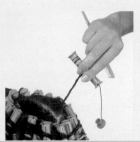
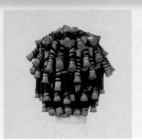

1. Twist each section before you spiral it.

2. As you spiral, twist the rod to add tension, if needed. Your instructor can show you the proper amount of tension. Excessive tension is not required or desirable. The amount of tension will relate to the hair type, the desired result, and the waving system selected.

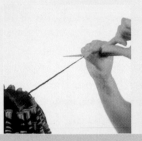
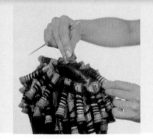

3. Subsection, twist, and spiral the hair according to the directional flow you desire. Fasten at the bottom of the rod.

4. This technique gives more expansion and volume to the hair than the conventional spiraling technique—and on extra long hair, it's a technique that will allow the rod to accommodate the length.

Practice is the best of all instructors.

Publilius Syrus

*If you do little jobs
well, the big ones
tend to take care of
themselves.*

Dale Carnegie

ℛecord keeping is often the least-favorite task of the creative individual—but if you spend time learning about clients and you don't write down what you learned, you're going to have to do it all over again the next time. Worse yet, there may not be a next time, because you missed something important and you made a very big mistake with a client. Recording client responses during the consultation is the only way to ensure that you make the right decisions.

The client card is also important to other salon employees who are providing different services to the same client. For example, the facialist or esthetician may need to know about reactions a client has to certain products—the client may have told you about these or you may have discovered certain product sensitivities in the course of your service. By the same token, the facialist may discover something about the client's skin that will help you make the right product selections for your hair care services. If you don't tell each other immediately, these vital facts can slip your mind, and then good customer service slips away.

Write down what you learn, and reread your client information cards, files, or computer printouts every time you see a client. Always keep your records up to date, and write them so that others can read and understand them.

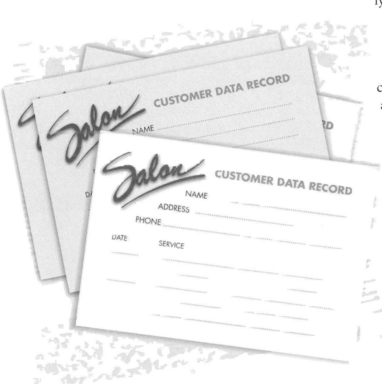

piggyback/double stack

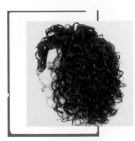

*T*his is a quick way to set long internal lengths for waving. You'll stack rods on top of each other, positioning two rods along each strand of hair.

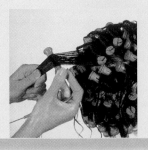 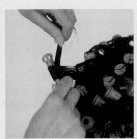

1. The perimeter of this hair has been set with a conventional spiral technique. In the interior, part out base sections that reflect the width and diameter of the rod you're using. Place the rod at mid-strand.

2. Revolve the hair ends around the rod toward one side.

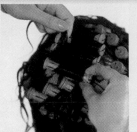 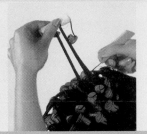

3. Now begin to roll toward the base area, letting the loose ends follow as you roll.

4. Place double end papers on the ends, and position a rod to roll from the ends toward the base area. This rod will rest on top of the rods at the base area. Use the tail end of your comb to secure the base-area rods and adjust tension before you roll.

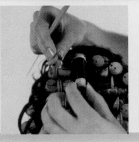 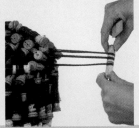

5. Roll the rod to rest upon the rods at the base area. Maintain it straight out from the base area as rolling.

6. It is possible to join and roll three end strands together, depending on the length of the rod you're using and the area you're working on.

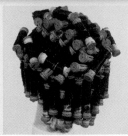 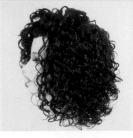

7. The perimeter here was conventionally spiraled while the interior was double stacked. This technique is quite adaptable to changing diameters between the base and the end rods.

8. Use the twisted spiral and double stack rolling techniques to create voluminous texture designs on long lengths of hair.

tool insertion method

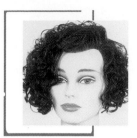

*T*he texture created to complement this haircut is unique and very natural in appearance, yet another way to not only add texture to longer hair, but to mix the texture up as well. Active movement around the exterior of the shape progresses to an interesting mix of textures throughout the interior. This allows for the style to be expanded a great deal around the weight area, while the surface has a soft, languid wave texture.

1., 2. Here's the finished set in different views. Note the placement and size of the rods—from the smaller rods bricklayed through the nape area, to the mid-size rods set vertically backward through the central area encircling the head, and to the double rods throughout the interior area. Also, note the parting pattern.

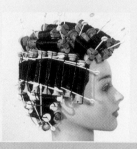
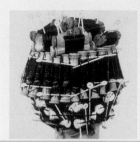

3. Begin by sectioning out the different areas for varying techniques. Section out the interior by parting out from the recession area on one side—around through the center crown area—and curving back around to the recession area on the other side. To section out the panel that encircles the head through the sides and back, use the length of your rod.

4. Begin at the front by taking a vertical part. Hold lengths straight up from the base, to create a halfoff-base rod position. Roll the hair from ends to base.

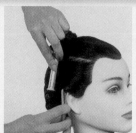
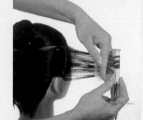

5. Fasten the rod. Direct all rods backward off the face on each side.

6. Continue to hold the hair straight out from each base for rolling to a half off-base position.

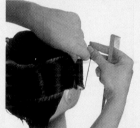
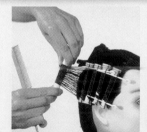

7. Place picks under the bands as you go, to alleviate band pressure on the hair. Or you may prefer to insert picks after the section or set is complete.

8. Continue to work toward the center back area. Note the clean vertical partings, and the use of a consistent rolling angle out from the base area.

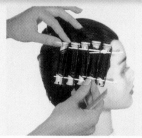
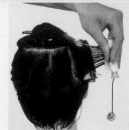

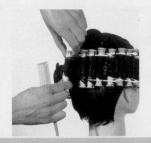
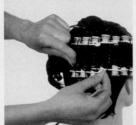

9. Roll smoothly and evenly from the ends to the base.

10. When you've completed the entire side to the center back, insert picks to secure.

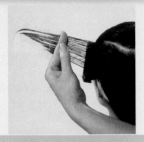
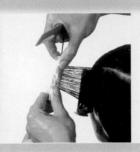

11. Begin the other side. Roll the hair; at that point where shorter lengths protrude from the original two end papers, one option is to place a new single end paper, with its end positioned along the top edge of the rod.

12. Continue to roll. The new end paper will engage the shorter lengths of hair. This is called a cushion wrap technique, used where lengths are strongly angled or contrasting in length. Continue to roll vertically toward the center back to complete this section.

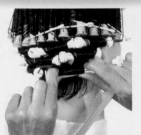
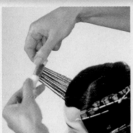

13. Set the nape area using a bricklay technique. The smaller rods here provide extra support through this graduated area of the cut.

14. Now set the interior area using the double rod insertion technique. Part out along the natural side parting. Part the first bases on an angle off the side parting; this is on the lighter side of the part. Measure the base to the size of the larger of the two rods that you'll roll along the strand. Roll the ends of the hair on the smaller of the rods, up to the point at which you'd like to switch the texture to a larger wave pattern.

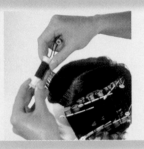
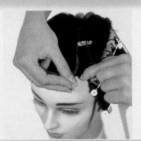

15. Insert a second rod underneath the first, partially rolled rod. Note how the bands are held out of the way with one hand. They will be fastened when rolled to the base area. Roll the two rods together to the base area.

16. Fasten the bands across the top of the rods.

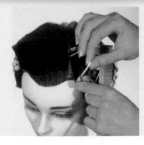
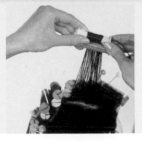

17. Insert two picks between these bands on each side, to support the rods and keep them aligned. Continue this same rolling technique throughout the interior. Section base areas out on an angle behind these first rods as you work back toward the crown.

18. When you finish working along the lighter side of the part, move to the other side. Part out at the angle opposite the one you used on the lighter side of the part. Use the double rod insertion method with the different size rods.

19. Here is a view of the same rods after they've been rolled to the base area. Note the angle of the base parting, and the rod positioning. Fasten along the tops of the rods and insert picks to secure.

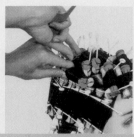
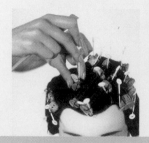

20. Complete rolling the interior area. Adapt base sections and rod lengths as needed to fit within the area.

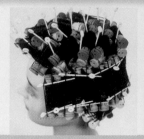
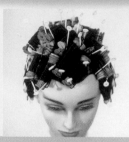

21. Here's the completed interior. You can see double rod insertion method and directional rolling throughout.

22. The progression of rod sizes and techniques from the perimeter toward the interior of the head will create a flow in the finished style.

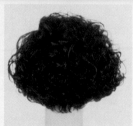

23. The better you understand the several techniques used in this wave set, the more you'll be able to adapt them to the various needs your clients will have. The finished texture embellishes the cut with movement, with volume, and with dimension that accentuate the shape of the cut's blunt and graduated areas.

Analyzing
the Condition of the
Hair

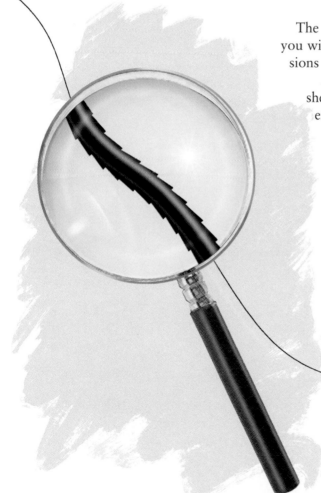

*A*s you gain experience and develop confidence, you will be able to recognize through observation and touch the following characteristics of each client's hair:

Porosity

Elasticity

Texture

Length

Shape

Density

Color treated

Previously textured

The more you work with clients, the more quickly you will recognize clues that will help you make decisions about products and services.

As you ask questions for the client record card, she may reveal other information that will help explain some of what you observe. For example, if a client says, "I take thyroid medication," or "I work in a place where many of my coworkers smoke," this information could help explain why her scalp or skin is dry, or her hair seems brittle. In turn, through your questions and explanations, you will help her understand how things in her environment and the things she puts into her body affect her hair, skin, and nails; and why, in turn, this will affect the recommendations you will make for products and services.

The hair and skin can tell you much about a client. Learn to read them well. And always explain to your client what you see and why you think certain products and services are necessary. She will appreciate your expertise. The willingness to share knowledge to help others is the mark of a true professional.

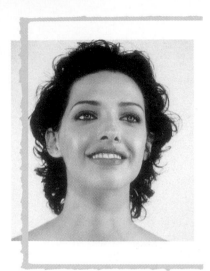

Curvature Set

Overview

This is a new, improved approach to block wrapping. The panels used throughout the head have a directional emphasis to them—they contour to the curve of the head. This curvature panel setting creates a seamless flow of texture throughout the lengths to complement the heavily layered cut. The flow of hair is very natural as well as extremely manageable for the client.

Connect

Block Setting versus Curvature Panel Setting

The examples here should make clear the differences between block and curvature panel setting. Essentially, the curvature panel setting takes into account the desired style lines—and how the client will wear her hair—making styling very easy for her. Yet the style has built-in versatility given the flow of one panel into the next, particularly through the interior. In addition, the area framing the face is set within a curvature motion. Contrast this to block setting, in which lines are rigidly set in a downward direction throughout the exterior of the set.

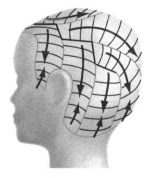

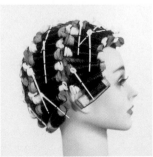

Connecting Panels

The movement created throughout the interior allows for the hair to blend beautifully from the front forehead area to the back.

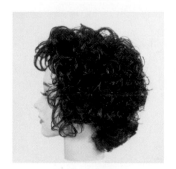

Volume Versus Indentation Rolling Method

In the volume rolling method, you lift hair from the base area up and out to roll the hair. The result, depending on the base control you use, will be varying amounts of lift and volume coming out from the scalp area. In the indentation method, however, you keep the hair at the base area flat as you roll the rod upward to rest on the base area. The indentation technique is generally used around the perimeter hairline area to create a very natural-looking result.

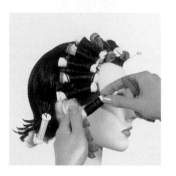

Focus

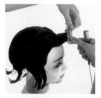

Positioning/Presectioning of Panels—Prepare for the set by using rods of the desired size and length to presection the panels throughout the head. As you become more proficient at this setting pattern, you will be able to begin setting right away.

Curvature Movement at Front Hairline—In this design, panels curve around the front hairline off a side part. Set rods in a gently curved movement to frame the face.

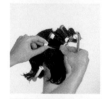

Alternation of Rod Sizes—Alternate two different mid-sized rods throughout this set to create greater visual interest in the resulting texture. Set the perimeter hairline with the larger of the two, for consistency in this area.

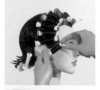

Volume/Indentation Method—Use volume rolling throughout the entire set, except for the perimeter hairline area—which you'll set with the indentation technique.

Base Control—Use the on-base rod position throughout the interior, and the halfoff-base position throughout the remainder of the set—until you reach the perimeter area, where you'll use the indentation method.

Apply

Curvature Set

After your consultation, drape the client, shampoo, and cut the hair according to the directions for the Heavy Layers cut.

1. The finished curvature panel set. incorporates a directional backward movement off the face within panels that curve around the head. Rod sizes alternate within the panels. Roll the rods for volume until you reach the perimeter of each panel, where you use an indentation application to create a more closely contoured effect.

2. Panels flow one into the next throughout the central region of the head, from front hairline to nape.

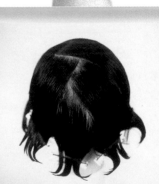

3. Begin by sectioning out the curvature panels throughout the entire head. Comb the hair in the direction that the hair will move, then section out individual panels to match the length of the rod you'll use. Begin this procedure at the front hairline area off of the side part area.

4. Alternate from side to side as you section out the panels. Here is the finished sectioning pattern from the back.

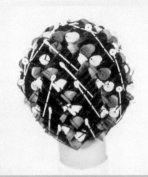

5. Presectioning of the curvature panels you'll use to roll this texture set will allow you to set neatly and in clear directions—it'll give you a road map or blueprint, if you will.

6. Begin the curvature setting at the front hairline area, next to the side parting. Part out a one-diameter base size and roll the rod to the on-base position.

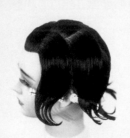
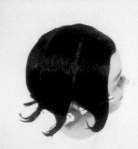
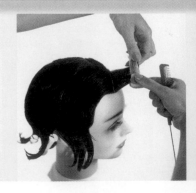

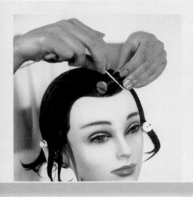
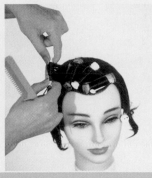

7. Stabilize your rods as needed while you roll.

8. As you work through the panel, continue parting base sections that are expanded around the outside area of the panel—the area farthest away from the face. The base areas should remain one diameter around the front hairline area. When you reach the crest area working over the curve of the head, distribute the hair straight out from the base area to position the rod half off-base.

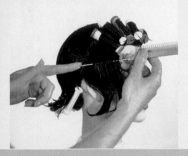
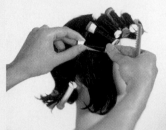

9. Note how the base is being parted out of the panel so as not to disturb the surrounding hair. Lift it out and around in a curve.

10. Alternate rod diameters as you work toward the perimeter.

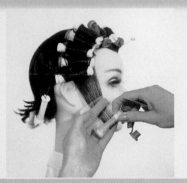
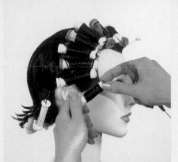

11. When you reach the last rod to be rolled, comb the hair flat at the base and position the rod in preparation for rolling up and away.

12. Roll the rod up and toward the base while keeping the base area flat. In this set, use the larger diameter rod to roll perimeter lengths in the indentation technique. This will maintain closely contoured movement within this area.

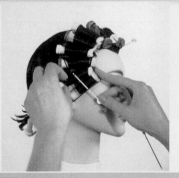
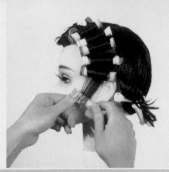

13. Because of the flat base you get with an upward-rolled rod, insert the pick in an upward direction.

14. Move to the other side of the head and set the panel around the hairline on the lighter side of the part, using the same technique.

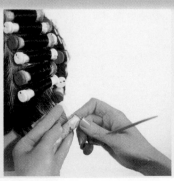
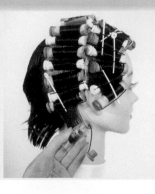

15. Move to the panel behind and next to the first one you set. Roll rods with an on-base rod control throughout the top area of the head; change to a half off-base control toward the exterior, until the perimeter area. Set the last two rods in each panel in the indentation technique to accentuate the effect.

16. Add a pick after rolling because the upward directed rod requires support..

17. Return to the panel on the opposite side of the head and roll for volume using the same technique alternating rod sizes within the panel. Here's the back of the head with two panels left to roll.

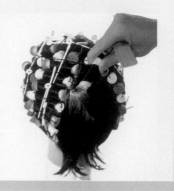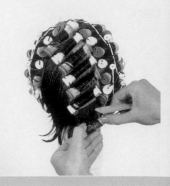

18. Roll all rods for volume in this panel until you reach the perimeter area, where you roll the rods upward.

19. Insert picks to secure the rods and ease any band tension on the hair.

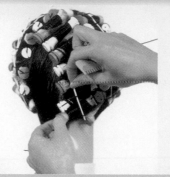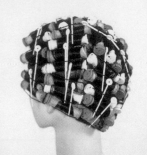

20. Complete the last panel. Note that the directional movement within this panel should remain consistent with the pattern you've already established.The directional movement throughout the back flows around and contours to the perimeter hairline area.

21. Note how all panels fit the curvature of the head, and how the rod alternation is consistent within the panels up to the perimeter rod. The panels all connect and blend into surrounding panels.

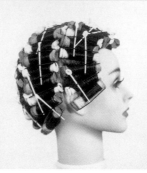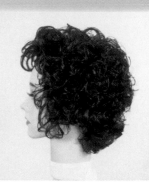

22. Here the finished texture has been diffused dry— this is the most representative finish of the wave set. Note the flicked-out areas around the perimeter, which combine and harmonize with the mix of voluminous texture throughout the interior of the style.

Reflect

Explore

Apply this technique to different lengths, colors, and cuts for almost endless possibilities.

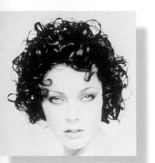

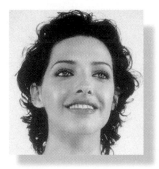

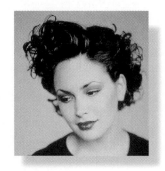

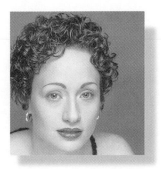

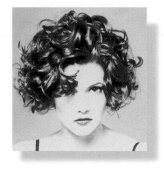

partial curvature set

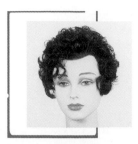

*T*his texture expression provides the client with the versatility to achieve extra volume and softness around the face. Here it has been diffused naturally; it can also easily be molded, for a closer effect. And when the hair is blown dry smoother with a vent or round brush technique, this textural effect can serve as a style support only.

1. This partial curvature set frames the frontal area around the face.
2. Hold the hair straight out from the base area and roll to position the rod half off-base. Continue to part out base sections that curve around toward the face in this panel. The base sizes and shapes should be slightly wider at one side, tapering to smaller at the other. Continue to roll in a curvature movement toward the front hairline, using a single bookend wrap. Roll to the base area to finish this panel and fasten to secure.

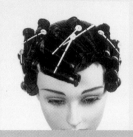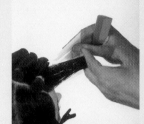

3. Into the side panel, part out a one-diameter base size and begin rolling large-diameter rods. Part out tapered base shapes to curve around within the panel. These will expand at the outside edge of the panel farthest away from the curving area near the front hairline, which uses a one-diameter base size. Roll rods while holding the hair stright out from the base. This will position the rods half off base. Roll the last tool off-base to diminish base volume.
4. Complete the other side with the same technique.

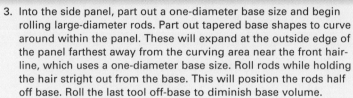
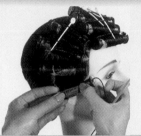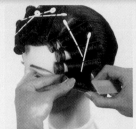

5. When you've completed the partial curvature set, insert picks to secure the rods and ease band tension on the hair. Place protective conditioning cream around the outer perimeter of the set area. Place ample cotton around the perimeter of the set area as well. Replace this cotton as needed after saturating with solution and rinsing.
6. The finished style has been dried with a diffusion technique. The results are very natural, enhancing the cut shape. Given the softness of the texture created, it blends with the surrounding unwaved hair quite smoothly.

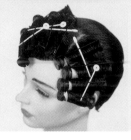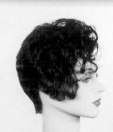

Client
Orientation

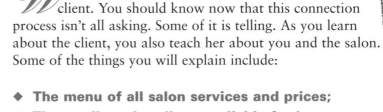

*Act as if what you do
makes a difference. It
does.*

William James

We've talked before about connecting with a new client. You should know now that this connection process isn't all asking. Some of it is telling. As you learn about the client, you also teach her about you and the salon. Some of the things you will explain include:

- ◆ **The menu of all salon services and prices;**
- ◆ **The retail product lines available for home care of hair;**
- ◆ **Salon hours; days that you are off; who else can service her if you are not there;**
- ◆ **Salon marketing programs (frequent client programs);**
- ◆ **Referral rewards and incentives; and**
- ◆ **Salon staff positions and "specialized" departments for color, skin care, and so on.**

Some salons create a "Salon Orientation" script to help stylists remember what important things to tell clients about how the salon operates and the services and benefits it offers for clients.

The keys to making this part of the consultation interesting for the client are to keep it brief but informative; show enthusiasm when speaking about the salon's offerings; and give the client a salon brochure, service menu, and retail product pamphlet, if these are available, to keep and refer to.

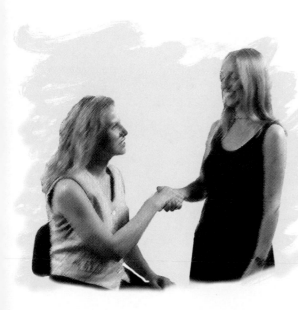

Another time you "orient" the client to the salon is when you are escorting her through it. Explain as you pass each area what takes place there and what services each employee performs: "This is Trish. She's our certified massage therapist. This is the private room where Trish gives half-hour and one-hour massages. Notice that the light is low. She always plays soothing music and uses aromatherapy scents to help her clients relax and get the most from the massage experience."

You are familiar with your surroundings. The client is not. Never assume that she understands. Always explain. If she is shy or embarrassed about asking, you will have denied the client an opportunity to experience a new service, and at the same time denied yourself the income from additional service and product sales.

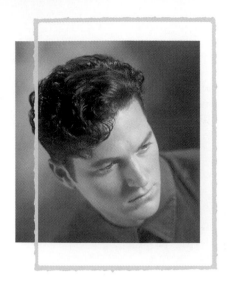

"V" Formation

Overview

In this design, an interesting technique creates an alternating wave movement throughout the side areas. It moves the hair back and off the face-as well as creating a very desirable volume through the interior that flows up and in toward the center.

What's unique about this set is the way tools are set in a V-formation. It creates a manageable movement and volume in this area—one that's particularly effective on shorter lengths of hair. You'll use the V-formation setting on the side areas to effect an alternating wave pattern, which will flow into the freeform curl through the back area. There, you'll use a bricklay setting pattern.

Connect

V-Formation Setting

The V-formation pattern is very similar to a herringbone pattern. And what's a herringbone? It's a pattern made of slanting parallel lines in rows. Adjacent rows form a V or inverted V and end up resembling the ribs of a herring's spine. This pattern is often used in textile weaves, embroidery, and masonry. When it comes to hair design, you can roll your V-formation tools all in the same direction—creating a voluminous style that covers a large area and blends beautifully. Or you can reverse the direction of your tools from row to row, which creates the alternating wave effect. The V-formation will be one of your most commonly used techniques for creating a very natural alternating wave pattern. This formation is what allows textured hair to flow and blend effortlessly. It's an alternative wave pattern that the block method through the top would provide.

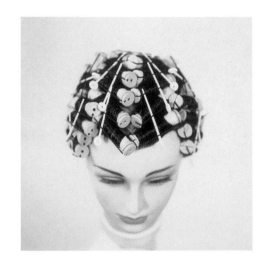

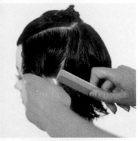

Sectioning—Here's the sectioning pattern you'll use: Part off a wide rectangle through the top of the head, from the front forehead area to the crown. Subdivide this down the center vertically for setting. Divide the sides from the crown to behind the ear on each side. The back will be bricklayed.

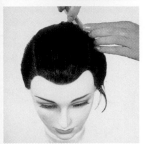

V-Formation Setting through the Top—The subdivided top area is set with diagonally positioned rods. These rods should meet each other in the center top to form a V that goes back and in.

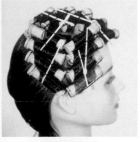

V-Formation Setting through the Sides—Create alternating directional movement through the side panels by using diagonal base and rod positioning to form a V.

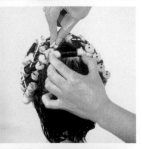

Beginning the Bricklay—Begin the bricklay setting in the crown area with the triangular section left over from setting the top rectangle area.

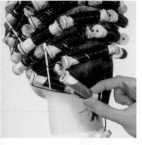

Volume/Indentation—Use the volume technique throughout the entire set—except for the hairline area in the nape, where you'll use the indentation technique.

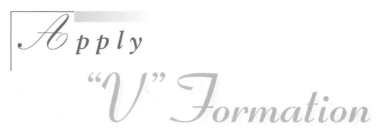

Apply "V" Formation

After your consultation, drape the client, shampoo, and cut the hair according to the directions for the Full Layers cut.

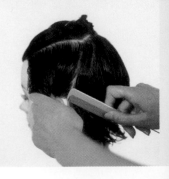

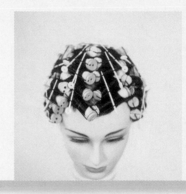

1., 2. In the finished wave set, rods are positioned through the top area in a V-formation to move the hair up and away from the front hairline. On the sides, set panels with rods positioned along opposite diagonal sections.

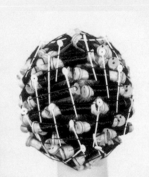

3. Begin by sectioning out the interior area from the sides and back. Use shorter rods positioned in a V at the front hairline to determine how wide to section off the top.

4. Section from the front hairline area back to the crown area.

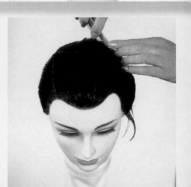

5. At the crown area, section across the center of the crown horizontally, to complete the top section.

6. Section out each side by extending the parting through the crown down to behind the ear.

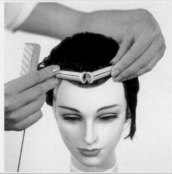

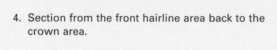

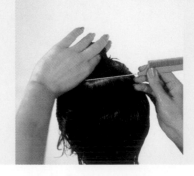

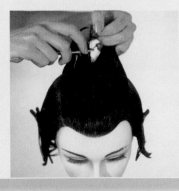

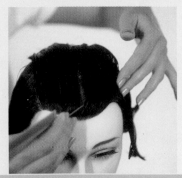

7. To begin setting, divide the top area vertically down the center.

8. Part out a one-diameter base size of the rod you're using (in this case, a mid-sized rod).

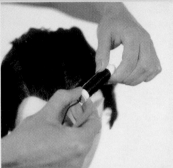

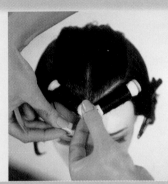

9. Roll this hair to position it on-base. This requires distributing the hair at 45 degrees (.785 rad) above the center of the base area.

10. Roll the first rod at the hairline in the other panel. Note the V-pattern developing. This will be the procedure you'll use to set rods throughout the top area-alternating back and forth between the panels as you set toward the crown area.

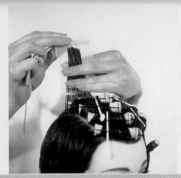

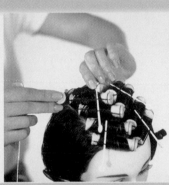

11. Continue back toward the crown area, rolling the rods within the V-formation.

12. Note the pattern developing—a herringbone pattern.

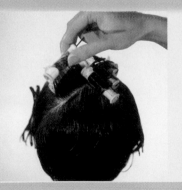

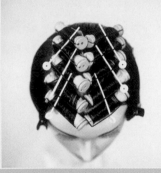

13. This is the last rod you'll roll within this area. You'll roll the small triangular area backward when you set the bricklay technique through the back.

14. The completed top area. Adapt rod sizes and lengths as needed to accommodate your client's head size and shape.

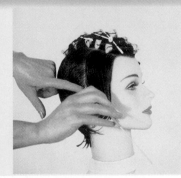

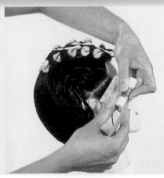

15. At the sides, divide the area in half.

16. Set the direction up and back in the panel closest to the front hairline. Comb this hair upward. Part the first base area out along a diagonal, as shown. Roll the rod to position it on base; you'll roll all rods to position along diagonal bases through this panel.

17. Continue to part out diagonal base areas and roll rods upward.

18. In the panel directly behind the first one, roll rods downward along diagonal partings opposite those you used in the first panel at the sides. It is this change in your direction of rolling along opposing diagonal partings that will create the alternating wave patterns at the side.

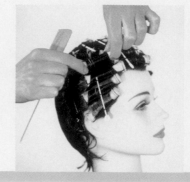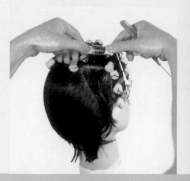

19. Continue to roll the rods diagonally through the panel to above the ear.

20. The completed side. You can see the two panels rolled in alternating directions. Complete the other side using the same technique.

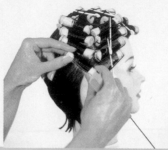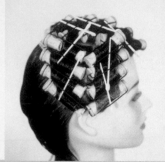

21. At the crown area, roll the first rod to begin the bricklay through the back. This first rod is positioned at the triangular area left over from the top V-formation.

22. Continue to bricklay rods throughout the back, using the volume technique. Adjust rod lengths as needed to accommodate the space.

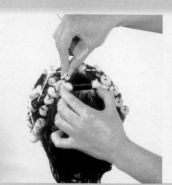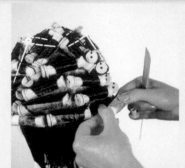

23. When you reach the nape area, roll the rods upward in the indentation technique. Work from the outer hairline area of the nape into the center on both sides.

24. With one side complete, begin to roll the other side into the center area.

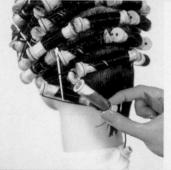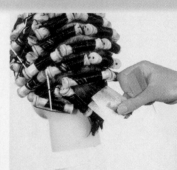

25. Adjust the diagonal parting and base positions, as well as rod lengths to fit within this area.

26. Roll all rods upward at this perimeter hairline area to create a closer contour at the base area, with a flicked-out texture on the ends.

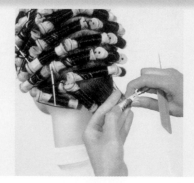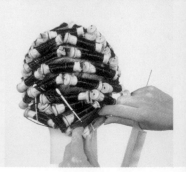

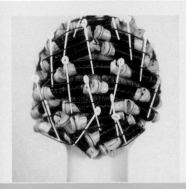

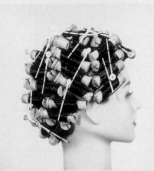

27. The completed bricklay through the back area.

28. From the side view, you can see how the different areas of the set fit together.

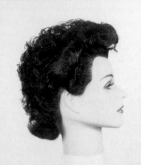

29. The finished dramatic style shows the directional movement, volume, and textural interest created through the setting technique. Here, the hair was styled by applying the appropriate styling product, then combing the hair lengths into the directional movement around the top and side areas while diffusing. The back area was diffused for full expansion and curl movement. You can also make the style and waves more dramatic and exaggerated by molding with gel—or make them soft, freeform, and voluminous with other styling techniques.

Patience, persistence and perspiration make an unbeatable combination for success.

Napoleon Hill

Explore

Apply this technique to different lengths, colors, and cuts for almost endless possibilities.

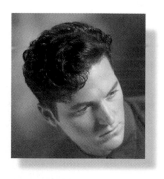

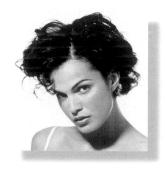

Restate
and
Confirm

Success doesn't come to you...you go to it.

Marva Collins

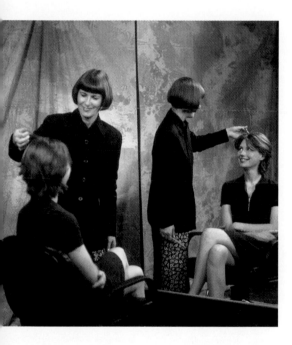

Whether you're in a special consultation room or simply asking the client questions as she sits in your chair, once you have the answers to all the questions you have asked, the next step is to confirm your understanding. Take a minute to review what you wrote about what the client told you and ask more questions if necessary—to clear up any confusion you might have. It's easier to show you than to tell you about this, so let's look in on the end of a stylist/client consultation.

STYLIST: "Brittany, let me just go over this with you to make sure I have everything correct: Your last perm was in March; you have never colored your hair, but you're interested in some highlights in your natural color. You'd like a shorter style, but not a whole lot shorter than the way you're wearing it now. Is that right?"

CLIENT: "That's right. I want something that's easy to care for, but I still like having hair around my face. I don't want a really short cut."

STYLIST: "And do you prefer it curly?"

CLIENT: "More like wavy."

STYLIST: "And you said that you feel comfortable with styling tools such as a blow-dryer, round brush, and curling iron . . . is that correct?"

CLIENT: "Yes, but I've never gotten the hang of styling gels and mousse and that sort of thing. I could use better hold, but I've never learned what to use and how much. I just don't seem to get it right."

STYLIST: "Don't worry, I'll work with you on that. Let me make a note of that so I can take a few extra minutes while I'm finishing your design today to let you practice some simple techniques. Okay, that's about it—now we're ready for the next step. Let's decide together how you want to look when you leave here today!"

CLIENT: "Okay, well, I was looking at this book that I found in the waiting room and..."

directional wave set I

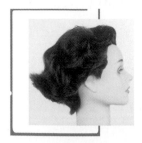

*T*his texture set gives clients a range of styling options and great versatility.

1., 2. In the finished wave set, hair is set back off the face around the front hairline, while lengths through the top and back move in alternating directions toward the nape. Do not set rollers in the nape area, where lengths are short. The texture from the rollers you set through the lower back will blend into the nape area effortlessly.

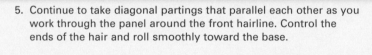

3. Section out a panel around the front hairline off a side parting. Part out a base area using a diagonal part. Take all base sections around the front hairline on a diagonal, to direct hair back off the face. Roll the hair to position on-base, maximizing base lift.

4. The on-base roller position will allow the self-gripping roller to engage the hair at the base and stay in position. If needed, you can insert a clip or pick. Section out base lengths that will enable the roller to sit within its base area and not engage surrounding hair.

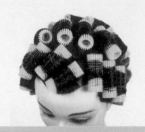
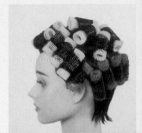
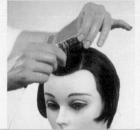
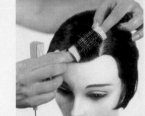

5. Continue to take diagonal partings that parallel each other as you work through the panel around the front hairline. Control the ends of the hair and roll smoothly toward the base.

6. At the area above the ear, change to the next smaller-diameter roller to accommodate the lengths.

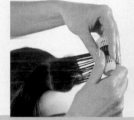
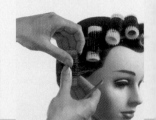

7. Here is the completed side off the side part. You can see that all rollers have been rolled back off the face.

8. Set the other side using the same technique. Take diagonal partings and roll the hair back away from the face.

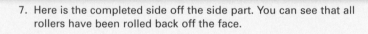
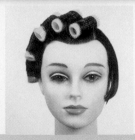
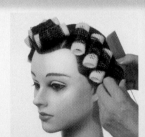

9. At the top area of the head, section out a panel in which you'll roll the self-gripping rollers along diagonal partings. The movement from the panel at the front hairline will turn and blend into this top panel.

10. Section out the next panel across the crown area. Reverse the direction from the previous panel. Part out diagonally across the panel and roll the roller parallel to the base area.

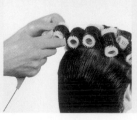
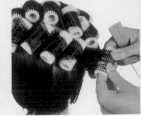

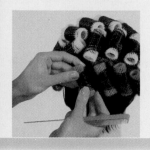
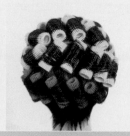

11. Section out the next panel to travel across the occipital area. Set the rollers in the direction opposite the previous panel. Note that the diameter size is smaller through this panel to accommodate the shorter lengths.

12. The completed back area. Three panels move in alternating directions from the top of the head to the nape area.

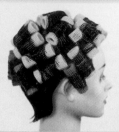
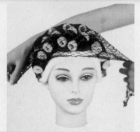

13. This profile view of the wave set shows how the directional movement around the front hairline will flow into the panels throughout the back area of the head.

14. After saturating the rollers with wave solution, apply a durable netting around the wave set to secure the tools in position before rinsing.

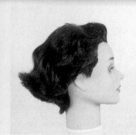

15. The finished style accentuates the cut shape with soft wave movement, and the texture provides the client with tremendous versatility in her styling options.

directional wave set II

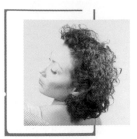

*T*his texture service will result in soft lift and body for the client. It will also provide width and volume around the sides.

1. The hair designer determines that a mid-length graduated cut coupled with a directional wave will create the client's desired result.

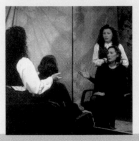 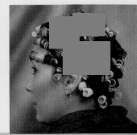

2. Begin the wave set at the fringe. Mold a C-shape, then section out a panel that's the depth of the rod. Part out the base areas by parting through the panel along a diagonal line. Roll and place rods diagonally.

3. Continue to part out diagonally through this panel, working toward the other side. Roll all rods to position half off-base-parallel to the base parting.

4. Mold a C-shape all the way around the head and section out this panel, using a rod placed at an angle to measure depth. Begin setting at the temple area by parting through the panel diagonally for a one-diameter base size. Roll the rod and pick to secure. Continue throughout this panel. Switch to the opposite direction in the next panel. Change to rods one size smaller than in the previous panel.

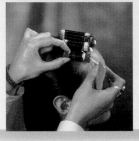 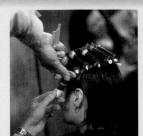

5. Begin the bricklay pattern at the occipital area. Again, change to a smaller rod to complete the progression within the overall set.

6. Complete the nape area with the bricklay pattern. Adjust rod lengths as required to fit within the space.

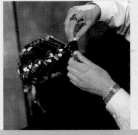 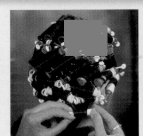

7. Position a towel around the neck, with the cape over it; place another towel over the top of the cape, and clip it to secure at the neck area. Apply protective cream to the skin around the perimeter hairline area. Apply a strip of cotton around the edge of the set. Apply solution along the top and underneath areas of each rod to thoroughly saturate all hair. Replace the cotton strip around the perimeter area.

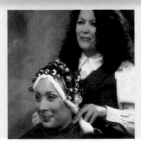

Consultation
Step 2:
Direction

If you develop the habits of success, you will make success a habit.

Michael Angier

In step 2, the consultation shifts from gathering information about the client to using that information to help her make decisions about the hair and skin care services she will receive that day, and in the future.

Use the tools at your disposal to assist you in this phase. Most salons have style selector books, hair design magazines, and even videos that clients can look at to get ideas. Familiarize yourself with what these contain, and help clients use them to make choices that are good for them.

Some salons even have computer systems that use a photograph of the client's face, matching it with different hairstyles and colors to show the client what she would look like with that choice. Typically, there is a separate charge for this service.

As you grow in your job, continue to learn and gather information to help each client find the best look. It doesn't have to be today's style. It just has to be her style.

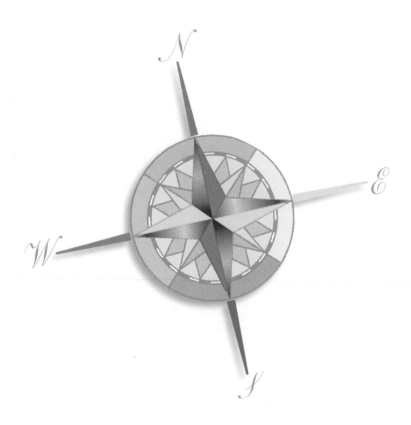

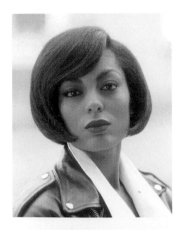

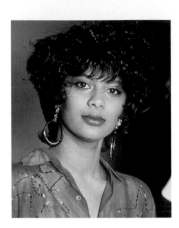

Chemistry of Hair Relaxers

Today's world is a beautiful mosaic of different ethnic groups— and chances are, that a cultural mix of women and men will be among your clients, looking for expert care of their textured hair. Here, you will find out how to focus on ethnic hair according to its specific type. Hair is either extremely curly (kinky), curly, wavy, or straight. And when you look at it in those terms, you will make the best decision in order to achieve the best texture results, whether adding or removing texture. You've already learned about many multicultural hair procedures—cutting hair dry, the press and curl, and the wrapping procedure among them. In this next section, you'll gain insight into modern methods of straightening hair and of treating textured hair in its virgin state.

The relaxer of old was looked upon strictly as a straightener. The modern approach to relaxers is to look at this service, not only as a straightener, but also as a retexturizer and a conditioner. A retexturizer means that you may want to smooth the texture to a certain degree but not fully straighten it. A conditioner means that a relaxer service can make the hair softer and more manageable. This depends on the initial condition or state of the hair. Uncontrollable, frizzy, and/or coarse hair types would greatly benefit by a relaxer as retexturizer/conditioner. Relaxers may even be used on straight hair as a bodifying treatment. Open your mind to the many possibilities that the relaxer service may fulfill. Ultimately it is the artist's technique that determines the result.

This service category is incredibly lucrative in the salon and growing tremendously. Communication and focus are integral to success. You're not just here to do hair. This is a business. To earn the amount of money you desire you must provide the best and most professional service possible to all of your clients.

Types of Relaxers

The relaxer market today features hundreds of products in varying strengths, and in a varience in ingredients. The following is a list of some of the primary ingredients used in permanent hair relaxers.

▶ **Sodium Hydroxide**

▶ **Ammonium Thioglycolate**

▶ **Ammonium Bisulfite or Ammonium Sulfate**

▶ **Calcium Hydroxide (no lye)**

▶ **Potassium Hydroxide**

Each of the above chemicals works on the cystine disulfide bonds. The disulfide bond is formed with a strong attraction between two sulfur atoms in the amino acid cystine (the primary sulfur-containing amino acid in hair). These bonds are responsible for approximately one–third of the hair's structural strength and can be broken only by the action of the reducing agent. The reducing agent will soften and swell the hair fiber, which in turn causes the cystine disulfide bond between the first sulfur atom and the carbon atom to break.

The most widely used chemical hair relaxer in the salon has traditionally been a sodium hydroxide base. Sodium hydroxide is an alkaline product which may range from a pH of 10 to 14; generally the pH is in the range of 12. The advantages of sodium hydroxide relaxers are:

▶ **fast processing time**

▶ **good straightening**

▶ **more permanent straightness with less likeliness of reversion**

(Note: It is important to remember that the chemical action of sodium hydroxide is irreversible and cystine bonds cannot be reformed.)

Extreme care must be used if the chemical relaxing process is to be successful, without causing hair damage, skin or scalp burns. The action of smoothing is of the utmost importance, along with the creme relaxer to achieve a successful chemical relaxer or retexturizing service. Insufficient realingment of the cystine bonds will occur if the hair is underprocessed, causing the hair to revert to its naturally curly configuration. If the chemical is left on the hair longer than recommended, it could become overprocessed causing brittleness, breakage or even dissolving the hair completely.

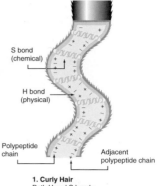

1. Curly Hair
Both H and S bonds holding polypeptide chains in position.

S bond (chemical)

H bond (physical)

Polypeptide chain

Adjacent polypeptide chain

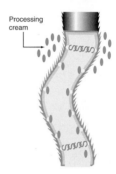

Processing cream

2.Hair Being Processed
All H bonds broken, most S bonds broken. Hand and comb manipulations starting to relax wave. (Polypeptide chains shift)

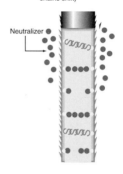

Neutralizer

3.Hair Being Neutralized
The neutralizer fixes polpeptide chains in a straight position after hair has beeen fully relaxed.

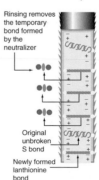

Rinsing removes the temporary bond formed by the neutralizer

Original unbroken S bond

Newly formed lanthionine bond

4.Straightened Hair...
after rinsing and proper drying. Lanthionine cross links now exist between polypeptide chains, keeping the hair in a permanently straight form. Drying reforms the physical bonds.

Sodium Hydroxide Relaxer

Ammonium thioglycolate or "thio" as it is commonly known, has traditionally been used primarily in permanent wave solutions. The pH can range from a level of 7 to 9.5. When used as a relaxer, the "thio" causes the hair shaft to soften and swell. The cystine linkages are broken and the bonds slip past one another to reform the curl configuration into a straight configuration. Through the use of a neutralizer, the bonds are permanently realigned into the new straight position.

The advantages of "Thio" are:

▶ **excellent retexturizer for partial relaxation**

▶ **"Thio" has little, if no tendency to irritate or sensitize the scalp**

When used on hair that is more than moderately curly, continuous combing and stretching is necessary to achieve the desired straight results. Care must also be used in order not to overstretch the hair and to avoid breakage.

Ammonium bisulfide is a slower acting chemical relaxer with a pH in the range of 7--7.5. This type of relaxer requires heat to assit in softening the hair. The advantages of sulfide are:

▶ **effective straightening**

▶ **little hair damage**

Hair straightened with sulfide has a greater tendency to revert to its naturally curly state upon shampooing and wearing than hair straightened with sodium hydroxide. However, a well–formulated bisulfide relaxer can be used frequently on hair without much hair damage.

Strive to learn as much as possible about this lucrative salon service. Manufacturers provide educational material and informative classes to help you expand your knowledge.

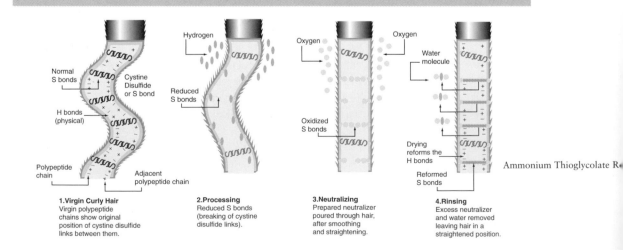

Ammonium Thioglycolate R◀

1. Virgin Curly Hair
Virgin polypeptide chains show original position of cystine disulfide links between them.

2. Processing
Reduced S bonds (breaking of cystine disulfide links).

3. Neutralizing
Prepared neutralizer poured through hair, after smoothing and straightening.

4. Rinsing
Excess neutralizer and water removed leaving hair in a straightened position.

Style
Selection

Well done is better than well said.

Ben Franklin

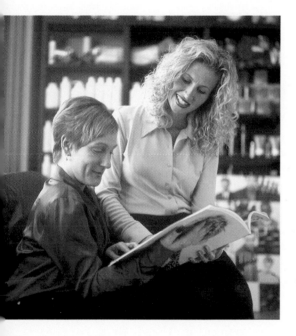

$\mathcal{S}$tyle selection is the core of Consultation Step 2-Direction. During this time the client and stylist review what they've discussed so far and decide on a hairstyle or other service. It's easier to show you than tell you about this:

STYLIST: (looking at photo client has selected in style book): "Yes, Brittany, that is a style that works well with your face shape and your hair's texture. I just want to make sure you realize that the length in back [she lifts client's hair] will need to be cut about four inches to right here [with the fingers of her other hand, the stylist mimics scissors cutting hair, while the client watches in the mirror] to achieve the shape in the back. It will fall to the nape of your neck in the back and just below your ears on the side, but it won't touch your shoulder as it does now when it's styled. Is this okay with you?"

CLIENT: "Yes, I guess so. I know I said I didn't want it cut very much. But I like the way this style looks, and if it takes cutting off four inches, that should be okay. I just wanted to make sure you wouldn't cut it drastically and change my whole look, which is what my last hairstylist did. I had a hard time even making an appointment to get my hair cut again after that experience."

STYLIST: "I completely understand. With this style you have selected, you'll look like you want to, but your hair will be easier to style and it will keep its style better with some of this weight off the bottom. Are we in agreement, then?"

CLIENT: "Okay, I can deal with four inches cut off. Let's do it."

Reread this section carefully and review the way the stylist communicated with the client. She explained, demonstrated, reassured, and confirmed to make sure she understood what the client really wanted.

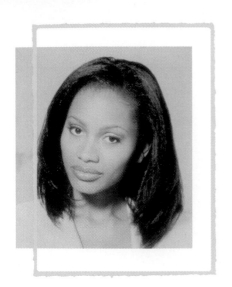

Consultation & Analysis on a Virgin Head for Permanent Relaxer

Overview

During a virgin relaxing service, you straighten hair with a relaxing product and a minimal amount of mechanical action. Remember this important concept. The manipulation is the key to successful relaxation. The processing technique when performed properly will yield superb results. However, when the processing has gone beyond necessity, irritation and over processing will result. Your action should be limited to smoothing hair with the glove-covered fingers, or pressing with the back of your comb. Manufacturers have improved the quality of relaxers so much that you could actually apply product without gloves, but it is not recommended. Always wear gloves to protect your hands, and place a protective cream around your client's entire hairline. Your hands can indeed become sensitized over a period of time to the chemicals, creating vulnerability toward contact dermatitis.

Connect

Virgin Head

Hair that has not undergone any chemical treatment is known as virgin hair.

Permanent Relaxers

These chemicals affect the hair strand by permanently rearranging the basic structure of curly hair into a straight form. Excellent products are available on the market today that come in a variety of strengths, with varying ingredients.

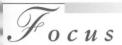

Focus

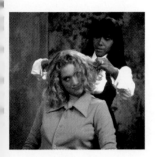

Analyzing the Hair—Remember to analyze the hair and strand test for porosity and elasticity. Test a few strands at the nape of the neck and the top of the head before you perform a relaxing service. Make certain the hair is completely dry.

Also analyze for different textures on the same head. Remember that it is our ethnicity that determines our hair type, textures, pattern, etc. It is your professional expertise in determining these factors plus the condition, porosity and elasticity that determines the relaxer formula, strength and process to be used for a successful result. Remember to analyze the scalp area for any adverse signs.

When you're servicing a Caucasian client who has naturally curly or wavy hair, evaluate her hair visually and by feeling. Also, do an elasticity test. Do not use any products near the scalp until you have gone through the entire head at least once.

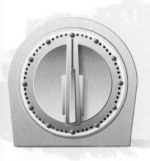

Relaxer Strengths—Most permanent relaxers come in three strengths, mild, regular, and super. Always evaluate the texture as related to kinky, curly, or wavy hair before selecting what strength to use. Keep in mind the manufacturer's recommended time for the product to remain on the head (from application to rinsing). The hair will not fall out if it is left on a few minutes longer! It is important to talk to your client the minute you start applying the relaxer. Do not wait until you are halfway through to ask how she is feeling. Phrase your question to her in "feeling" terms, and let her tell you whether she feels any discomfort, tingling sensations, etc. For relaxer clients, it is recommended that you base the scalp until you become quicker and more proficient in your applications.

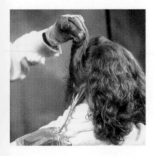

Application Process—Depending on the client's hair type, curl pattern, etc., you may work through initially placing the relaxer 1/2 inch up to 11/2 inches away from the scalp. On the Caucasian client with moderately curly hair that you are about to see in the following procedure, the relaxer was applied 1 to 11/2 inches away from the scalp initially given the base area was not as curly. Your service will begin either at the front or nape areas.

Do not use any products near the scalp until you have gone through the entire head at least once with the smoothing process. This process requires two smoothings before working product toward the scalp.

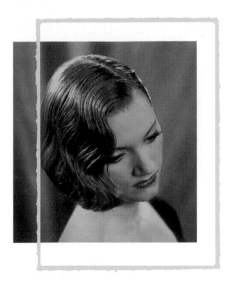

A pply

Consultation & Analysis on a Virgin Head for Permanent Relaxer

After your consultation, drape the client. Your shampoo and cut will occur later in this technical.

1. Consult with your client on the style she wants.

2. Perform a strand test on various areas of the head. Move to the back crest of the head and take one hair strand.

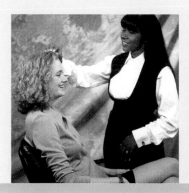
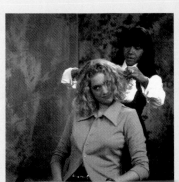

3. Hold the strand of hair firmly at the scalp and wrap it around one of your fingers to gently stretch it. If the hair stretches and does not return to its original form, or worse yet, breaks, this hair has poor elasticity and should not be relaxed at this time. Also, run your fingers down the hair strand to check for porosity.

4. The strand test will tell you what condition the hair is in relative to porosity and elasticity, as well as whether it's weak, strong, dry or oily. It will also help you determine what products to recommend.

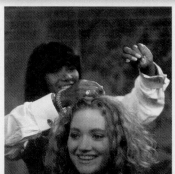

5. Evaluate the strand test. This will be the client's first relaxer, and you use a different technique in applying a new relaxer than in applying a touch-up.

6. Wear gloves when you apply the relaxer, and place a protective cream around the client's entire hairline.

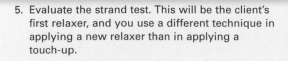
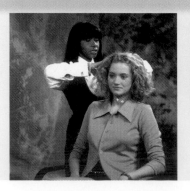
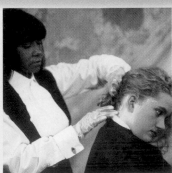

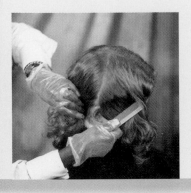
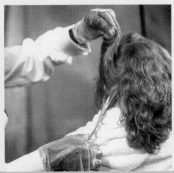

7. Divide the client's hair into four sections, from front forehead to center nape and from ear to ear. Starting in the left back at the nape area, Take 1 1/2" (3.75 cm) horizontal partings.

8. Relaxer is applied with fingers about 1" to 1 1/2" (2.5 to 3.75 cm) away from the scalp, bringing it down the entire hair strand. Work as neatly as possible in the parting, applying, and spreading of the relaxer. Continue this process as working up through this section of hair. Part out, at least a couple of inches away from the scalp to prevent product from getting on the scalp.

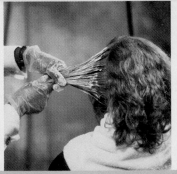
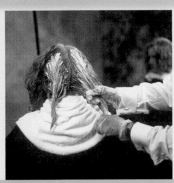

9. After applying relaxer to the first section, take that section and bring it together, smoothing it without allowing the relaxer to touch the scalp. Bring the smoothed hair away from the scalp.

10. In the next section, use the same technique. Applying time and initial smoothing should be done as quickly and efficiently as possible. Whether it's the first, second, or third time working through the complete head section by section, you should apply more relaxer to the area closest to the scalp as needed. Follow the manufacturer's suggested application and processing times.

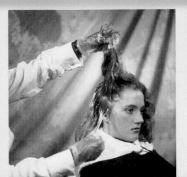
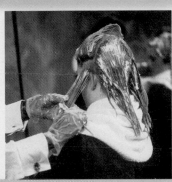

11. Apply the relaxer to the third section of hair.

12. Continue into the fourth section—proceed to part out approximately 1 1/2" (3.75 cm) partings with the fingers. Then apply the relaxer through the lengths.

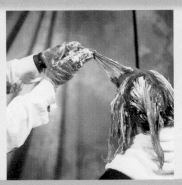
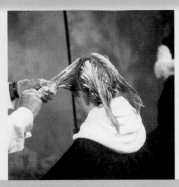

13. Complete the application technique with the relaxer.

14. Squeeze and smooth the fourth section of hair.

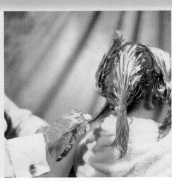
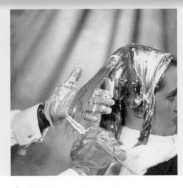

15. Move to the back nape area. With a comb, take a 1 1/2" (3.75 cm) section and comb and smooth through the hair. Be as gentle as possible. Continue combing and smoothing, moving up the entire section of hair. While combing, place any excess relaxer from the comb onto the hair and continue smoothing.

16. Move to the next section using the same technique with your comb.

17. Use a tail comb so that you can part or section the hair with its tail end. After combing it through, there will be excess relaxer; reapply it to the hair.

18. Move onto the third section. Smoothing is very important. Smoothing utilizes the heat from the head, helping to relax the hair.

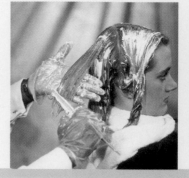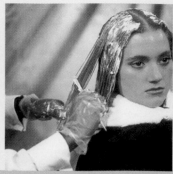

19. Work the relaxer toward the scalp and smooth through all the sections for a third time.

20. Continue smoothing and working through the sections with relaxer.

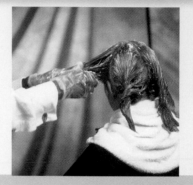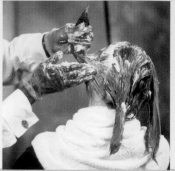

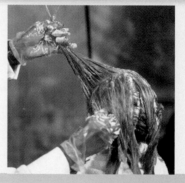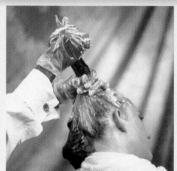

21. The relaxer should cover the entire head as you work through the sections as shown.

22. Squeeze and smooth the sections together. Again, always reapply excess relaxer to the head.

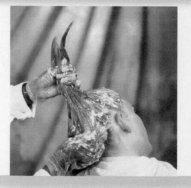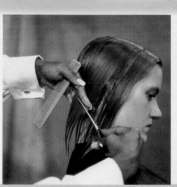

23. Smooth and bring sections together. The relaxer is now ready to rinse out.

24. Cut hair to the desired length and style. In this case, the graduated blunt cut. The hair around the front hairline is then molded into waves.

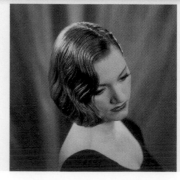

25. The finished style features soft, alternating waves framing the face to harmonize with the smooth, sleek, relaxed hair.

Reflect

Explore

Apply this technique to different lengths, colors, and cuts for almost endless possibilities.

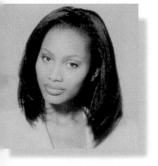

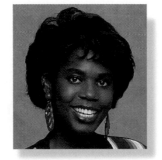

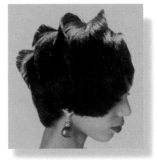

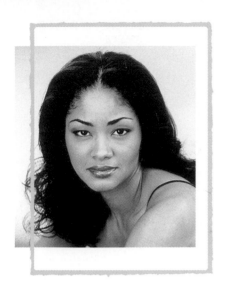

Retouch with a Sodium Hydroxide Relaxer

Overview

Sodium hydroxide relaxers are generally preferred by professional stylists for the ultimate straightening. Any client who wants to reduce kink, curl, or wave is a perfect candidate for this service. Here for illustrative purposes we will demonstrate, on four different parts of the head, four different methods of application. Each, method has its own unique application and processing time; each displays your presentation and technical skills in a different way. Presentation, of course, has a significant impact on your financial earnings!

Connect

Retouch

Six to eight weeks after a client has received a permanent relaxer service, new hair will have grown in, and this new growth will have the same texture characteristics as the hair before straightening. To make this new hair just as straight as the grown-out hair, requires a relaxer. Applying permanent relaxer to the new growth only is called a retouch.

This client's hair was previously relaxed by a different designer which presents many variables from the new service being performed. Therefore, initial application will treat this service as a retouch. However, the relaxer will be brought through the hair towards the end of the processing time to equalize the texture.

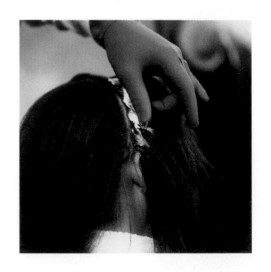

Shampooing the Relaxer Out of the Hair

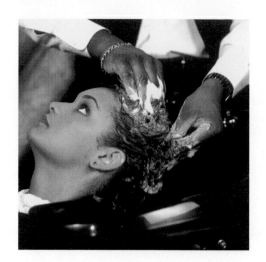

Removal of the relaxer, treatment, shampooing and conditioner take on new twists with today's products. The key is to properly rinse the chemical out of the hair, which also normalizes the hair.

Modern-day salons use back-wash, adjustable shampoo bowls. These put less stress on the client's back, and you can adjust them to maintain her comfort. After you rinse the relaxer out of the hair, try the new deep penetrating treatments, which you apply before you shampoo. Follow the manufacturers recommendations. Treat the hair for moisture and strength right at the shampoo bowl, with a variety of shampoos that can "normalize" and create more luxurious hair. This also gives the salon an opportunity to increase retail sales.

Focus

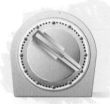

Retouch Timing—Always follow the manufacturer's suggested processing time. In general, though, a retouch requires four to eight ounces (120 to 240 ml) of relaxer, with an application and processing time that varies according to the strength of the product used, the amount of manipulation used, the hair type and condition, and the desired results. Apply as quickly and efficiently as possible.

Hand and Comb Smoothing Techniques—Combing and smoothing the hair with your hands or a comb helps to relax it. You can use a tail comb to section the hair. Essentially, the amount and type of manipulation determines speed and amount of relaxation achieved.

Processing Technique—After you apply the relaxer, use the teeth or back of your tail comb to maintain consistency as you spread it. Then go through the hair a second time with the comb, using your fingers to smooth and work the kink or curl out of the hair by applying light pressure. You can repeat this step a third time throughout the entire head if necessary.

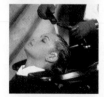

Rinsing—Rinse with warm tepid water and strong water pressure for two to three minutes to remove the relaxer from the hair. This begins your normalizing process. Always give the best conditioning treatment possible after a relaxer service and before drying and styling. Then place your client under a heat cap for approximately 15 minutes.

Shampoos—Three shampoos are recommended after a relaxer service. This ensures that the hair has been thoroughly cleansed of the relaxer base or cream. It also will normalize and return the hair to a normal pH.

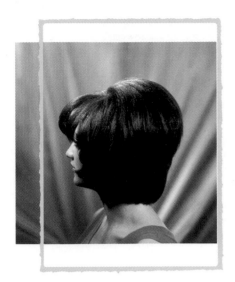

Apply

Retouch with a Sodium Hydroxide Relaxer

After your consultation, drape the client. Your shampoo, and style will occur later in this technical.

1. Prepare your client for the relaxer service.

2. Section the hair into four parts, or sections.

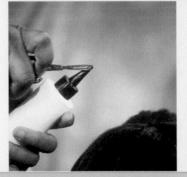
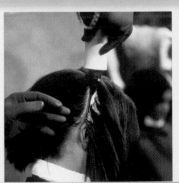

3. In the first section you'll apply relaxer from an applicator bottle. Use utility scissors to cut the tip of the applicator diagonally.

4. Put on protective gloves. Keep the applicator bottle inverted, and begin outlining. Place the tip of the applicator bottle 1/4" (.625 cm) from the scalp. Continue to outline the section. Squeeze the bottle gently to flow and apply the relaxer.

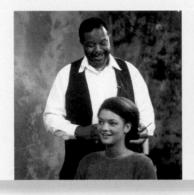
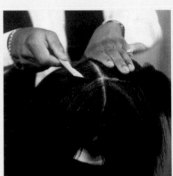

5. Use your thumb to gently spread the relaxer through the regrowth area. Do not apply pressure—this could push relaxer through the hair and possibly onto the scalp, which might be uncomfortable for your client.

6. Continue to outline. Apply relaxer around the outer perimeter of the entire section using the same application technique, maintaining the tip of the applicator in a downward position.

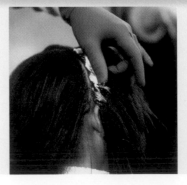
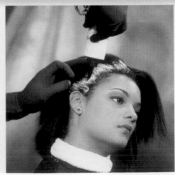

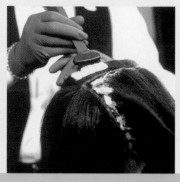

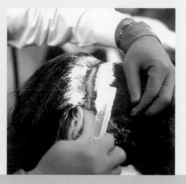

7. In the second section, begin the retouch process with an applicator brush. Remember to keep the product 1/4" (.625cm) from the scalp.

8. Now you'll outline and apply relaxer for a retouch with a tail comb. Outline the outer perimeter of this section applying product 1/4" (.625cm) away from the scalp. Note how neat and meticulous the application is.

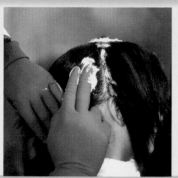

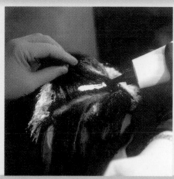

9. In the fourth section, use a finger application technique. Using your fingers is not as controlled, therefore it is most often used on virgin applications of relaxer.

10. Go back to the first section, and proceed to work through the interior. Use diagonal partings 1/4" to 1/2" (.625 to 1.25 cm) thick to apply the relaxer near the base or scalp area.

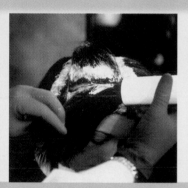

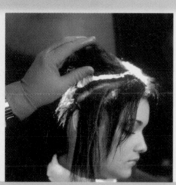

11. Continue the application, working from the crown down to the hairline. Apply then, gently smooth the relaxer with your fingers, repeating this process on either side of the part as shown.

12. Continue to gently smooth the relaxer with your thumb.

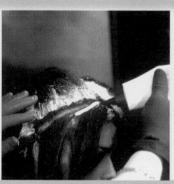

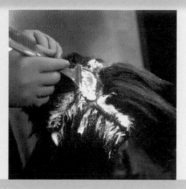

13. Finish this section. Note that using an applicator bottle for a relaxer service involves the same technique as applying a tint, you apply it 1/4" (.625 cm) from the scalp. After the product has been on the hair for approximately eight minutes, body heat should soften the relaxer and help draw it closer to the scalp.

14. Modern technology allows you to part, comb, and apply with one brush. Note that the relaxer touch up was started in the frontal area of the head. Begin your service wherever you determine the hair to be most resistant.

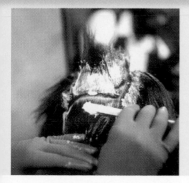

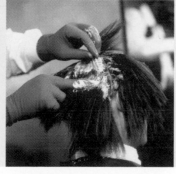

15. Work through the back section with the tail comb. Make horizontal parts, beginning at the top of the crown and progressing down to the neck area. Moving each section in an upward motion toward the crown prevents hair from resting on the neck.

16. Apply within the interior of the fourth section using horizontal partings.

17. After you've thoroughly applied your sodium hydroxide relaxer to all four sections, go back to all of your partings and check the application to make sure that no product is resting on the scalp.

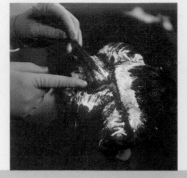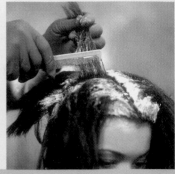

18. After the comb application is complete, straighten the hair repeatedly combing with the teeth or the back of your comb and smoothing the hair. This will cause unwanted curl or kink to decrease.

19. Now you are ready to begin smoothing. Using the teeth or back of your tail comb, go through all of hair, applying a small amount of pressure. This will smooth the hair, removing unwanted kink, curl, or wave. Go through the entire head of hair once or twice as required.

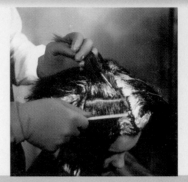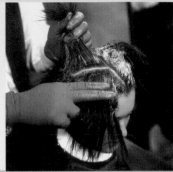

20. Your final comb through for a retouch involves smoothing the hair with your fingers. Work through all four sections using this technique.

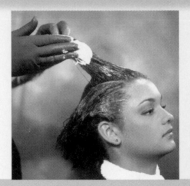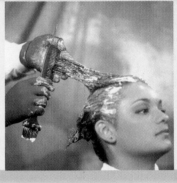

21. Spread the relaxer throughout the shaft during the last three to five minutes of the relaxer service. This ensures consistency in texture given that this client's previous end texture was somewhat different having been done with a different formula and by another service provider. On her next visit she will not have the relaxer brought through the ends.

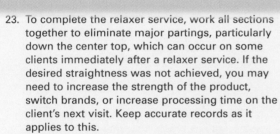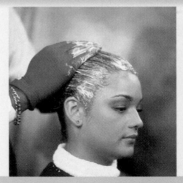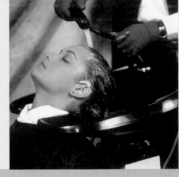

22. Using a wide-toothed comb, comb the relaxer throughout the shaft at least once.

23. To complete the relaxer service, work all sections together to eliminate major partings, particularly down the center top, which can occur on some clients immediately after a relaxer service. If the desired straightness was not achieved, you may need to increase the strength of the product, switch brands, or increase processing time on the client's next visit. Keep accurate records as it applies to this.

24. Adjust the bowl and the water temperature before you begin rinsing your client. Start with any areas causing her discomfort, or else with the section of hair that you applied the relaxer to first.

25. Keep the spray nozzle pointed away from the face and into the bowl.

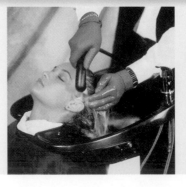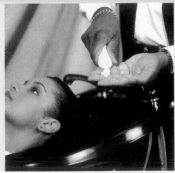

26. When you've removed all of the relaxer from the hair, the processing stops. Now the bonds of the hair are still open. This is an excellent time to use a deep penetrating treatment. Apply approximately one ounce (30 ml) into the palms of your hands.

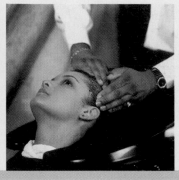

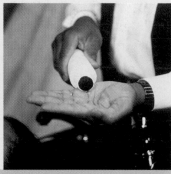

27. Massage the treatment into the hair shaft.

28. After you've applied the treatment, place your client under a heat cap for approximately 15 minutes, then rinse. Now you are ready to begin your shampoo system.

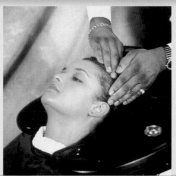

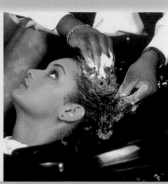

29. Use a normalizing shampoo. This will lower the pH and ensure removal of relaxer. This first shampoo is simply a deep cleansing. Second and third shampoos are recommended.

30. These shampoos may be luxurious and moisturizing for particular hair types. Rinse thoroughly.

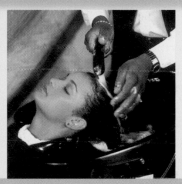

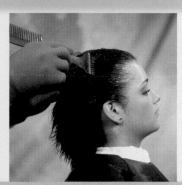

31. After three shampoos, apply a moisturizing conditioner or detanglerand rinse it out. Rinse thoroughly.

32. Using a semipermanent vegetable-based haircolor and tint brush, paint on haircolor for highlights. Leave on until processed and rinsed.

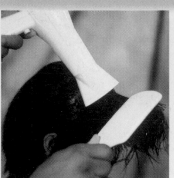

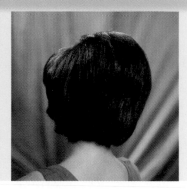

33. Begin to blow-dry. Control tension on the hair through the angle at which you hold and maneuver your brush. This is the first step in preparing the hair for cutting.

34. The glamorous finished style! The relaxer touch up and refresher or retexturizer through the ends of the hair have harmonized the texture in this design. Color and conditioning treatments create tone, gloss, and shine.

Apply this technique to different lengths, colors, and cuts for almost endless possibilities.

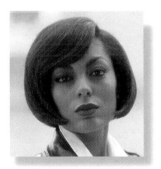

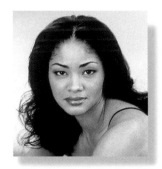

The Client
Service Plan

You can only become a winner if you're willing to walk over the edge.

Ronald E. McNair

$\mathcal{L}$et's look at something that will help keep your clients coming back: the client service plan.

When you consult with a new client, you have two purposes:

1. **To decide what services the client will receive today, and**
2. **To create a plan of services for the future.**

During the consultation, you discover what the client wants. Then you recommend to her what steps are required to achieve the desired look she wants. For example:

CLIENT: "I hate the way this old perm is growing out. My hair feels like straw. I want an easy style to manage and I want to get rid of this gray."

STYLIST: (restating the client's wants): "I understand that you want to change the way your hair feels, and to achieve a style that's attractive and easy to manage, without the gray. We can do all of that, but I don't recommend we do it all at once. Here's what I think would be an ideal plan for you:

"First, I recommend we use a special conditioner today before we cut. Here's a style [show photo] that you liked that we can create today. Deep conditioning is essential, though, before future chemical services.

"There's a great conditioner I recommend you use regularly at home before your next visit. When you come back in six weeks, we can perm and cut. Depending on the condition of your hair then, we may also be able to color to blend the gray away."

You have set the stage for future services, and you've shown the client that your main concern is her satisfaction, not your immediate income. You've also introduced the subject of the right products to use at home. You've created a service plan, and you're on your way to a lasting relationship with this client.

Haircoloring
An Art and a Science

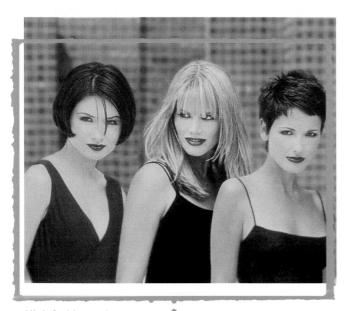

High fashion colors

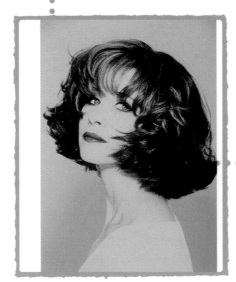

Dimentional color

*H*aircoloring is an art, and you are taking the first steps toward becoming an artist. This chapter will get you under way, in a practical and easily understandable manner. By working your way through hands-on techniques, taken from real-life salon situations, you'll prepare yourself to assess your clients' hair and make sound haircolor recommendations.

From fundamental principles, such as defining primary and secondary colors, to understanding categories and uses of haircolor, mastering formulation, mixing, timing, and—most important—the client consultation, this chapter clearly outlines various application procedures. You'll learn how to achieve a variety of looks by adding dimension to the hair using highlighting techniques such as balayage, paneling, and foil placement. These skills are essential to the mastery of haircoloring.

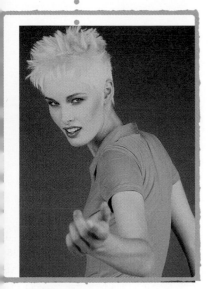

High lift blonde

Haircolor is now looked at as the "cosmetic for the hair." Clients are no longer afraid of color—all the more reason why it is such a necessary skill in this industry. And taking the time to learn haircolor is fun and easy, and not as complicated as it seems. You will be highly rewarded financially for your efforts.

So if you want to know how you can lift dark hair to a pretty shade of blonde, what is the best way to add dimension, or how to deal with chemically treated hair, you'll find out here. Exploration of theoretical fundamentals is also offered in the Haircoloring chapter of *Milady's Standard Textbook of Cosmetology.*

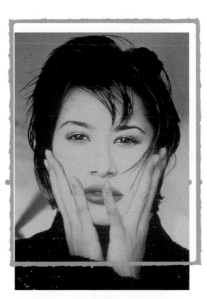

Dramatic color effects

What You Will Learn

This chapter will give a whole new meaning to the word "haircolor." You'll explore all the information you will need to succeed as a salon colorist. Let's take a look at some application skills that you will explore and learn during this chapter. You will learn about:

- Making a color decision with a client.
- Placement of color at the base area—initial glaze and retouch application.
- Placement of color on the shaft and ends—full head application.
- Creating a double process blonde.
- Adding dimension as:
  - Blockings
  - Balayage
  - Slicing
  - Weaving

Growing Service

Below list why people color their hair.

_____

_____

_____

_____

_____

_____

_____

Haircolor Service Menu

Once you start your career working in a salon, you will learn to identify how different color services are offered to the client. These names will all be new to you now; after you go through this chapter, however, you will have a much better understanding. Most salons offer a color menu for the clients that list descriptions and pricing. Most color services take up a specific amount of time. Here's an example of how a salon might list color services in its brochure:

- **Single-process color/color enhancement**— A single-process color service is an application of color that is put all over the head or just on the base area or the regrowth. This color is done when a client wants to lighten, cover gray, or enhance her natural hair color. This service usually processes for 20 to 45 minutes, depending on the situation. Time between appointments—4 to 6 weeks.

- **Single-process retouch color with a glaze**—A single process with a glaze means that there are two steps to the color service. The first color is put on the base area or the regrowth and processed for 30 to 45 minutes. The second color is the glaze. This is a non-ammonia color that adds shine and tone to the hair. The glaze is applied at the sink after the first color is rinsed and processed for 10 to 15 minutes. Time between appointments—4 to 6 weeks.

- **Double-process color**—A double process color is color desired by someone who wants to be very blonde all over. Her hair is pre-lightened with a lightener and then toned with a toner or glaze. This process can take anywhere from 45 to 90 minutes to lighten. Time between appointments—4 to 5 weeks.

- **Double-process retouch**—This process is lightening the base (regrowth area) only with a lightener and then toning or glazing the entire head to refresh the color. Time between appointments—4 to 5 weeks.

- **Dimensional haircolor**—This type of haircolor service is when you are isolating certain strands in the hair with foil or free hand painting to create dimension or a variety of different colors in the hair. It is also referred to as highlighting. Following are a variety of dimension services:

FACE-FRAME HIGHLIGHT—A face-frame highlight is framing the face with foils from ear to ear. This service is an easy way to introduce a client to the highlighting service. A glaze is included to add tone and shine to the new highlights and existing hair. Time between appointments—8 to 12 weeks.

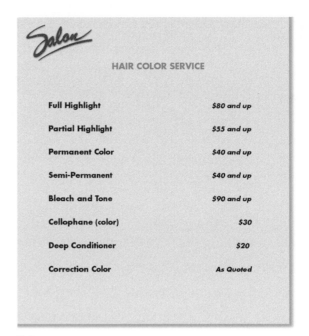

Color menu

HALF-HEAD HIGHLIGHT—This highlighting service is placing foils on the sides and top portion of the head. A glaze is included to add tone and shine to the new highlights and existing color. Time between appointments—8 to 12 weeks.

THREE-QUARTER-HEAD HIGHLIGHT—This highlighting service is placing foils on the sides and top portion of the head down the back to the occipital bone. A glaze is included to add tone and shine to the new highlights and existing color. Time between appointments—8 to 12 weeks.

FULL-HEAD HIGHLIGHT—This highlighting service is placing foils all over the head. A glaze is included to add tone and shine to the new highlights and existing color. Time between appointments—8 to 12 weeks.

- **Special effects**—Any service that is not mentioned above. A consultation is recommended and a price will be determined at that time.

- **Corrective color**—Corrective color or color adjusting is any color situation that requires special attention along with a series of visits. A consultation is advised to determine time and cost.

Application Times for the Colorist

Now that you have reviewed how haircolor services are offered in a menu to the salon—it is also important to understand that you will have a specific time for applying this color. This is known as a booking pattern—how that service is booked by a salon coordinator to allow for the proper amount of time to build into your daily schedule when you are working. Processing time is separate. All new clients will have an extra 15 minutes for consultation.

Here are some examples of booking patterns. As you start out as a junior colorist, you will have more time for application. As you become more experienced, your speed will automatically build and you can reduce your time. As a result, you can see more clients, and in turn make more money in the course of a day.

◆ Single-process color/color enhancement (15 to 30 minutes)

◆ Single-process color with a glaze (15 to 30 minutes)

◆ Single-process retouch (15 to 30 minutes)

◆ Double-process color (30 minutes)

◆ Double-process retouch (15 to 30 minutes)

◆ Dimensional haircolor:

  * Face-frame highlight (30 minutes)

  * Half-head highlight (30 to 45 minutes)

  * Three-quarter head highlight (45 minutes to 1 hour)

  * Full-head highlight (1 hour to 1 hour and 15 minutes)

These booking times are defined as the amount of time the colorist needs to apply the color. Processing time is started after the color application is complete.

When you start practicing these color services, refer back to the booking patterns to test yourself on your speed.

Hair Structure

Understanding the science behind haircolor is very important. Before we start talking about how color works, it is important that you have a thorough understanding of hair structure, porosity, and texture. Each of these areas gives you important information about how the color will react on the hair. Every haircolor service will affect the structure of the hair. Some haircolor products will cause a dramatic change, while others affect it very little. The key thing to remember is that the hair strand will be altered or weakened by the products applied to the hair. Hair can also be weakened when proper procedure is not followed.

Let's Review the Three Layers of the Hair

Cuticle

The cuticle is the outermost part of the hair structure. This layer protects the cortex. If the cuticle is abraded or weakened, it will affect the haircolor as it is processing. Processing time is usually shortened because the color will develop darker and faster since there is damage to this protective layer.

Medulla

The center structure of the hairshaft, this is sometimes absent in fine or very fine hair. It plays a very minor role in the hair with haircolor as it processes.

Cortex

The cortex is the most important layer as it relates to haircolor. It is the layer of the hair that contains all of the natural pigments or melanins, which is what determines whether we become red, brunette, blonde or gray.

Natural Hair Pigments

Learning to identify natural color pigments is the most important step to becoming a good colorist. This is where your work begins. Nature produces endless varieties of hair colors.

Natural pigments are called melanins. These melanins are classified into two groups.

Group One

Eumelanin is a black-brown pigment. It can be found in brunettes and blondes. When it is found in blondes it may appear as very dark, almost black strands of hair mixed with blonde. This melanin breaks up easily and lightens quickly when haircolor is applied. That is key when you are coloring blonde hair. If it looks like it has these dark strands without a lot of gold or yellow to the hair, it will lighten quickly without a lot of warmth or gold to the final result.

Group Two

Pheomelanin pigments are red and yellow. Very dark hair and most brunette hair contains pheomelanin pigment. This pigment leaves orange behind in lightened hair. This pigment can be difficult to break up in the hair, because it is very strong.

Natural hair color is composed of these melanins scattered throughout the cortex of the hair. Some hair color can be a combination of both types of melanin. We refer to this as mixed melanin.

Gray Hair

When hair turns gray, it retains the same basic structure but loses its melanin. When this happens the hair turns white in color. Most hair starts turning white around the hairline and the top of the head. When the white hair is mixed with the pigmented hair we refer to it as salt and pepper.

Refer to *Milady's Standard Textbook of Cosmetology* for further details.

Do an Experiment

Take salt and pepper shakers. Think of salt as gray hair, pepper as pigmented hair. Mix them together to create percentages of gray from 10 to 100 percent. This is a good visual example of pigmented and non-pigmented hair.

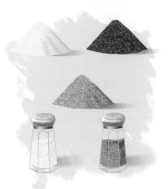

Salt and pepper exercise

Natural Hair Color

Natural hair color ranges from black to dark browns to reds, and from dark blondes up to light blondes. The human eye has a varying perception of how we see color due to light reflection. This is why no two colors will ever look exactly alike.

When coloring hair, your environment will play a key role in how color is perceived. Surrounding colors such as paint, wallpaper, or a client's blouse can alter your perception of her hair color. Placing a client in natural light or in a white room will give you the best option to identify her color. Salons generally have lighting in the color area to accommodate a realistic color identification.

Coloring Brown Hair

Brown hair has a high concentration of red and gold underlying pigments known as pheomelanin pigments. These pigments are sometimes difficult to lift if a cool brown is desired. In a case like this a colorist would use a cool base, such as blue, or a violet base to balance this warmth. Brown hair is the most common natural color.

Coloring Red Hair

Red hair can be difficult to lighten to a blonde color because of its strong natural red tones. Occasionally when you highlight red hair to a golden blonde, it can revert back to red within 24 hours due to the strong red pigments in the natural color. If this happens re-highlight.

Coloring Blonde Hair

Blonde hair will lighten easily, especially if the hair is fine in texture. Sometimes dark blonde hair can hold a lot of gold tones, making it more difficult to lighten to a pale blonde containing little tone. In this case you would choose a violet base to balance the unwanted yellow or gold in the hair.

Coloring Gray Hair

Gray hair is caused by the reduction of any pigment in the cortical layer. Therefore, it often takes more time for color to develop on gray hair, since you are starting with less pigment. Formulating a color for gray hair is easy: Simply pick the exact level and tone of the desired color.

Porosity

Hair porosity is the hair's ability to absorb liquids. Porous hair will always accept haircolor darker and faster. It is important to be able to identify porous hair. The longer the hair, the more porous it can be. The cuticle of porous hair can look like there are many "split ends" present. Overall, the hair will look dull in appearance, because abraded cuticles absorb light, while smooth cuticles reflect light.

Some experimenting with wet and dry sponges might help you understand porosity. Take a dry sponge and add water to it; this is how liquids are absorbed into the hair.

Now take a wet sponge and add more water to it. This is how hair can become over-porous. It can't accept any more liquids. Over-porous hair results when someone has had too many chemical services. These wear away the cuticle. Color will then soak in quickly, but the hair can't retain it. The color may go off tone or darken, or it may just wash out of the hair within a few shampoos, since there isn't any hair structure to support it.

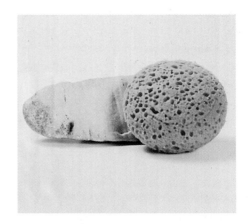

Texture

The diameter or thickness of the individual hair strand is referred to as texture. Common terms such as fine, medium, and coarse are used to describe different textures in the hair.

Within each texture different amounts of natural pigment are distributed in the hair. For example, in fine hair the color pigments are packed close together, because of the hair's smaller diameter. This means that fine hair can lighten faster. It may develop darker, however, because there is less area to color.

Medium hair has an average response to haircolor. Remember, the hairline is sometimes made up of finer hair that can grab on to color faster.

Coarse hair will have the longest developing time because it has the largest diameter. It is slightly less resistant when you're lightening hair. It may take longer to process, and the haircolor result can be warmer or more golden than expected. We will review this more later on when we talk about choosing the right tone for the haircolor result.

 Fine textured hair

 Medium textured hair

 Coarse textured hair

Hair textures

Learning Levels and Tones

Learning to read levels and tones is an important first step to hair coloring. Reading haircolor levels means learning to look at the depth, lightness, or darkness of the haircolor, which is your starting point. There are ten levels, from dark to light. To understand this, think of watching a black and white television, where all you can see are the depths of black to white.

Haircolor Levels

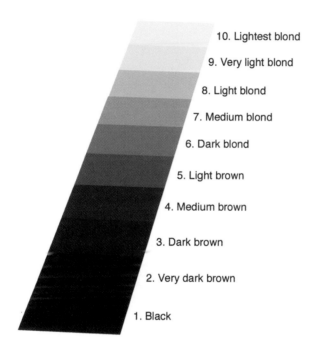

10. Lightest blond

9. Very light blond

8. Light blond

7. Medium blond

6. Dark blond

5. Light brown

4. Medium brown

3. Dark brown

2. Very dark brown

1. Black

Haircolor Levels

It is important to understand that natural hair color has a level. Think of a level 6, which is a dark blonde. Haircolor manufacturers also identify their haircolor with a number, which indicates the level, and a letter, which indicates the tone (example, 6B—Level 6—Dark Blonde, Base—blue). When the natural hair color reacts with the artificial color, this processes as the final haircolor result.

Sometimes manufacturers provide colorists with tools to identify natural levels—such as natural level finders. These tools are generally a set of labeled swatches that you can match up to the client's hair. Remember, at this point you are only looking for depth of color. It is important to fan out this swatch when you place it next to the scalp. This will diffuse the color and make it easier to identify the level you are starting at.

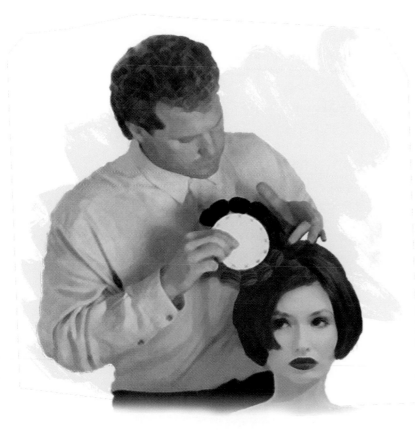

Stylist using color swatches

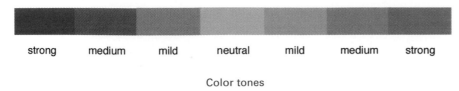

Natural cool tones show
no red or yellow

Natural warm tones
contain red or yellow

strong   medium   mild   neutral   mild   medium   strong

Color tones

All About Tones

Tone refers to the highlight or the hue of color seen in their hair. These tones can be described as warm, cool, or neutral.

Warm tones reflect light, so they always look lighter than the level that they are at. These tones are golden, orange, red, and yellow. Some haircolors may use more descriptive words, such as "auburn," "amber," "copper," or "bronze." These are the tones that you
will use to describe the effect to the client. Base colors used when formulating a haircolor will be gold, red, and red-orange, to create a warm tone.

Cool tones are colors that absorb more light, so they can look deeper than their actual level. These tones are blue, green, and violet; more descriptive words for cool tones would be "drab," "ash," and "smoky." Base colors used when formulating a haircolor will be blue, blue-violet, violet, or green to achieve a cool result.

Neutral tones are a cross between cool and warm tones. Neutral tones can be looked at as "sandy" or "tan." They're used for covering gray or to balance a formula so it is not too bright. Using neutral tones is a way to become a good colorist. Mix them with stronger tones to learn how natural hair color is affected by artificial color. Base colors used when formulating a haircolor will be neutral or
natural base to create a neutral tone.

Remember, it is very important to use descriptive words with the client that define what the haircolor will look like. It is also a good idea to use pictures to have a clearer understanding.

Color intensity is the strength of tonality (term used to describe the warmth or coolness in color) in a color. You can make a color as intense or as soft as you like, depending on the amount of a certain color that you mix. Color intensifiers exist to serve this purpose as well.

Do an Exercise

Cut out pictures from magazines to create a level and tone chart. Separate each level into warm and cool colors.

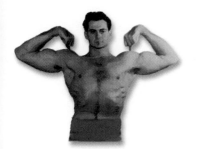 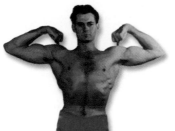 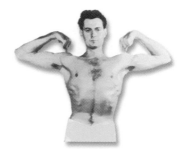

Primary color strength

Color Theory

The law of color is a system for understanding the relationships of colors. When you combine these colors, you will always get the same result.

Primary Colors

Primary colors are pure pigments that cannot be created by mixing any other colors together. The primary colors are blue, red, and yellow. This is also the order of their strength.

Blue is the darkest and coolest primary.

Red is the next strongest in tone. It is often said that red is the strongest, most vivid pigment to get in the hair and the hardest to get out.

Yellow is the lightest and warmest primary. It will brighten up any haircolor formula.

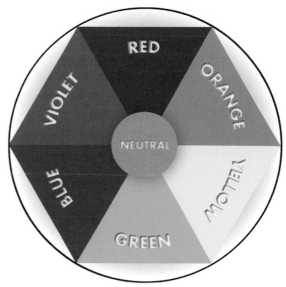

Color wheel

Secondary Colors

Secondary colors are green, orange, and violet. They are created by combining two of the primary colors together in equal proportions.

Do an Experiment

Mix red, blue, and yellow Playdough in equal proportions to create secondary colors. Mix:

Blue and yellow = green

Red and blue = violet

Yellow and red = orange

Red, blue, and yellow = neutral

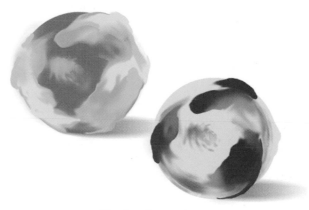

Playdough exercise

Complementary Colors

These colors neutralize one another. It's important that you know and understand these colors when you're doing color adjustments or corrective work.

Tertiary Colors

Tertiary colors are blue-green, blue-violet, red-violet, red-orange, yellow-orange, yellow-green. They're made by mixing a primary color with an adjacent secondary color on the color wheel.

Find the Missing Primary

Green = yellow and blue
Adjust with red

Missing primary = red

Orange = yellow and red
Adjust with blue

Missing primary = blue

Violet = red and blue
Adjust with yellow

Missing primary = yellow

Understanding Underlying Tones

Now, that you have been introduced to identifying haircolor levels, tones, and color theory, the next step is to learn to identify what underlying tones are underneath natural hair color at each level. This is very important because these underlying tones are exposed when natural color is lightened. This means you will have to adjust the haircolor formula to help balance the final result.

Important Reminders

◆ Always look for underlying tones when identifying the natural level.

◆ Always expect underlying tones when you lighten the natural hair color.

◆ Always use the Law of Color Theory to add a color that will help counterbalance these tones.

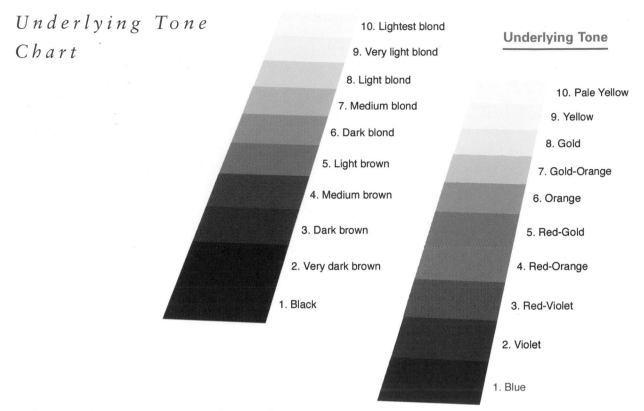

Underlying Tone Chart

Level

- 10. Lightest blond
- 9. Very light blond
- 8. Light blond
- 7. Medium blond
- 6. Dark blond
- 5. Light brown
- 4. Medium brown
- 3. Dark brown
- 2. Very dark brown
- 1. Black

Underlying Tone

- 10. Pale Yellow
- 9. Yellow
- 8. Gold
- 7. Gold-Orange
- 6. Orange
- 5. Red-Gold
- 4. Red-Orange
- 3. Red-Violet
- 2. Violet
- 1. Blue

Classifications of Color

Haircolor falls into four main categories: temporary, semipermanent, demi-permanent or deposit only, and permanent. For more information, refer to the Haircoloring chapter of *Milady's Standard Textbook of Cosmetology*. These classifications refer to the lasting power, but also reflect the actions on the hair.

To create most haircolor results, the color must be mixed with some sort of catalyst or developer to provide oxidation. During this process the natural color will work with the artificial color to produce a new haircolor result. Developers must be mixed with color or lighteners to produce final result.

Developer Strengths

- ◆ 10 volume—will lighten the hair a minimum of one level.

- ◆ 20 volume—is the standard volume that will lighten haircolor two levels of lift. It is also recommended for gray coverage.

- ◆ 30 volume—will lighten the haircolor three levels.

- ◆ 40 volume—will lighten the haircolor four levels. 40 volume is used with most high-lift blonde series to produce the blondest results.

Most non-ammonia or demi-permanent colors come with their own developers that range from 10 to 13 volume, to open and swell the cuticle to process the color.

Consultations

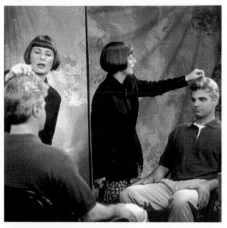

Stylist/client consultation

A haircolor consultation is the most important part of the color service. This time allows you a chance to establish a relationship with a client. It is their time to communicate to you their wants and desires for a haircolor, and it is your time to listen and properly assess the situation to make a proper haircolor recommendation. Taking this time for consulting can result in clients that leave the salon happy with their new haircolor.

The communication process that takes place during this time is key to the end results. The following steps will help you conduct a successful consultation:

1. Use an area that has proper lighting to assess the client's hair.

2. Book out 15 minutes extra to have a proper consultation. Introduce yourself and welcome the client to the salon. Offer her a beverage. During this time with a new client there should be no interruptions.

3. Have the client fill out an information card. This allows you to gather history on her hair, as well as what type of color service she is looking for.

4. Look at the client directly. Do not look at her through the mirror. Ask her what she's thinking about doing with her hair color. Try to get as much information as you can by asking leading questions. Let her talk. Keep her on track by discussing the recent history of her hair.

5. Give her haircolor options. Recommend at least two different options.

6. Review the procedure, maintenance, and cost of the service.

7. Be honest and don't overpromise. If you are faced with a corrective situation, let the client know what you can do today, and how many visits it will take to achieve what she's looking for.

8. Gain approval from client.

9. Start the haircolor service.

10. Follow through during the service in educating and informing client about home care, products, and rebooking.

Formulation

After the consultation is complete, you are now ready to formulate the haircolor. Refer to the manufacturer's directions and formulation grid to choose the color. Remember, when you are using a permanent color, select a color no more then 2 levels from the client's natural color. When you are formulating a non-ammonia or demi-permanent color, select a color 2 levels lighter because they deposit only and can appear darker.

There are three questions that always have to be answered before a haircolor is applied:

1. What is the natural level?

2. What is the desired level and tone the client wants to see?

3. What color do I mix to produce this result?

If you refer to these questions and use a natural level finder guide, underlying tone chart, and the tonal chart from the manufacturer, you will be on your way to becoming a good colorist.

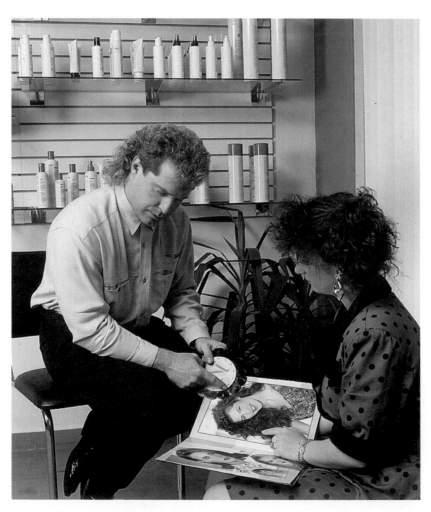

Stylist using color charts

Common Haircolor Adjustment

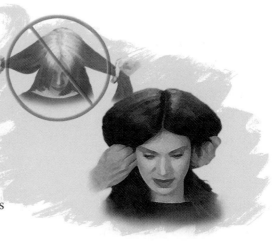

Bad and good color jobs

What the client sees is reality. The haircolor can be technically excellent, but if she doesn't like it, you have to fix it

One of the most important things you can learn as a colorist is how to do color adjustments or more commonly called corrective haircolor. Reasons for color adjustments range from a poor consultation, color not coming out the way you had expected it to, to a color being off tone, to a client coming in with black ends and blonde roots. This service can also be very lucrative. Some colorists gain a reputation by specializing in this kind of coloring.

Take time to look at the situation in front of you. Consider the logical steps to correct the problem. Always ask yourself, "What do I have to take out of the haircolor or what do I have to add to the color to get the result I want?"

Green Cast to the Hair

You may have to use a product to purify the hair to see if that will remove some of the green. After this step, you must mix a non-ammonia color with a light red-orange (warm) base to neutralize the remaining green. Apply the color all over the head, and process up to 10 minutes, checking it every 5 minutes.

Overall Color is Too Light

This is a result of an incorrect formula being applied to the head. Choose a non-ammonia color one level darker than the current color. Apply all over the head as quickly as possible and process up to 10 minutes, checking it every 5 minutes.

Poor Gray Coverage

Most of the time when gray doesn't cover it is a result of formulating too light a color and not leaving it on the hair long enough. For the next application, apply a deeper color. Add 1/2 to 1 oz(15 to 30 ml) of a neutral base to the formula to help the gray cover, and let it process for a full 45 minutes.

Overall Color is Too Dark on First Application

Use a gentle color remover to lift some of the unwanted color from the hair. Apply the remover all over the head for 10 minutes, then rinse. Check to see if you have to reapply the color. Make sure you towel-dry the hair to get an accurate read on the color.

Color That is Bright at the Base

This occurs when the heat from the body makes the color process faster. Mix and apply a deeper color to the base and process for 10 minutes. Formulate the color one to two levels deeper than the formula you originally selected.

Highlights That Are Too Light

Highlights can end up looking white if they are processed for too long. Choose a light blonde, non-ammonia color in a neutral or gold base to add color back into these highlighted sections. Apply the color all over the head and process for 10 minutes.

● ● ● ● ● ● ● ● ● ● ● ● ● ● ● ● ● ● ● ●

Blonde Who Wants to Go Back to Natural Color

(Refer to the Underlying Tonal Chart to add missing pigments.) Deepening haircolor can be tricky. The first step is to use a non-ammonia color with a very light red-orange base to add some of the missing pigments that have been removed. Apply this color on the lighter pieces of hair only. Process for 20 minutes.

After 20 minutes, rinse out the color. Formulate a final color 2 levels lighter than the client's natural color.

When you are formulating non-ammonia colors, remember that they can seem darker than they really are. Apply this formula to the pieces you just colored. Process for 15 minutes, then work the rest of the color all over the head for the last 5 minutes. The key here is to always put the color where it is most needed first, and then work it through to the other areas if necessary.

Highlights That Were Not Lifted Light Enough

Highlights can get stuck at the orange stage if they are not processed long enough. To correct this, you will have to deepen the hair first with a non-ammonia color to deposit color back into the hair and then re-highlight. Process highlights to desired results and glaze ifnecessary.

Haircolor Tips

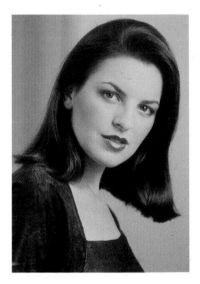

Brunettes

Always use a cool base such as a blue or violet when you are lightening brown hair with a permanent color to avoid warm or brassy tones.

It is advised not to lighten a brunette more than two levels away from her natural color – thi will result in allowing a very warm tone to be visible in the hair.

When adding highlights to brown hair, keep them very deep or caramel in color. If you make them too blonde, they will contrast too much with the brown hair. Even though this is possible, it is considered more of a high fashion or avant garde look.

Create rich red highlights by mixing red-viole and gold base colors together.

Always add 1oz.(30ml) of a neutral base into the formula when covering gray on brunette hair. This will ensure good gray coverage.

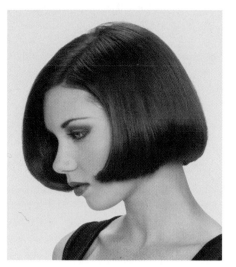

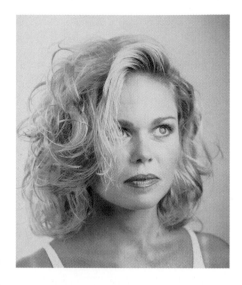

Redheads

To create warm coppery reds, use a red-orange base. To create deep reds use red-violet or red bases.

If you are putting red on gray hair, mix 1 oz. (30 ml) of a neutral base into the formula. This will prevent the red from coming out too bright.

Blondes

When lightening blonde hair, remember that there may be underlying gold tones in the hair.

To achieve a cool blonde result, use blue and violet bases.

Double-process blonding is the best way to get the lightest, most sheer blonde haircolor.

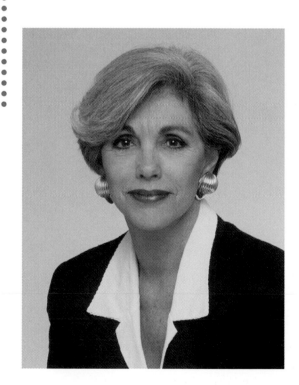

Gray Hair

Always mix gray coverage formulas with 20 volume developer and process for 45 minutes for maximum coverage.

Always add 1 oz. (30 ml) of a neutral tone to ensure complete gray coverage, especially if the hair texture is resistant.

Always use colors that are level 8—light blonde or deeper to cover gray.

High-lift blonde colors are not recommended for gray coverage. They are developed for maximum lightening and gray hair will appear not covered.

Colleen Hennessey

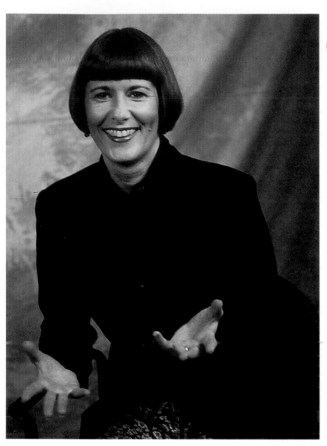

*C*olleen Hennessey, the author of the haircoloring education in this course, is a nationally known and respected educator and gifted colorist, the former Director of Education for the world's largest haircolor product manufacturer. Where did it all begin for Colleen, who now owns her own haircolor education consulting business and trains and manages a staff of 70 in one of the country's largest and most successful salons?

"I knew from the time I was a little girl that I wanted to work with haircolor and makeup. I was always cutting my dolls' hair and playing with make-up," she reminisced. Colleen's parents weren't thrilled with her plans to become a cosmetologist, but they agreed that she could study cosmetology as part of her public high school education, provided she would also take all the required college preparatory courses and enroll in college. And so she did. Colleen took the New York State Cosmetology Board exam just a week before graduating from high school, and went to work in a salon as a hairdresser at the same time she was enrolled as a full-time student at Buffalo State University, majoring in chemistry. "My dream was to learn all about the science of cosmetology so that I could someday create cosmetics and haircolor products," she added.

Shortly after she began her freshman year in college, Colleen landed a night job teaching cosmetology in a nearby private cosmetology school, a job that helped pay her way through college. She earned a bachelor of science degree with a minor in secondary education, and began teaching math and science to seventh and eighth graders that fall.

Colleen kept her "night job" at the cosmetology school, too. That winter, she attended a haircolor seminar, where a manufacturer's technical specialist so impressed Colleen with her presentation and skills that Colleen said, "I want to do that." She sent a resume to the company but heard nothing, so she kept on with her other two jobs...and nurtured her dreams.

"After a month or so, I got a call from the company telling me there were no openings at the time, but they would keep my resume on file. I thanked them, and then the following month I sent them another letter telling them I was still interested. The next month, I got a call and was asked to come in for an interview."

Colleen was hired and began to travel around the country, introducing new color products, training hairstylists, presenting at shows, seminars, and workshops. She was promoted through the company's upper management until she became the Director of Education, responsible for creating all the company's product education geared to professional stylists. And, she worked with the company's chemists on the product formulations. "I realized then that I had achieved my dream to help make products that would make people look and feel better."

Having achieved her goals, Colleen decided it was time to step down from the ranks of upper management and do what she loved best, work with people. She divides her time between a full client schedule; hiring, training and managing 70 assistants, stylists, and colorists in a salon that employs 140 people; and her consulting business that provides advice to product and education companies about haircolor and haircolor education.

And what is the one thing Colleen would tell the hundreds of thousands of aspiring stylists and colorists who are reading this book? "Be patient, because it's all worth it. Learn, practice, work hard . . . and you'll be there before you know it.

"Oh, and one more thing: Enjoy the journey. Do what you like to do every day, and have fun doing it."

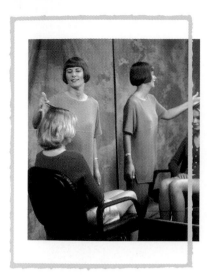

Patch Test

Overview

The most important part of the client consultation is to find out all you can about her. Take down necessary information so that you can always have it on record. When working with chemicals such as haircolor, you will have to find out if the client has any sensitivities or allergic reactions to anything. Use the patch test on a client who has never had a haircolor service to see if she has any reaction.

Connect

Some people have allergic reactions after taking certain medications or foods. That is why it is important to get as much information about the client before you perform a haircolor service.

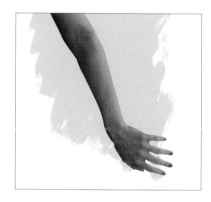

Focus

Mixing—Mix a small amount of product for the patch test.

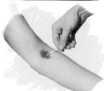
Applying—Make sure you apply the product to the inside of the elbow.

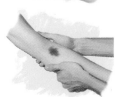
Examining—Check the results.

$\mathcal{A}pply$

1. Explain to your client that this test must be done to see if she has any sensitivities to color.

2. Determine the product for the haircolor service.

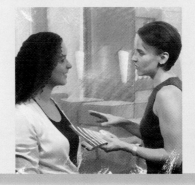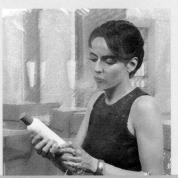

3. Mix a small amount of this product in a bowl.

4. Apply it to the inside of your client's elbow with a cotton swab.

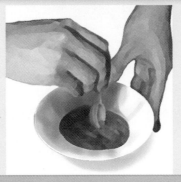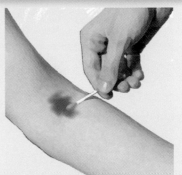

5. Let the color dry.

6. Examine the results in 24 hours. If there is no irritation on the area, you can move forward with the service.

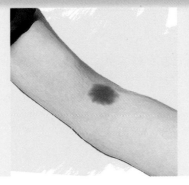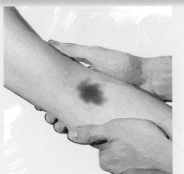

The best way to predict the future is to invent it.

Alan Kay

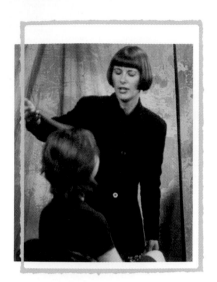

Strand Test

Overview

Now that you have learned the different categories of haircoloring products, along with the different characteristics of hair, you are ready to begin strand testing. This is the most important part of the haircoloring process. It establishes what the haircolor result is going to look like. It's especially vital with new clients or hair that is chemically challenged.

Connect

Primary and Secondary Colors

Review the importance of these colors to haircolor bases (the predominant tonality of existing colors).

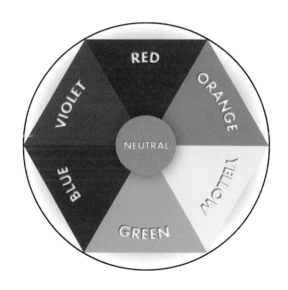

Porosity

Porous hair always accepts colors darker and faster. Always make sure that you add some warmth into the formula to balance. Refer to the Underlying Tone Chart.

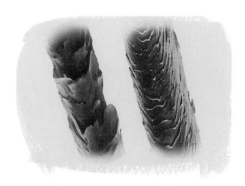

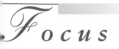

Focus

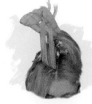

Strand Testing—Use strand testing to double-check the haircolor result before you apply it all over the head.

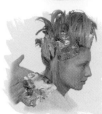

Small Strands—Use small strands of hair underneath the nape area.

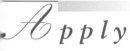

Apply

1. During the client consultation, explain why it is necessary to strand test the hair before starting.

2. Determine and mix the formula.

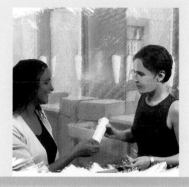
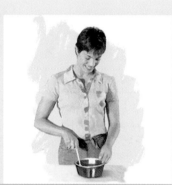

3. Apply the formula underneath a strand of hair in the back of the head. Wrap that piece of hair in foil.

4. Set a timer for ten minutes.

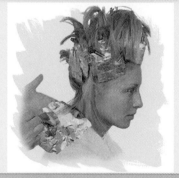
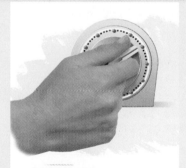

5. After the timer goes off, wipe the area by using a water bottle and a towel.

6. Check the resulting color development.

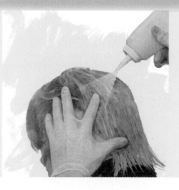
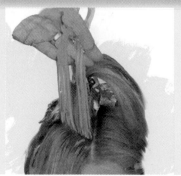

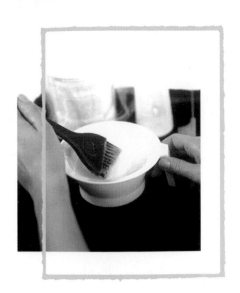

Mixing

Overview

Learning to mix haircolor is a very important skill. It will generally be mixed in equal proportion (1:1), or 2:1, meaning 2 parts developer to 1 part color. (This is most often a high blonde formula.) Most of these products combine a color and a developer. Most are mixed in equal proportions, although some are not. Lighteners are mixed completely different from color products. In the steps below, you'll mix combinations of different products.

Connect
Tools

If a chef works with the wrong tools in the kitchen or deviates from a proven recipe, the finished product may not be successful. In the same way, haircolorists must learn all the tools and products they are working with to create the best results.

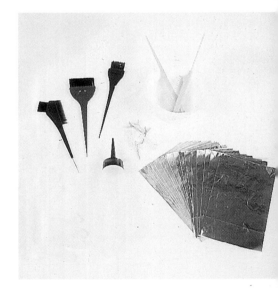

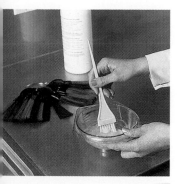

Reading Directions—Always read the manufacturer's directions.

Mixing—Use accurate measurements. Always keep the bottle on a level surface when mixing. Be careful. Make sure the product is mixed thoroughly before it is applied.

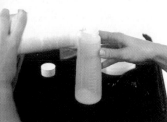

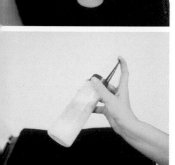

Apply

Mixing

Applicator Bottle (1:1 Mixing)

1. Pour 2 oz. (60 ml) of the developer into the applicator bottle.

2. Add 2 oz. (60 ml) of the color.

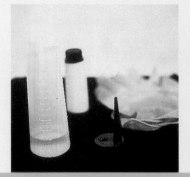
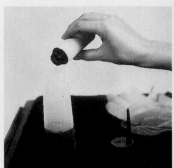

3. Put the top on the bottle and shake gently until mixed.

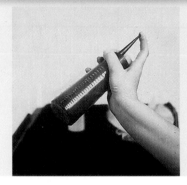

Applicator Bottle (2:1 Mixing)

1. Here, 2:1 mixing is shown for a high-lift blonde color formula. Pour 4 oz. (120 ml) of developer into the applicator bottle.

2. Add 2 oz. (60 ml) of color into the bottle. Use all contents in the 2 oz. (60 ml) tube of cream color.

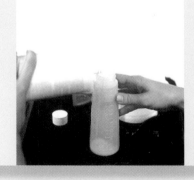
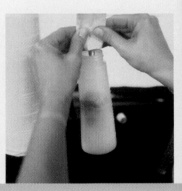

3. Put the top on and mix gently and thoroughly.

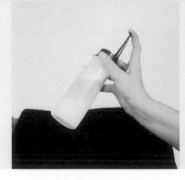

Bowl and Brush (1:1 Mixing)

1. Pour 2 oz. (60 ml) of developer into an applicator bottle. Pour the developer into bowl.

2. Squeeze 2 oz. (60 ml) of color into the bowl.

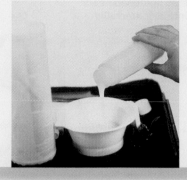 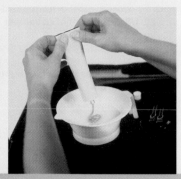

3. Mix to a creamy consistency.

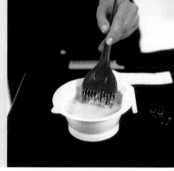

On-The-Scalp Lighteners (2:1 Mixing)

1. Pour 4 oz. (120 ml) of 20-volume developer into the applicator bottle.

2. Add one to three lightening activators according to the amount of lightening desired. Follow the manufacturer directions.

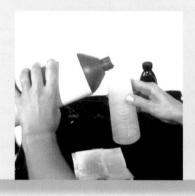 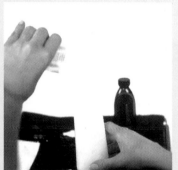

3. Put on the top and shake gently.

4. Add 2 oz. (60 ml) of lightener into the bottle.

5. Put on the top and shake gently.

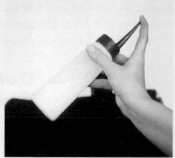 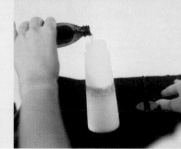

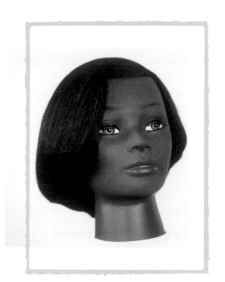

Color Enhancement for Relaxed Hair

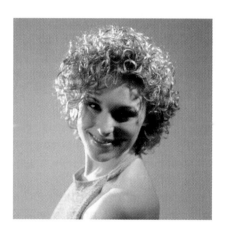

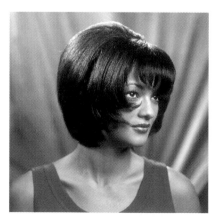

Overview

Color enhancement is a great way to introduce a client to color services. Enhancements add tone and shine in one easy step to any haircolor—without lightening the hair. The total color service takes about 20 minutes. In the following steps you'll enhance the color of brunette hair, both textured, and relaxed. A color enhancement may complement a wide variety of hair types, whether blonde, red head, brunette, or black hair.

Mastering color enhancements will build a strong foundation for other haircolor situations you will encounter. Learning good formulation and application skills is very important.

Connect

Mastering New Skills

The first discipline to master in becoming a good haircolorist is proper formulation and application skills. Think of it as learning a new board game. Always read the instructions along with the rules before you start.

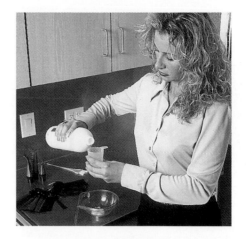

Importance of Application

Use the color chart provided by the manufacturer to review all the base colors and choices you have available.

After you select your color, review the mixing and timing for the color process. The way you apply the color will determine how well the color takes on the hair strand. Improper saturation can lead to an uneven haircolor result.

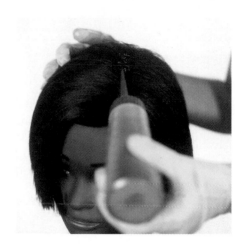

Focus

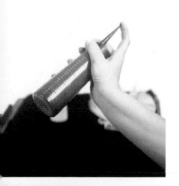

Formulation and Mixing—Remember that non-ammonia colors deposit only, so they may appear deeper to the eye. Select a color one to two levels lighter than your client's natural color. Follow the mixing instructions. Always refer to the manufacturer's color chart to formulate the color. Be sure to know what desired result you are looking for. Pick the proper tonal family and the proper volume of developer.

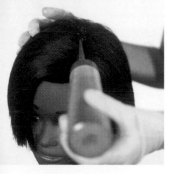

Application—Work with the tip of the bottle and spread the color with the nozzle. Use fine, even sections to ensure even application and proper saturation of the product. Then work the color in with your hands making sure the head is covered.

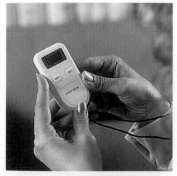

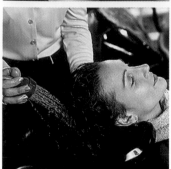

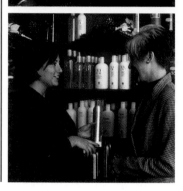

Processing and Timing—Some color-enhancing products are processed with dryer heat. If you're working with one that does, place cotton around the client's hairline, and cover with a plastic cap. Set the timer for processing. Most color enhancements process in 20 minutes, but follow the directions recommended by the manufacturer.

If there are signs of porous hair or if hair has been chemically relaxed or waved, less processing time may be needed. Never bring color through to the ends until the last five minutes, and watch the color carefully, until you achieve your desired result.

Color Removal—Rinse until the water runs clear. Shampoo and condition.

Color Results and Home Maintenance—Check the haircolor result to make sure the client is satisfied. Recommend proper retail products to maintain this color until her next visit, i.e., shampoo and conditioner for color treated hair or color enhancing shampoo. It is very important to schedule her next appointment before she leaves.

Your blessings come back to you based upon how you give them out.

Oprah Winfrey

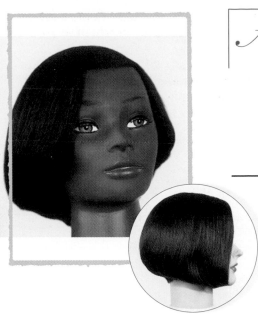

Apply
Color Enhancement for Relaxed Hair

1. Mix the formula, 1:1 proportions of 2 oz. (60 ml) 3R Medium Red Brown with 2 oz. (60 ml) of demi-permanent developer. Wear gloves when you apply color. Section the hair with the tip of the applicator bottle.

2. Outline the hair into four sections—from ear to ear and from front forehead to center nape.

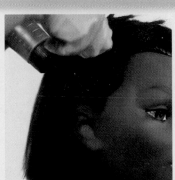
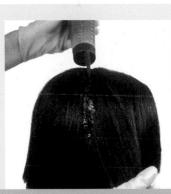

3. Begin applying where it is determined that the hair is the most resistant. Here, you'll start in the front right section. Take 1/2" (1.25 cm) partings and apply the color to the base area, working neatly, precisely, and efficiently. Bring all sections out away from the head to allow air to circulate. Move to the front left section and apply color to the base area, again taking 1/2 (1.25 cm) partings. Continue until the section is complete.

4. Move onto the back section of the head, following the same method. Work neatly until this section is completed.

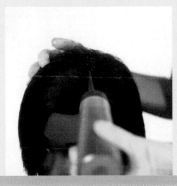
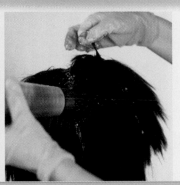

5. After all four sections have color on the base area, work the color down the hairshaft to the ends, making sure the hair is saturated with color. Gently massage the color through all of the hair. Do not rub or work aggressively. Set the timer for up to 20 minutes, to process the color.

6. Previously drab in tone, now note how the rich color accentuates this relaxed hair. Coloring and relaxing services can both be done successfully on the same day with non-ammonia, color-enhancing products.

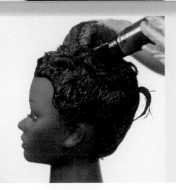
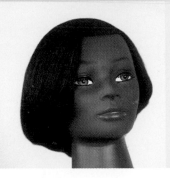

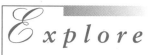

<table>
<tr><td></td><td></td><td></td></tr>
<tr><td></td><td></td><td></td></tr>
<tr><td></td><td></td><td></td></tr>
</table>

Apply this technique to different lengths, colors, and cuts for almost endless possibilities.

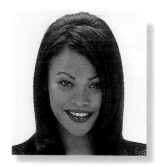
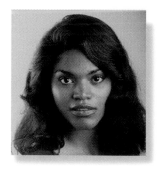
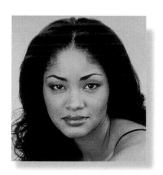

color enhancement
on textured hair

*O*n this, the Textured Light Layered Shape, a color enhancement formula is used to add rich warmth and dimension to the hair.

1. Mix the formula, 2oz. (60ml) of 6R, Dark Red Blonde, with 2oz. (60ml) of demi-permanent developer. Wear gloves when you apply color. Section the hair with the tip of the applicator bottle.

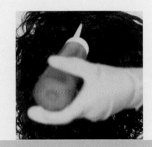

2. Outline the hair into four sections-from ear to ear and from front forehead to center nape. After all sections have color on the base area, work the color down the hair shaft to the ends, making sure the hair is saturated with color. Gently massage the color through all of the hair. Do not rub or work aggressively. Set the timer for up to 20 minutes to process the color. Remember to shorten the processing time for porous hair.

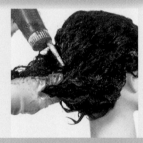

3. The finished color adds richness and dimension to the textured hair. Coloring and texture services can be done successfully on the same day with non-ammonia, color-enhancing products.

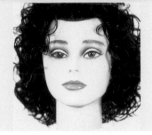

Shampoo Bowl
Etiquette

If you've finished shampooing a client and all she feels is wet, you haven't done your job correctly. The shampoo is the first opportunity you have to "touch" your client and demonstrate both personal service and technical skills at the same time. Follow these shampoo pointers to make sure the experience is one that your client enjoys. A good shampoo service can strengthen the rapport she feels with you:

◆ *Position*: Make sure the client is comfortable in this position. If she's clutching the arms of the chair to keep from falling, or twitching and moving her head around, ask if you can adjust the position of the chair to create a more comfortable "fit" for her.

◆ *Temperature*: Always ask if the water temperature is too hot or too cold. Your hands will feel temperature differently from the way the client's scalp will feel it. Different people have different temperature tolerances. Don't trust your own sense of hot and cold; ask clients about theirs.

◆ *Spray*: A personal service professional always pays attention to what she's doing. Clients hate getting their clothing and face wet. Be aware of an errant spray, and don't give your client an unwanted shower!

When love and skill work together, expect a masterpiece.

John Ruskin

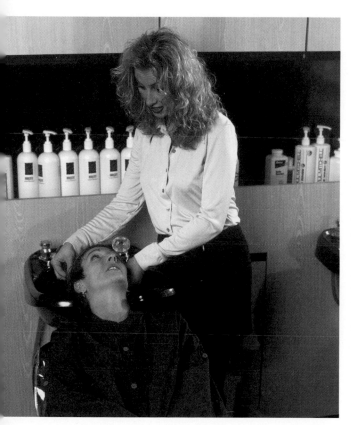

◆ *Touch*: The sense of touch can work to your advantage during the shampoo service like no other time during a hairstyling! Practice your shampoo technique until you can judge, based on your clients' reaction, that you are scoring personal service points. A scalp massage is a surefire retention tool—for most clients. It stimulates and relaxes, and puts the client in a better mood. Take your time during this phase of the service. An extra minute or two invested here will pay generous dividends in client retention.

Warning: Occasionally you'll have a client who isn't comfortable with touch. If you see a frown or other sign that she's uncomfortable when you perform a scalp massage, try saying, "The purpose of massaging the scalp is to stimulate the hair follicles, which results in better-looking, better-conditioned hair. If this makes you uncomfortable, please tell me and we won't massage your scalp when we shampoo."

Remember the client card—and if you find that a client does like something (or likes something particularly well), write it down. When she comes back, she'll be impressed that you remembered her special needs.

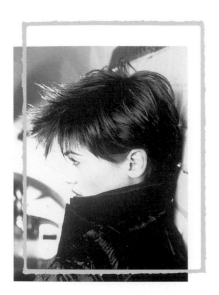

Permanent Haircolor

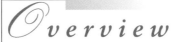

Overview

Now that you've worked with non-ammonia color-enhancing products, it's time to graduate to the next phase of haircolor: permanent haircolor. This can lighten natural color, change tone, cover gray hair—the possibilities are endless

You'll begin permanent haircoloring by lightening natural pigment. This is referred to as a virgin application going lighter. It's a popular service with clients who want to lighten and change the tone of their existing color.

Connect

The Applicator Bottle and Bowl-and-Brush Method

Mastering these two ways to apply color will give you a variety of options. The two application procedures are the same, except for the different tools they use.

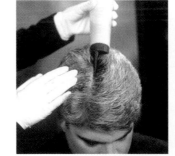 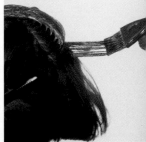

Base Area and Shaft

With permanent haircolor, you must treat the base area and the shaft differently. The base area of the head always processes color faster, so it needs less time to process.

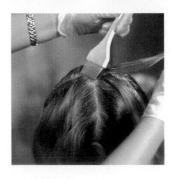

Selecting the Formula

Get out your color chart and look at the possible haircolor choices for your client. Understand that several formulas can be used to create any one result. It is best to use no more than two colors in one formula. Review the natural level chart. When you formulate the color stay within two levels lighter from the natural color. This will give the most controlled results. Then choose the proper tone and review the underlying tones in the natural color. Formulate the color once you have looked at these items.

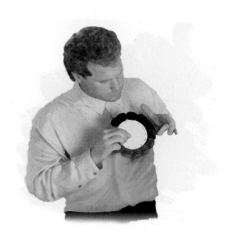

Focus

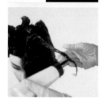

Product Selection—Select the right formula according to the manufacturer's recommendation.

Mixing—Always add the developer first, and then add the color.

Application—Apply the color starting 1/2" (1.25 cm) away from the scalp, and work the color through the shaft to the ends. Do this in all four sections. Set the timer for 20 minutes.

Processing Time—After 20 minutes, apply the color to the base area. Do this in all four sections. Set the timer for an additional 25 minutes. The total processing time is 45 minutes.

Color Removal—Rinse the hair with warm water until the water runs clear. Shampoo, condition, and style.

Color Results and Home Maintenance—Analyze the color result and recommend home maintenance products.

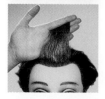

The Base and Shaft—In a virgin application, it is recommended to apply the color 1/2 inch away from the scalp. Because of the heat from the body the color will process quicker so less time is needed after the color is applied to the shaft of the hair. Set a timer for 20 minutes. After the timer goes off, apply the color to the base area. Set the timer for an additional 20 minutes.

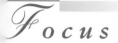

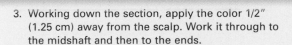

Apply *Permanent Haircolor*

phase 1—virgin applications

The graduated blunt cut will be dramatically transformed with the application of permanent color throughout all of the hair. The deep brunette color will be lightened to a warm red brown.

1. Mix the formula—pour the 4 oz. (120 ml) of 20 volume developer in first, then add the color, 2 oz. (60 ml) of 12, Lightest Golden Blonde.

2. Divide the hair into four sections—from ear to ear, and straight down the back of the head. Take a 1/2" (1.25 cm) subsection beginning in the top area of the head, apply the product 1/2" (1.25 cm) away from the scalp, and work the product down to the ends.

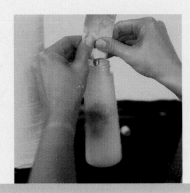

3. Working down the section, apply the color 1/2" (1.25 cm) away from the scalp. Work it through to the midshaft and then to the ends.

4. Continue around the head with the same application technique. Note how the tip of the applicator bottle is multi-purpose in that it neatly parts out the 1/2" (1.25 cm) sections, then dispenses the product on the hair, as well as spreads the product along the length of hair.

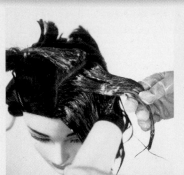
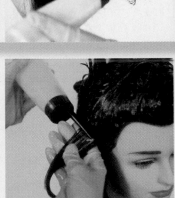

5. For illustrative purposes, a bowl and brush will be used to apply through the back area of the head. Mix the formula following the manufacturer's directions.

6. Apply the color to the back of the head taking 1/2" (1.25 cm) subsections, and applying 1/2" (1.25 cm) away from the scalp.

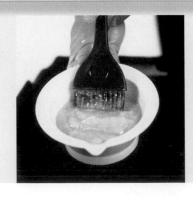
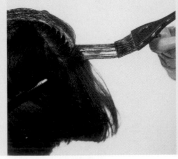

. 7. Work precisely and quickly through each section. Use the brush and the fingers to work the color formula into the hair.

8. Next, complete the fourth quadrant.

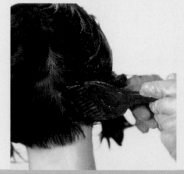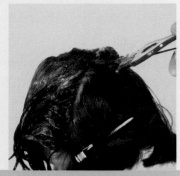

9. Continue the application process down to the nape hairline area. Where lengths are extremely short in this area, work color throughout.

10. Set the timer for 25 minutes.

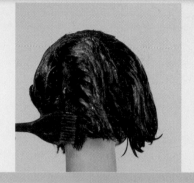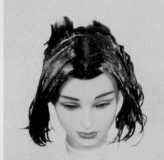

11. Apply the color to the base area in all four sections. Outline the quadrants first.

12. Take 1/2" (1.25 cm) subsections, working through each one until the head is completed. Work neatly and efficiently, dispense color along the base area then work in with the applicator bottle tip. Part out each new parting and dispense the color along the upper part of the parting as shown. Make sure to apply enough color as to thoroughly saturate the hair, including around the front hairline.

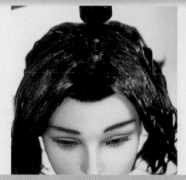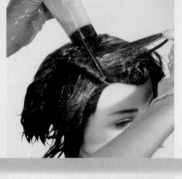

13. Work through the interior of the back quadrants using the brush method introduced earlier.

14. Set the timer for an additional 20 minutes. The total processing time is 45 minutes.

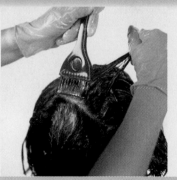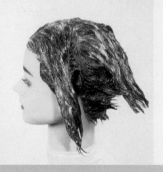

15. This permanent color change lightens brunette hair to a warmer brown with soft red tones.

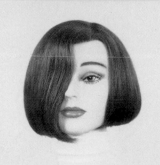

Apply this technique to different lengths, colors, and cuts for almost endless possibilities.

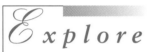

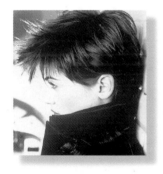

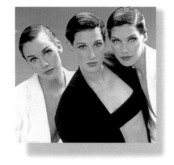

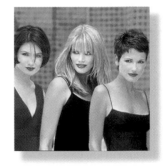

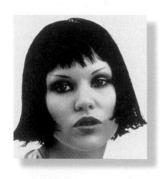

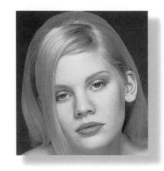

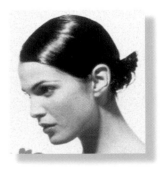

single-process
virgin redhead application

1. Greet the client by introducing yourself.

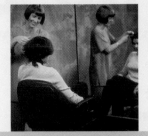
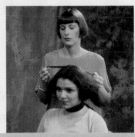

2. Discuss the type of haircolor the client is looking for. Mix 1 oz. (30 ml) 3RV Medium Red-Violet Brown and 1 oz. (30 ml) 4RO Light Red-Orange Brown and 2 oz. (60 ml) 20 volume developer.

3. Using the tip of an applicator bottle, divide the hair into four sections.

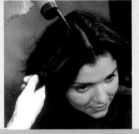
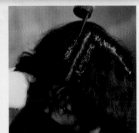

4. Apply the color 1/2" (1.25 cm) away from the scalp to outline the four sections.

5. Start at the right front section and apply the color 1/2" (1.25 cm) away from the scalp. It is a good idea to always start the application in the front sections of the head, to obtain maximum coverage through the front areas.

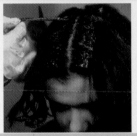
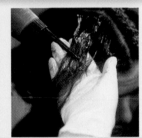

6. Take 1/2" (1.25 cm) subsections and continue applying color 1/2" (1.25 cm) from the scalp area down the hair strand.

7. Develop a rhythm of speed in working as to get the product on the entire head as quickly as possible. Thoroughly saturate each section of hair for thorough coverage.

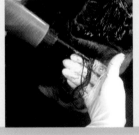
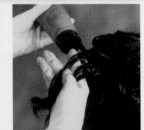

8. Continue around the head until all four sections are complete.

9. Set the timer for 25 minutes. Next, apply color to the base area. Work around the outline first, then work into the interior of each section.

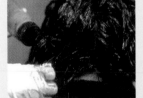
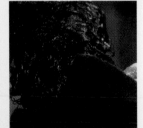

10. Continue applying color to the base area around the entire head. Work the color through the hair and set the timer for 20 minutes. Rinse. Shampoo and condition. Style and finish hair.

11. Check the color, record the color formula and recommend home maintenance.

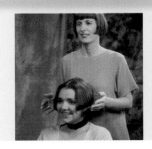
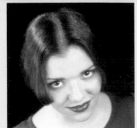

12. This finished look is a vivid high-fashion red.

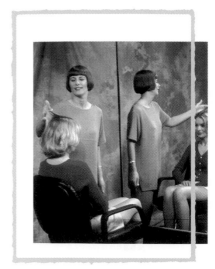

Permanent Haircolor

Overview

Once a client has had a color application, her next visit will involve retouch. This means you'll use permanent haircolor only to lighten t new growth at the scalp area. To refresh the ends, you'll formulate a non-ammonia color that adds shine and tone to the hair without lightening. This technique is proven to keep the hair in the best condition with minimal fading—because you don't use permanent color, which has ammonia, down the shaft and ends of the hair.

You've already learned how to use non-ammonia color and permanent haircolor products. Now you'll use them both on the sam head. This is called a single process with a retouch glaze. It is the most sophisticated way to use permanent color. .In a retouch application, you apply permanent color only to the new growth of th hair,. Formulate the color referring to the color chart. The color generally needs to process for 45 minutes. After rinsing and towel drying, the glaze will be applied through the lengths.

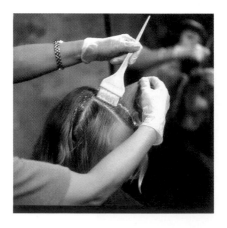
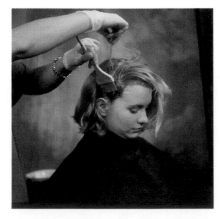

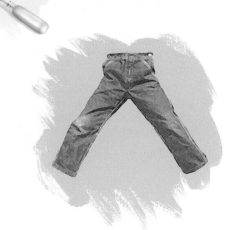

Connect

Base Area and Hair Shaft

Treat the base and shaft areas differently once the hair has been lightened with a permanent color. Permanent color should be applied to the base area only.

Fading

Once the hair has been lightened with permanent color, the permanent color should not be pulled through the ends again. This can cause fading.

Focus

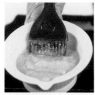

Mixing—Add the color to the developer, then mix.

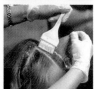

Application—Apply the permanent color to the new growth of the hair only. Use fine, even sections to make sure the hair is saturated.

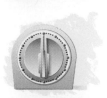

Processing Time—Set the timer for 45 minutes once the application is complete.

Formulation of Non-ammonia Glaze—When the timer goes off, check color development at the base area. Formulate a non-ammonia color. Sometimes this is referred to as a glaze. Remember, when matching the ends to the new color at the regrowth, always formulate the non-ammonia color at least two levels lighter because, these products deposit only. Work within the same tonal families for the best result.

Color Removal—Rinse the color from the base area. Towel dry. Apply the non-ammonia color to the hair. Set the timer for ten minutes to refresh the color through mid-shaft and ends.

Color Results and Home Maintenance—Check the color results and recommend home maintenance products. Schedule another appointment in four weeks.

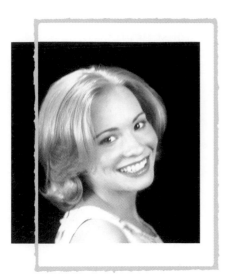

Apply
Single Process Retouch with a Glaze

1. Greet your client by introducing yourself. In consultation, discuss the haircolor result she's looking for. Mix the formula. Apply a high lift blonde formula at the retouch area first—2 oz. (60 ml) of 12G, Lightest Golden Blonde, and 4 oz. (120 ml) of 40 volume developer.

2. Using a color brush, begin by outlining all four sections of the regrowth. Then apply color to the regrowth area within each quadrant.

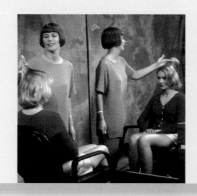

3. Starting at the front right section, apply the color with the color brush to the new growth at the base area.

4. Continue working down the right side, taking 1/4" (.625 cm) subsections and applying the color to the new growth.

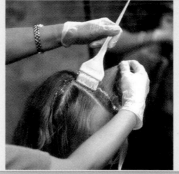

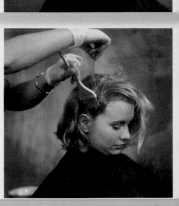

5. Continue around the head taking fine even sections.

6. Complete all four sides. Set the timer for 45 minutes. Rinse the color thoroughly.

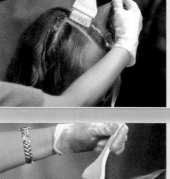

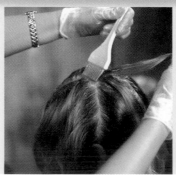

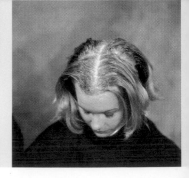

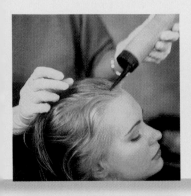

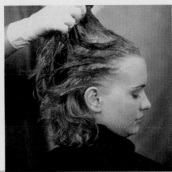

7. Mix the glaze—1 1/2 oz. (45 ml) 10 RO, Red-orange Blonde, and 1/2 oz. (15 ml) 8G, Light Golden Blonde, with 2 oz. (60 ml) of demi-permanent developer. Now it is time to apply the non-ammonia haircolor glaze. Start at the front hairline.

8. Apply the glaze in a base-to-ends fashion, moving it through the hair quickly. Set timer for up to 15 minutes. Rinse. Shampoo and condition.

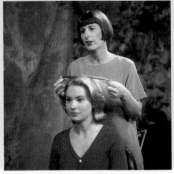

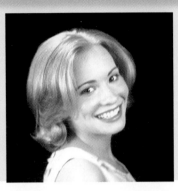

9. Check haircolor results, and recommend home maintenance to your client.

10. Here's the finished look: a light warm blonde color that is even from the base to ends, with lots of vibrant shine.

I like color to seduce and enchant people.

Jo Blackwell

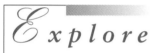

Reflect

Explore

Apply this technique to different lengths, colors, and cuts for almost endless possibilities.

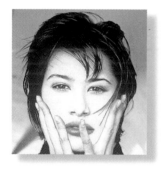

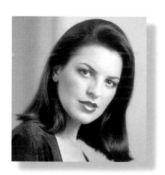

Clue #1

Set Personal and Professional Boundaries

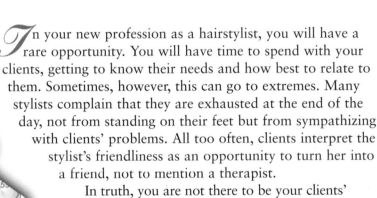

*I*n your new profession as a hairstylist, you will have a rare opportunity. You will have time to spend with your clients, getting to know their needs and how best to relate to them. Sometimes, however, this can go to extremes. Many stylists complain that they are exhausted at the end of the day, not from standing on their feet but from sympathizing with clients' problems. All too often, clients interpret the stylist's friendliness as an opportunity to turn her into a friend, not to mention a therapist.

In truth, you are not there to be your clients' friend. You're there to be a friendly, helpful professional. There are other people they can turn to for advice on relationships and problems. You want to be the one person they turn to for style and image advice.

Setting and maintaining boundaries is good for you as well as your clients. To learn how to do this, try a visualization technique. Visualize the salon as a place on a map, with lines drawn around it, and label it "Professional Me." Visualize everything outside of the salon as a totally separate place—a country called "Personal Me." Pretend the citizens of these two different countries speak different languages and have different customs; when you step across the line from one to the other, you use the language and observe the customs of the place you're in.

When clients begin to talk about their personal lives, listen actively and pay attention, but refrain from giving your opinion. Some clients love to gossip. Don't get drawn into that trap!

And just like a good doctor or lawyer is supposed to do, don't reveal information about one client to another. Such practices will destroy your reputation.

Whenever you begin to sense that boundaries between the personal and the professional are getting crossed, learn to step back and politely draw the boundaries again. Your clients have other friends. They should have only one top-notch, friendly—but completely professional—hairstylist.

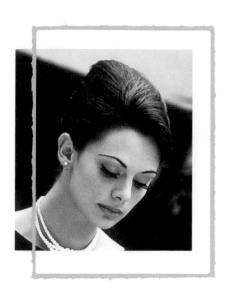

Permanent Haircolor

phase 3—covering gray

Overview

Gray hair is still the number one reason why people color their hair. To cover gray completely, your best choice is a permanent haircolor—but there are different ways to change gray hair to suit the client. Understanding the difference between blending and coverage is key to a successful consultation. When a client sees that he's faced with a few gray hairs, he usually wants to get rid of them. He'll say things like, "Can I try a color?" or, "Can I make the gray hair look highlighted?" This is when you reach for a non-ammonia color to blend the gray. This type of color service has a more sheer result, and it will also wash out faster, so it is less permanent. Once the client starts seeing more than just a few gray hairs, though, he's usually looking to get rid of them completely. Now you should reach for a permanent color to cover the gray.

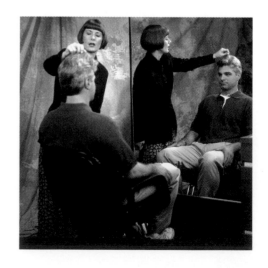

488

Connect

Pigmented versus Non-Pigmented Hair

Some people have more gray than others. The less gray your client has, the more you should consider blending. The more gray hair he has, the more you should consider covering.

Gray Hair Takes Color Differently than Pigmented Hair

Gray or white hair takes on the exact level and tone of the color that you apply; if you apply a bright red haircolor to white hair, it will come out bright red. And you already know that permanent color lightens pigmented hair. So when you are working on hair that is a combination of pigmented and gray, remember that the two types will take the color differently. The rule in formulation is to stay within two levels of the natural color. If you are creating reds, you must add some neutral to the formula to soften the red on the gray hair. Start with 1 oz. (30ml) of neutral mixed with 1 oz. (30ml.) of a red.

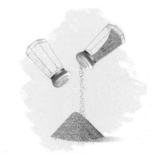
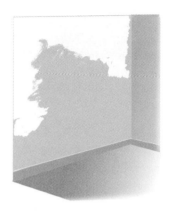

Focus

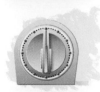 **Product Selection**—Select the color and mix with 20 volume developer. 20 volume is used most often for gray coverage.

 Application—Take fine, even sections to make sure that the gray is covered.

 Processing Time—The standard processing time for gray coverage is 45 minutes.

 Color Removal—Rinse the color. Shampoo and condition.

 Color Results and Home Maintenance—Check the color results and recommend home maintenance. Schedule the client's next appointment.

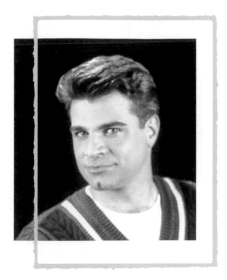

$\mathscr{A}pply$
$\mathscr{P}ermanent\ \mathscr{H}aircolor$
phase 3—covering gray

1. Introduce yourself to the client. Discuss the color result that he's looking for. The formula to be used is 1 oz. (30 ml), Dark Natural Blonde and 1 oz. (30 ml) of Light Golden Brown and 2 oz. (60 ml) of 20 volume developer.

2. Start the application down the front center part. Apply the color to the base area only.

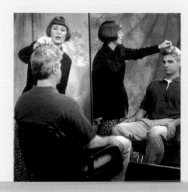
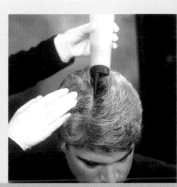

3. Part out 1/4" (.625 cm) subsections and apply the color to the root area.

4. Continue around the head using 1/4" (.625 cm) subsections.

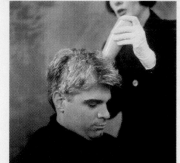
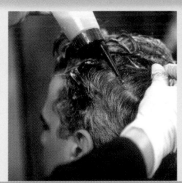

5. Once all four sections are complete, work the rest of the color through to the ends. Process the color for 45 minutes.

6. Record all formulas and recommend specific shampoos and conditioners for color-treated hair. Notice how one simple formula can make a client look more youthful!

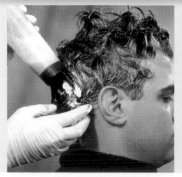
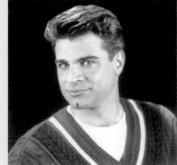

$\mathscr{R}$*eflect*

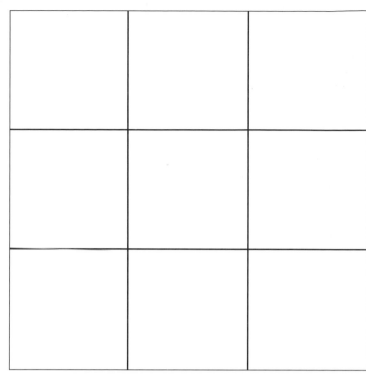

$\mathscr{E}$*xplore*

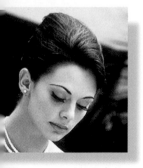

Apply this technique to different lengths, colors, and cuts for almost endless possibilities.

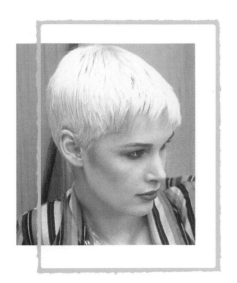

Double-Process Blonding

Overview

There are different ways to make people blonde. To create the lighte[...] blonde all over the head, especially on clients who have dark hair to[...] start with, a double-process is best. This involves two steps: lightening the hair, and then toning the hair.

In this segment you'll learn to identify how lighteners react on t[...] hair. In addition, once the hair has been lightened, it must be toned.[...]

In this lightening process, you'll first remove all natural pigment[...] from the hair with an on-the-scalp lightener. This haircolor service i[...] for the client who wants to be the blondest she can be.

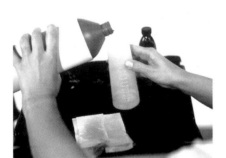

Connect

Understanding Lighteners

Lighteners remove natural and artificial pigment from the hair. They are mixed differently from regular haircolor products.

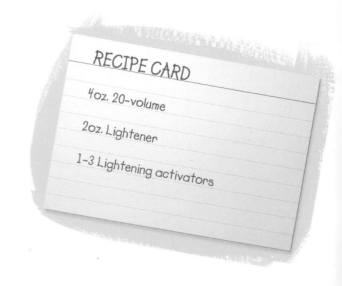

RECIPE CARD

4oz. 20-volume

2oz. Lightener

1-3 Lightening activators

e hair passes through different stages of lift as a
htener works on the hair fiber. Most double-
cess colors are processed to yellow or pale
llow—the lightest blonde result. Lighteners gener-
y process for 60 to 90 minutes.

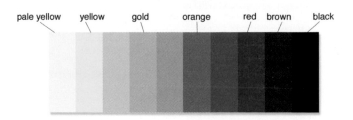

pale yellow   yellow   gold   orange   red   brown   black

*F*ocus

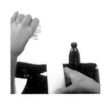

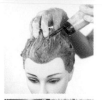
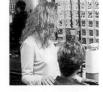

Mixing the Lightener—Pour 4 oz. (120 ml) of 20-volume developer into an applicator bottle. Add the lightening activators. Shake. Add 2 oz. (60 ml) of lightener.

Sectioning and Application—When you're applying lightener to a virgin head, it is important to stay 1/2" (1.25 cm) away from the scalp. An option to ensure this is to place strips of cotton in between each subsection, so the lightener doesn't bleed onto the scalp. After all four quadrants are complete, set a timer for 25 minutes.

Removing Cotton—After the shaft of the hair starts to reach the desired lightness, remove the strips of cotton. Now apply the lightener to the base area in all four quadrants. Once all quadrants are complete, go over the entire head and check for spots that you missed.

Proper Degree of Lightness—See if the hair is light enough. Most double-process blondings take at least 60 minutes to lighten. Generally, you want the haircolor to look like the inside of a lemon peel. If too much warmth—orange or gold—is left in the hair, the toner formula will not produce the proper result.

Lightener Removal—Rinse the lightener with warm water. Make sure you remove all of the product from the hair. Give one light shampoo. Do not use manipulations; the toner process still has to take place. Sometimes clients scalps become sensitive after their hair has been lightened.

Toner Mixing, Application and Processing—Select toner to deposit color onto the lightened hair. Most toner shades are available in very light delicate shades. The key is to apply the toner quickly to the hair. First, apply it to the base area in all four quadrants. Set timer for five minutes; after this, bring the lightener through to the ends. Toners usually process in ten minutes or less.

Color Results and Home Maintenance—Check the color and recommend home maintenance products. Schedule the client's next appointment in three to four weeks.

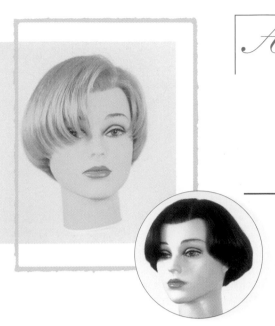

Apply Double-Process Blonding

1. Pour 4 oz. (120 ml) of 20-volume peroxide into a bottle.

2. Add up to three lightening activators, also called catalysts.

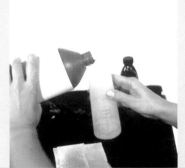 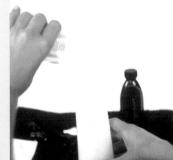

3. Shake gently until mixed.

4. Add 2 oz. (60 ml) of liquid lightener.

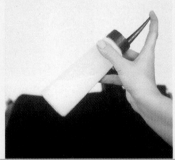 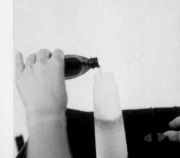

5. Place cotton in all four quadrants to protect the scalp. This is an option that may be used.

6. Starting in the left front section, apply lightener 1/4" (.625 cm) away from the scalp. Work it down through to the ends with the gloved hand.

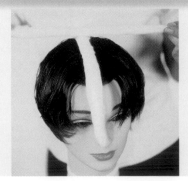 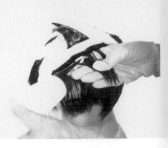

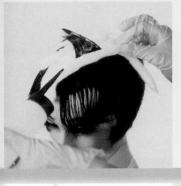

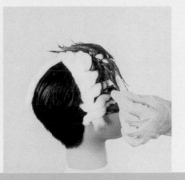

7. Place a strip of cotton in between each section so that no lightener bleeds onto the hair nearest the scalp.

8. Take 1/4" (.625 cm) sections and work until the side is complete.

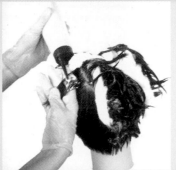

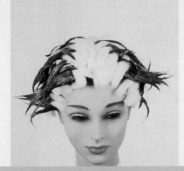

9. Through the back, the technique of application will be shown without cotton strips. Continue 1/4" (.625 cm) sections starting 1/2" (1.25 cm) away from the scalp, work the lightener down the ends.

10. Complete all four sections, and set the timer for 25 minutes.

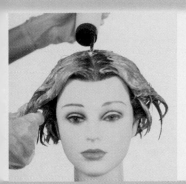

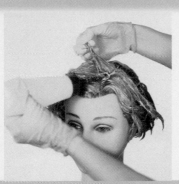

11. After the 25 minutes are up, remove the cotton. Start applying the lightener to the base area.

12. Continue to apply the lightener to the base area within the interior area of all sections.

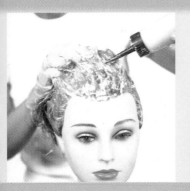

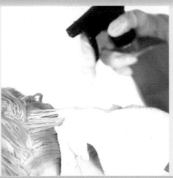

13. After all the sections are complete, work the rest of the lightener through the hair so it is completely saturated. Set the timer for 30 minutes.

14. Do a strand test to check for desired lightness. Place a strand on a white towel—spray with a water bottle and remove the lightener. When complete, rinse and shampoo. Now, you are ready to apply the toner.

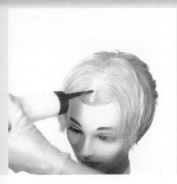

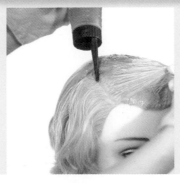

15. Lightened hair should be handled delicately. Towel dry the hair thoroughly. Be gentle to the hair as you divide it into four quadrants. Begin outlining with the toner mixture—2 oz. (60ml) 8N Light Neutral Blonde and 2 oz. (60 ml) of demi-permanent developer. Hair that has just been lightened is fragile.

16. Starting at the front, apply the toner to the base area.

17. Continue moving quickly around the head.

18. Set the timer for five minutes.

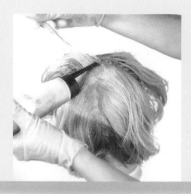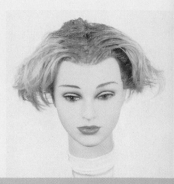

19. After the five minutes are up, start working the remainder of the toner down to the ends.

20. Let the toner process for another five to ten minutes. Strand test to see if the color result is there.

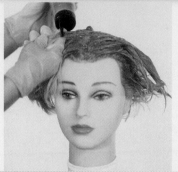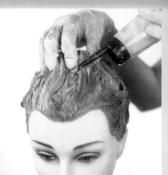

21. What a dramatic transformation—from the Level 3 (Dark Brown) to this dramatic blonde tone! Here's the clarity you can create with a double-process blonding.

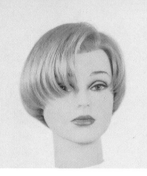

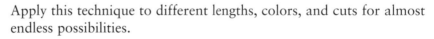

Apply this technique to different lengths, colors, and cuts for almost endless possibilities.

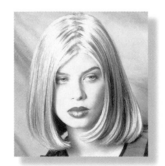

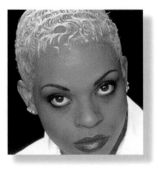

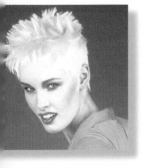

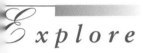

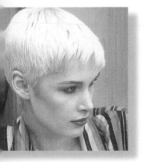

Lose
the You

A simple communication technique that can greatly improve your relationships with clients, co-workers, supervisors, teachers, and friends is to break the habit of starting your sentences with the word "you." "You messages," as they are called, are the spoken equivalent of pointing your finger at someone while you talk (another communication no-no).

Sentences that begin with the word "you" put the other person on her guard; she feels she's being blamed for doing something wrong and, as a result, she becomes defensive. When this happens, good communication doesn't. Try turning the "you" into an "I" (and sometimes a "we") and see how much better you get along with others in all areas of your life. For example:

NOT THIS: "You really shouldn't have used that color on her.

THIS: "I think this product would have worked better. I can reapply a color if you would like."

NOT THIS: "You don't know what you're talking about!"

THIS: "I disagree, but I'm willing to compromise. Can we work this out?"

NOT THIS: "You weren't supposed to do it that way!"

THIS: "I wish you had tried doing it the way we originally discussed."

NOT THIS: "You asked for this color!"

THIS: "I thought this was the color we agreed upon."

NOT THIS: "You are late again!"

THIS: "Didn't we agree that you would come to work on time?"

Remember, never use a "you" when an "I" (or a "we") will do.

Dealing with Difficult People

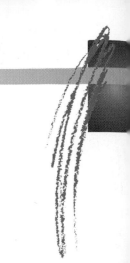

The pessimist sees difficulty in every opportunity: the optimist, the opportunity in every difficulty.

J.P. Jacks

Wherever you go in life, there will be difficult people, and the salon is no exception. You may have cranky, hard to please clients. You might find your station next to that of a co-worker who has made it his mission in life to make other people miserable. Your boss may seem to have two personalities: one for the clients and the other for the employees.

This happens everywhere. It doesn't have to ruin your life or take away your enjoyment of work, however, if you remember one simple rule: Don't take it personally. Often, people are cranky and hard to please because of other problems in their lives. They just happen to direct their misery at whomever is handy.

Another thing to keep in mind is that many of your clients may be in positions of authority in their own work. They demand excellence from their staffs—and expect to receive it. They don't turn that personality trait off when it comes to how they look. As their stylist, you become one of the people they pay to give them what they want.

You do not have the power to change anyone—except yourself. You can choose to deal with difficult people in a way that makes life more pleasant. All it takes is a little understanding on your part. As you work with people, try to become a "student" of personalities and communication styles. When someone comes across in a way that seems offensive or critical, don't react by becoming defensive. Stop for a minute. Think about what you know about communication. Try to figure out what is making this person "tick." And then use your professional language and manners to help you get over this "communication challenge."

Every communication challenge can be turned into an opportunity–an opportunity to make a customer happy and keep coming back. With each challenge you face successfully, you become a more competent, professional, in-demand, and successful hairstylist.

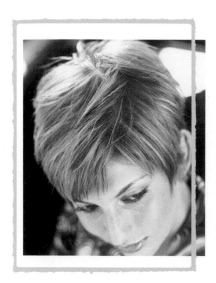

Dimensional Haircolor Services

Overview

Dimensional haircolor services—better known as highlighting—is one of the fastest-growing haircolor markets. This is where your creativity is endless. Here, you will learn some of the most popular techniques that are done in the salon today. We will focus on four different foil wrapping methods: face frame highlight, half-head highlight, three-quarter head highlight, and full head highlight. Foiling is the professional choice for highlighting the hair. It provides tremendous control in the application, and creates precision results. The specific application process may be recorded to ensure that you may reproduce results with the client's next visit.

Connect

Foiling

The foil technique involves weaving out (selecting) alternating strands from a sub-section. The selected strands are then placed over foil or plastic wrap, and the appropriate lightner is applied. The foil is folded to prevent lifting any unwoven hair. With this technique, the colorist can strategically place highlights. Foiling hair is like building a puzzle. Every section and every placement is important to the result. Putting this puzzle together the next time the client visits requires the use of a systematic process of application that is recorded thoroughly.

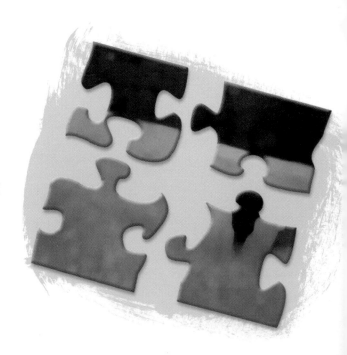

Sectioning, Slicing, and Weaving

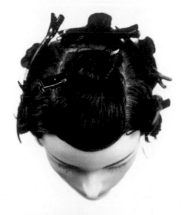

Placing foil in the hair is an art. It takes practice and discipline. To make it easier, start by working on creating clean section blocks on the head. Once you have perfected this, you will know the difference between a slice parting and a weave parting. The next step is to create different subsections in between the slices or weaves, to create a certain look. The difference between slicing and weaving is minute, but the end result can vary greatly. The end result of any method of highlighting depends on the size of the strand and the degree to which it is lightened. Slicing involves releasing a narrow section (1/8", .33cm) of hair by making a straight part at the scalp. To weave use a fine-tail comb and make a zigzag part to release a narrow section of hair. Hold the section, isolating only the upper points of the zigzag. The width of the section to be colored depends on the desired effect.

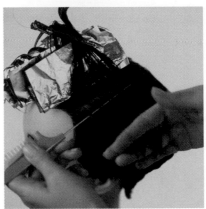

Product Formulation

All foil work in this section of the program was done with powder or gel lightener: 4 scoops of powder lightener mixed with 2 oz. (60 ml) of volume developer. This is for a half head to full head highlight—mix new product as needed on full head highlights as to keep the product fresh. Be guided by your instructor and follow the manufacturer's directions in mixing product for highlighting face-frame highlights or partial areas.

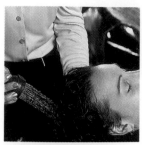

Wet Hair—All the highlights are done on damp hair, which is easier to work on. Wet the client down at the sink. Apply a leave-in conditioner, and detangle the hair. You are now ready to begin.

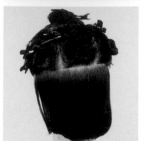

Sectioning—Practice parting out clean sections. Practicing these sectioning techniques will strengthen your placement patterns.

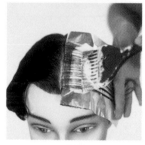

Applying—Apply the product with a brush, using very little pressure on the foil.

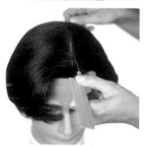

Highlights—When you are doing a face-frame highlight, part the hair down the center and work off the middle part. This technique will softly frame the face with highlights.

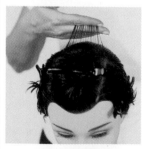

Half-Head—When you're doing a half-head, block off the three sections around the front area of the head surrounding the face: the top, and two sides.

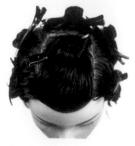

Three-quarter-head—Review the blocking for a three-quarter-head. This area covers the entire head down to the occipital bone.

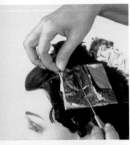

Book End Wrap—Practice a book end wrap. Refer to "Three-Quarter-Head Highlight" for more detail.

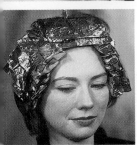

Full-Head—On a full-head highlight, place foils in all six sections down to the nape area—the bottom of the hairline.

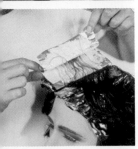

Remove Foils—Check the foils to see if you've achieved the desired lightness. Remove foils one at a time. Rinse the hair. It is very important to remove the foils at the shampoo area as to immediately rinse. This will prevent color from affecting surrounding unfoiled hair.

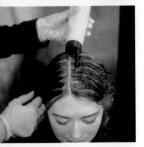

Finishing the Color Service—Having used a lightener to highlight, finish the highlight with a non-ammonia glaze to add tone and shine in one easy step. This step would not be necessary if a high lift permanent haircolor was used to create the highlights.

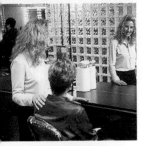

Check Color Results—Ensure that your client is happy with her highlight. Recommend the proper home maintenance products. Schedule her next appointment. Highlights are generally done every three months, or four times a year. If a client had a full-head highlight, her next visit should be for a half-head. This is an economic solution for your client.

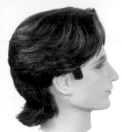

Face-Frame Highlights—Creating soft highlights that frame the face is a great way to introduce a client to highlight services.

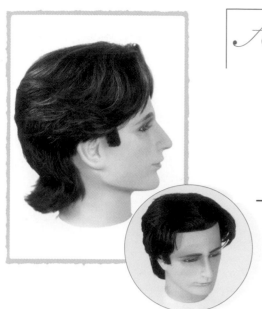

Apply Face Frame Highlight

1. With a tail or foil-tip comb, part the hair from ear to ear, with a part going down the center.

2. Starting at the center part, part out 1/8" (.33 cm) slice with the tail end of your comb.

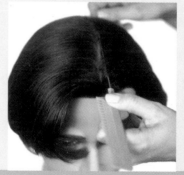
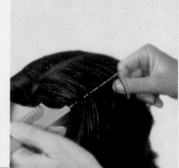

3. While holding the slice of hair, pick up a piece of foil. Fold the end of the comb under the foil and place it at the scalp.

4. Lay the hair on top of the foil, getting as close to the scalp as possible.

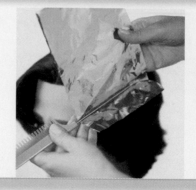
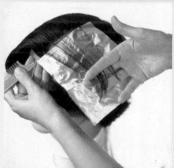

5. Slide the comb out from underneath. Hold hair taut to the foil.

6. Brush on lightener starting 1/2" (1.25 cm) away from the top of the foil and working the product down the strand. Once the product adheres to the hair in the foil, work it up to the top of the foil.

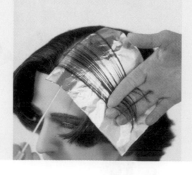
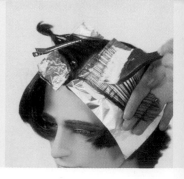

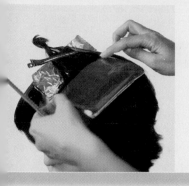 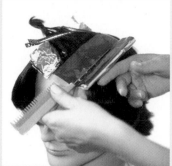

7. Fold the foil in half to meet the piece at the top.

8. With the metal end of your comb, crease the center of the foil.

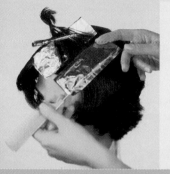 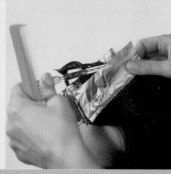

9. Fold the foil again and slide the metal end of your comb out.

10. Clip the foil up and out of the way.

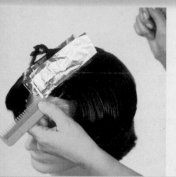 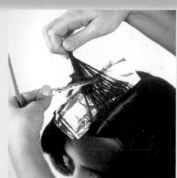

11. Part out 1/2" (1.25 cm) subsections of hair in between each foiled slice.

12. Clip each foil section up and out of the way.

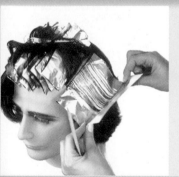 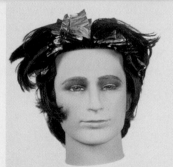

13. Continue working down the side in the same way. The foils on the side will go to the temple area. Once one side is complete, move to the other.

14. Here, all the foils are in.

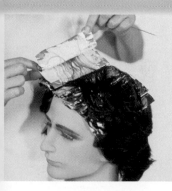 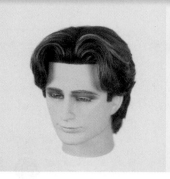

15. Open a foil to see if the color has reached the desired lightness. When complete, rinse thoroughly then shampoo and condition. Apply a glaze if desired

16. Notice how this service adds a subtle amount of dimension that frames the face.

Constructively

> *I can take any amount of criticism, so long as it is unqualified praise*
>
> *Noel Coward*

While we all know how hard it can be to deal with difficult people and their criticism, it's important to mention that there's a right way to give criticism, too. When you criticize carefully and constructively, taking the other person's feelings into account, you can actually accomplish something more than just making her mad.

It won't be long before you move up the salon ladder and someone else will be relying on you for training and guidance. When you're helping another person become a good stylist—or giving criticism for any other reason—try to remember what it was like to be on the receiving end of criticism, and do your best to communicate in a way that will help build the other person up rather than tear her down.

Follow these simple rules for criticizing constructively and fairly:

1. **Remember to keep the blaming, judging "you" out of your statements. Say "I think" rather than "you should."**
2. **Criticize the behavior or action, not the person. Someone who does something foolishly is not necessarily a fool.**
3. **Wait until you are alone with a person to discuss your criticism of her.**
4. **Try not to deliver criticism in the presence of others.**
5. **Do not criticize someone behind her back to a third party. This is cowardly and inappropriate.**
6. **Suggest workable solutions to the problem you are pointing out, and set a timeline for follow-up.**

For example:

SALON MANAGER TO STYLIST: "James, please come see me in my office when you've finished."

STYLIST, appearing in manager's office: "You wanted to see me, Anne?"

ANNE (looking up, smiling in a reassuring way, making eye contact): "Yes, James, please come in and have a seat."

JAMES: "What's up?"

ANNE: "Well, a lot of things, James. I'm very pleased with your progress. You're averaging two more clients each week and the work you're doing is very good. I have just one concern."

JAMES: "What is that?"

ANNE: "I noticed that when you've finished with your clients, you're letting them go to the desk to pay without your help. Remember that we discussed how important it is to stay with the clients after the service, making sure they understand what products you've recommended they use at home, and helping them reschedule their next appointment? It's worth the extra five minutes it takes, James. The stylists who follow through with clients have, on average, 50 percent higher rebooking rates and earn 25 percent more in retail commissions."

JAMES: "I know. I guess I was just getting caught up in making sure my station was clean and the hair was swept up."

ANNE: "Those are important jobs, James, but so is this. How about if I give you some help? Let's say I ask Melissa, our new assistant, to help you with station sweeping and cleanup for just one week so that you can make sure you see each client through to the door. After all, you're the only one who knows what you recommended for a home care regimen and future styling plans. When you see the results in your rebooking and retailing, I'm sure you'll agree that both are important ways of cleaning up.

JAMES (laughing at the pun): "Okay, I get the point. Are you sure I couldn't have an assistant to sweep up after me all the time?"

ANNE (smiling): "Now, James, do you want all the other stylists to hate you? No, I'm just giving you this extra help for one week so that you can concentrate on your client follow-up. Besides, when you get your income up as high as I think it could be, you can hire your own private assistant if you'd like."

JAMES: "Never mind. I'll take the week."

ANNE: "It's a deal. Let's schedule a meeting for one week from today to see how it's going. Say five o'clock? We'll go next door to the coffee shop, okay?"

JAMES: "Okay. Thanks for your time, Anne. I'll work on this."

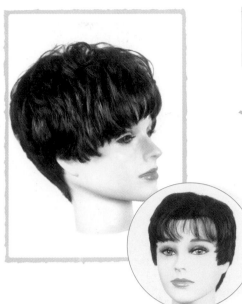

In this service, you highlight the top and sides of the head.

1. Block off sections. The three main sections are the top and the sides. Take a fine 1/8" (.33 cm) slice starting at the crown of the head.

2. While holding the slice of hair, pick up a piece of foil. Fold the end of the comb under the foil and place it at the scalp.

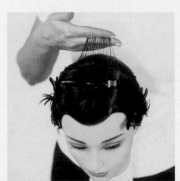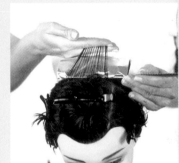

3. Brush on lightener starting 1/2" (1.25 cm) away from the top of the foil, working the product down the strand. Double fold the foil.

4. Release the next 1/2" (1.25cm) section and clipout of the way Continue working toward the front of the head.

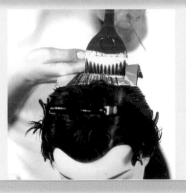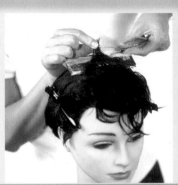

5. To create a chunky look toward the front, take the metal end of your comb and weave it back and forth through the strand.

6. Slide your comb from underneath the foil. Notice the hair in the foil.

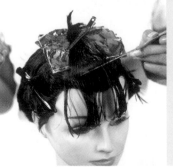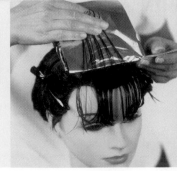

7. Apply the product to the hair.

8. Bend the foil once over the hair, and then fold the foil again. Fold the foil and clip it out of the way.

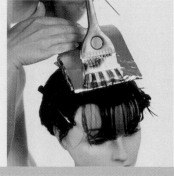
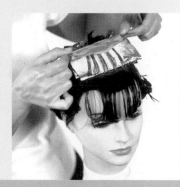

9. Part out approximately a 1/2" (1.25 cm) section to leave unfoiled, then part out a 1/8" (.33 cm) section for the next foil. Complete up to the front hairline.

10. The top of the head is complete. It is now time to do the sides.

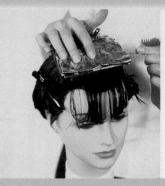
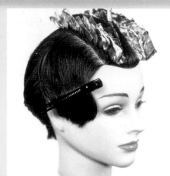

11. Take a fine 1/8" (.33 cm) slice at the top section of the right side.

12. After placing the foil, apply the product, working down the entire strand.

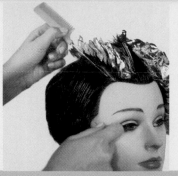
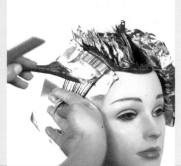

13. Clip the foil up and out of the way. Clip a section out of the way to go unlightened between each foil.

14. Complete both sides.

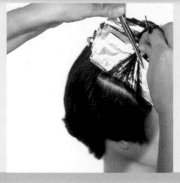
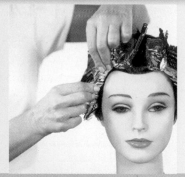

15. This half-head technique covers the entire front portion of the head.

16. This haircolor technique adds dimension that covers a fairly wide surface of the head.

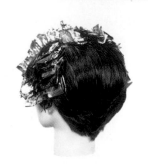
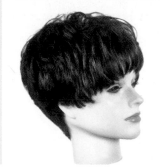

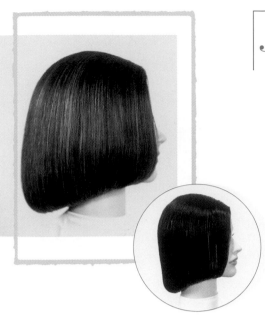

Apply Three-quarter Head Highlight

In this service, you'll provide highlights over the entire head, all t[...] way down to the occipital bone in the back.

1. After blocking off the head into six sections or panels. Start at the center back crown area. Part out a fine slice, place the foil as shown, apply the lightener. Enclose the hair with a double fold method.

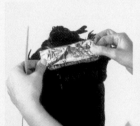
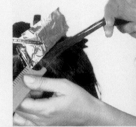

2. Take a 1/2" (1.25 cm) subsection between each foil. Clip this section up and out of the way.

3. Continue placing the foils down to the occipital bone using the procedure as outlined. Upon completion release all of the clipped up foils. Turn the edges of the foil on either side.

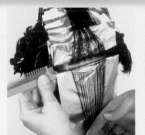
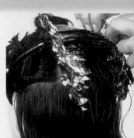

4. Here's the completed back section.

5. Move to a side section. You'll place these foils with a book end method. Take a fine slice. Place hair in the center third of the foil.

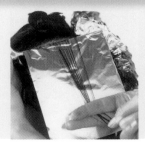
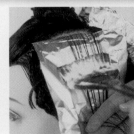

6. Apply the product to the hair in the foil.

7. Fold the foil in half until the ends meet.

8. Fold the right side of the foil in halfway, using your comb to crease it.

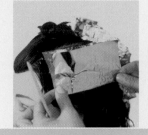 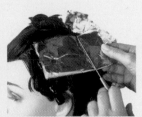

9. Fold the left side of the foil in halfway.

10. Clip the foil upward. Notice the book wrap effect.

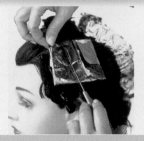 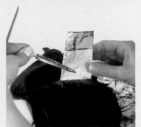

11. Take a 1/2" (1.25 cm) subsection in between the foils.

12. Clip the hair up and out of the way. Continue working down the back side until you reach the occipital area. Complete this section on the opposite side.

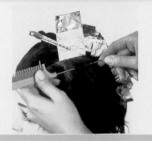 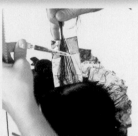

13. Move to the front sections and continue foiling. Use the same technique as outlined.

14. After completing both sides, continue wrapping the top portion of the head, taking a 1/2" (1.25 cm) subsection in between the foils. Alternate the process of fine slices with 1/2" (1.25 cm) left unfoiled.

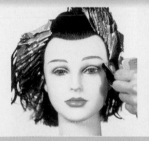 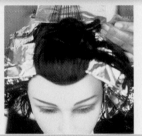

15. Finish the last foil at the hairline. Fold the sides of the foil up on each side to secure them in place.

16. This finished look gives a very desirable and natural dimensional effect throughout, accentuated further by the unlightened nape area. Apply a toner to create a harmonious blend of highlights to natural hair.

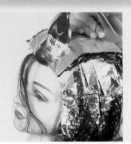 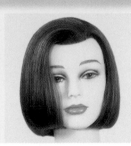

*Y*ou're nearing the end of a great client visit. As you complete the final design now, remember to stay focused on your goals and objectives with this client. Restate the decisions the two of you made earlier, and point out how you've achieved them.

For example:

STYLIST: "Here, take the mirror and look at the back of your hair. See how nicely it is shaped? We haven't shortened it all that much, but isn't it nice how it blends from around your face to the back? I think this is a much more flattering look for you, ar oh, the color really brightens you up!"

CLIENT: "You were right. I'm really happy with it. just hope I can take care of it properly at home."

(Aha! A gift! The client gives you your opening . . so go for it!)

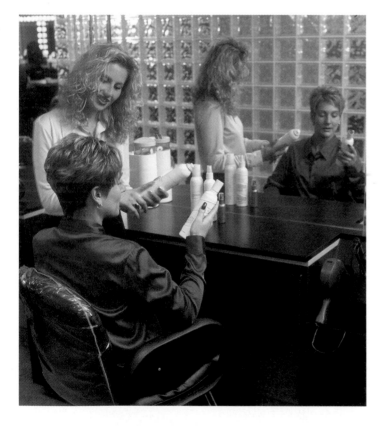

STYLIST: "Of course you can. Remember how I showed you the round brush technique? Do you have one of those at home? Don't worry, we're having a special on all our hair tools this week—you can get a great one right here at half off. Also, remember that I told you what shampoo would help the color last? Here, let me write these down for you."
"And you'll want to use this texturizing styling spray when you're blowing it dry and using the brush. See, like this. You jus come with me and I'll get you all set up."

CLIENT: "Okay, lead the way."

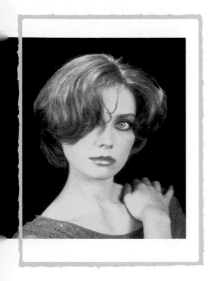

Apply
Full-Head Highlight

Highlights all over the head give the brightest look to a client.

1. Consult with your client on her haircoloring wishes.

2. Take a slice of hair at the lower crown area of the head.

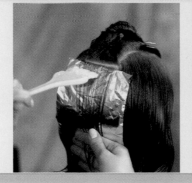
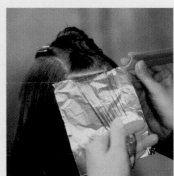

3. Holding the hair taut, brush lightener onto the hair in the foil.

4. Double fold the foil and clip up and out of the way.

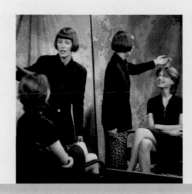
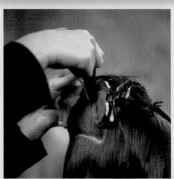

5. Take a 3/4" (1.875 cm) subsection in between the foils.

6. Continue working down the back center of the head until the section is complete. Note the contrast in size between the foiled and unfoiled sections.

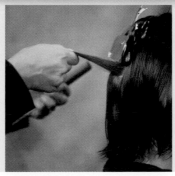
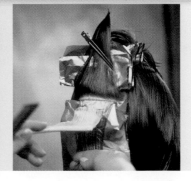

7. Once the section is complete, release the clipped up foil.

8. Working around the head, into the side area, divide the panel into two smaller sections.

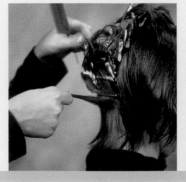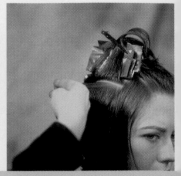

9. Continue working down the side by taking fine slices of hair into the foil. Continue through the center back. Clip everything up and out of the way. When complete, release the foils downward.

10. Move to the other side of the head and complete this same panel.

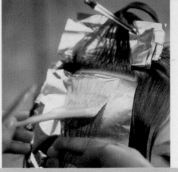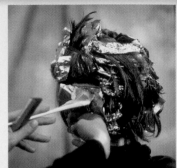

11. Finish the front panels on each side of the head with the same method.

12. Now it's time to do the last section—the top of the head. Take a fine slice of hair off of the top of a larger section and place it onto the foil.

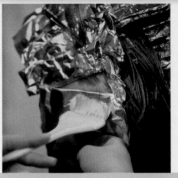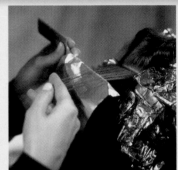

13. Apply the product to the hair.

14. Part out a larger section, then take a fine slice from the top of this section.

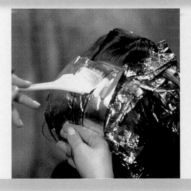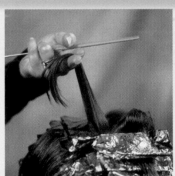

15. Continue to the front until the last foil is placed.

16. In this top view, you can see where the foils were placed. They were processed to a pale yellow. Note the alternation of light and dark.

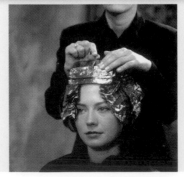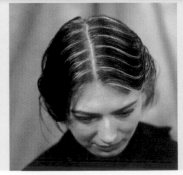

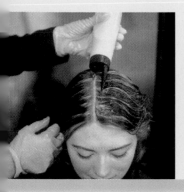

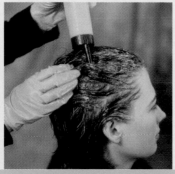

17. Apply haircolor glaze over the highlights. This will add tone and shine to the natural color, and tone the highlights. The target color is an amber light blonde. Mix 1 oz. (30 ml) of 10RO Lightest Red-Orange Blonde with 1 oz. (30 ml) of 10R Lightest Golden Blonde with 2 oz. (60 ml) of demi-permanent developer. Outline all four sections of the head.

18. Apply glaze all over the head in a base-to-ends fashion.

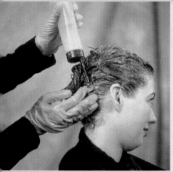

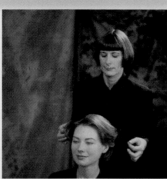

19. Work the color into the hair to make sure it is completely saturated. Process for ten minutes.

20. This finished look shows beautiful golden amber highlights all over the head. Discuss home maintenance.

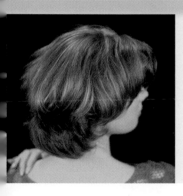

21. The finished look is dynamic, sophisticated, and glamorous. Some of the best color work is the most natural and this understated yet glorious color that accentuates the overall style is a fine example of this.

Reflect

Explore

Apply this technique to different lengths, colors, and cuts for almost endless possibilities.

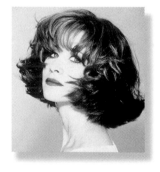

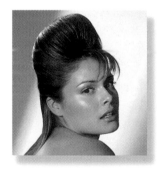

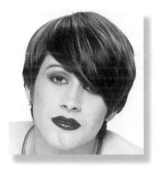

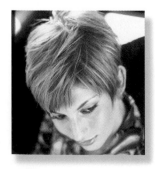

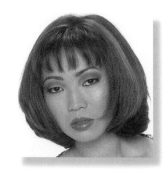

panel highlights

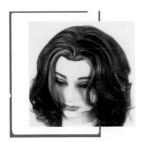

*I*n this service, you'll create a dramatic highlight effect throughout on the top portion of the head, featuring wider bands of highlights.

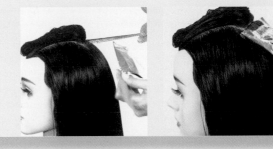

1. Part out the top portion of the head from the middle of the eyebrows. Starting at the crown area, take a fine slice and put it into a foil.

2. Apply the product to the strand and fold the foil.

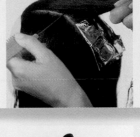

3. Without taking a subsection of hair to remain unlightened as in previous technicals, take another slice and place it into foil right behind the first one. This will make for thick highlights that process effectively. Here you can see two foils back to back. Part out a 1" (2.5cm) subsection to be left unlightened between the foils and work neatly and efficiently. Clip the hair not being worked on out of the way.

4. Part off a fine slice from the top of the section released.

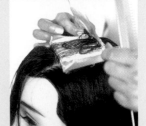

5. Place it into the foil and apply the product.

6. Continue working to the front of the head using the procedure as outlined—two fine slices foiled right next to each other with a 1" (2.5cm) subsection unlightened in between the foils.

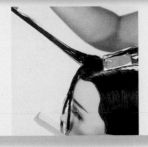

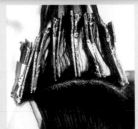

7. Take a 1" (2.5cm) subsection in between the foils.

8. You can see the two foil packets back to back, with a 1"(2.5cm) subsection in between.

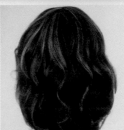

9. This look creates dramatic highlighted pieces of hair on the top surface of the head.

chunky front pieces

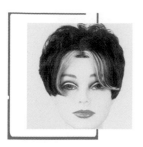

his is an easy way to add dramatic light pieces to the fringe area.

1. Take a 1″ (2.5 cm) subsection from the front hairline. Take a fine slice and put it onto the foil.

2. Double fold the foil.

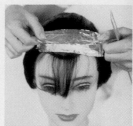 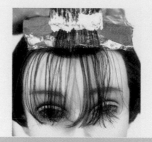

3. Take the next slice of hair back to back with the first one, and place it onto the foil.

4. Continue placing foils to the front hairline. Fold the edges of the foil back to secure.

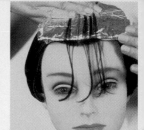 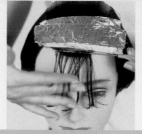

5. Here's the finished view of foils.

6. This look creates bold highlights right in the front fringe area. This is a definite statement for a more progressive look. You can also tone the hair if desired.

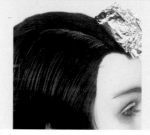 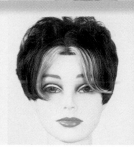

balayage technique for adding subtle highlights

*T*he word balayage means "to paint." Whenever you want to add subtle highlights to make the top surface of the hair sparkle, this is an easy, fun way to do so. The product you'll use here is a powdered lightener.

1. Apply the powered lightener to a tail comb or color brush and lightly paint the product down the strand.

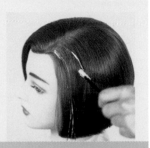

2. Work downward diagonally around the entire head.

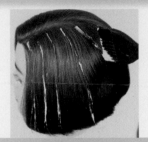

3. Once the balayage technique is complete, let it process for 10 to 15 minutes. Rinse and apply a color-enhancement formula over the highlighted hair if desired.

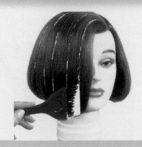

4. Haircolor highlights strategically placed are a dramatic, yet quick and practical, addition.

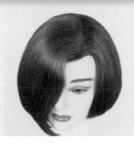

> **The man who does more than he is paid for will soon be paid for more than he does.**
>
> *Napolean Hill*

*T*his is a vitally important part of the service, as important as how well you styled the client's hair. Sadly, many stylists never take advantage of the client-satisfaction-building and career-enhancing opportunities available during the extension phase.

And what is his extension? It's the very close of every service, where you make sure the client goes home with the right products and tools to help her achieve the same look at home, makes an appointment for her next visit, and is happy with the results of today's service. This phase is too important to hand off to the salon receptionist. You want to stay with your client all the way, to a fabulous finish. (And don't forget to say thank-you.)

For example:

STYLIST: "Now, remember, I'd like to see you again in three weeks for an appointment. That's when we shampoo, deep condition, and style your hair to make sure everything's okay and you're happy with it. I want to check how the color is holding and make sure you are comfortable with styling it at home. We've made several changes today, and I want to help you adjust to them as much as I can. That's why we offer a free deep conditioning during the visit. If you're not happy with your hair or don't think you look good, we don't look good!"

CLIENT: "Oh, I appreciate that. You don't have to talk me into coming back. That scalp massage was great. I could stand one of those every day."

STYLIST: "Well, we can accommodate that! But for starters, how's Wednesday the 21st at four o'clock for you?"

CLIENT: "Can you make it four-thirty? I get off work at four o'clock and sometimes the traffic over here is terrible."

STYLIST: "Four-thirty it is, here's your appointment card; and here's the brush, the shampoo, the conditioner, the texturizing styling spray. Now, can I help you with anything else?"

CLIENT: "No, I think I have everything I need."

STYLIST: "Okay then, thank-you so much, Glenda. You have just been a pleasure to work with today. I look forward to seeing you again on the 21st, but if you have any questions at all in the meantime, you just call me. My name and number are on the appointment card."

CLIENT: "Oh, I will, and thank-you."

STYLIST: "Have a nice day."

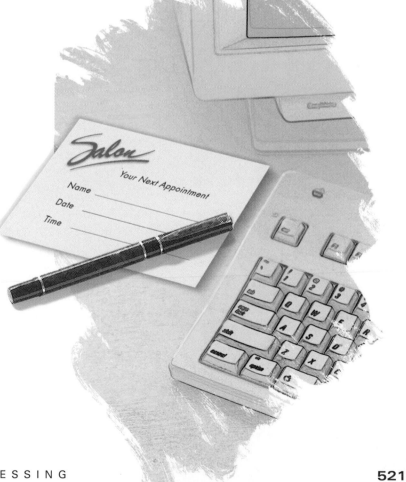

Men's Haircutting
A New Dimension

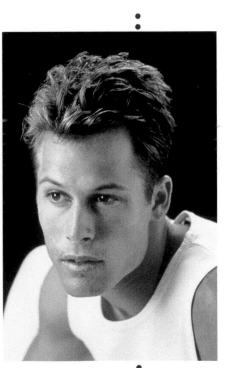

The term barber refers traditionally to the realm of men's haircutting techniques and styles. Men's haircutting has generally been viewed as different from women's, with training and techniques addressed under separate educational requirements. The same approach applied to the environment for clients, who were ushered into separate shops. Today, however, the lines are being blurred as more and more men are stepping into full service unisex salons, and stylists are borrowing from time honored, classic men's techniques by giving their female clientele barber-style cuts. Male clients now regularly have their hair textured, colored, and styled using a blow dryer, borrowing from the world of women's hair techniques.

What does this mean for you? It means that, if you want to be proficient at servicing a complete client base, learning the techniques of men's haircutting is essential. The information you will find in this section will help make that learning process clearer. This will enable you to work on your future male—and even give you a one-up on your female—clientele.

Many of the basic techniques and concepts used to cut men's hair are the same as those used for women's hair. For that reason, we recommend that you review the first part of the Women's Haircutting section, pages 26 through 51, before you embark on this section. Once you have those concepts in mind, you will begin learning to apply them to the male head.

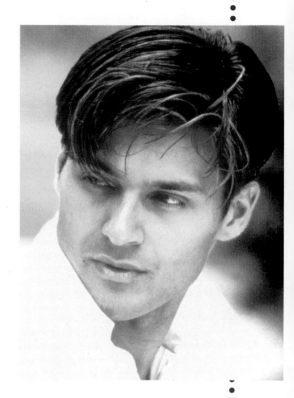

*Y*ou'll learn basic layering and apply it to long, medium, and short lengths; classic tapering for short, medium, and long graduated lengths; and precise graduated shapes, using clipper-over-comb and scissor-over-comb, as well as other comb-controlled techniques.

While many principles—such as holding, cutting, and scissor position—are the same for cutting men's hair as for women's hair, there are basic differences. They relate to classic techniques and terminology, which are derived primarily from the tools used, and some common barbering terms (scissor-over-comb, clipper-over-comb, fading, taper) are used specifically for male clientele. But more important is the realization that while the hair will fall the same once it's cut, the finished look will look different on a man than it does on a woman because of anatomy, head and face shape, bone structure, and facial features.

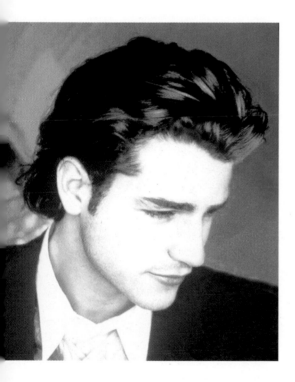

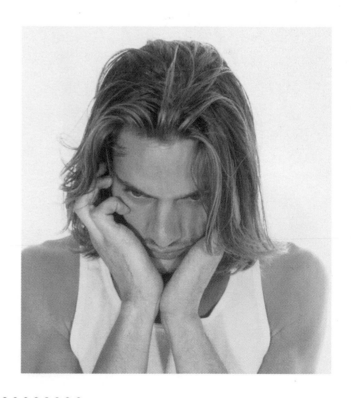

The cutting tools, which you can see here are (from left to right): the straight cutting scissors which you'll mainly use for removing length and detailing work; the blending or tapering scissors which have evenly spaced teeth along one side of the blades for removing lengths of hair in a section (excellent tools for removing excess bulk from the hair); the tapering comb with wider and narrower ends—a classic barbering comb that is essential for detailed cutting and often used in the nape and side areas, as well as above and around the ears. Note how much smaller the wide-spaced and close-spaced teeth are. The next tapering comb is not as tapered, and its teeth are farther apart. Again, the wider-spaced teeth are used for combing and cutting, while the finer-spaced teeth are used for detailed cutting and very short lengths using scissor- or clipper-over-comb techniques. The next tool is the wide-toothed comb, which you'll use for thicker and longer lengths of hair when fine detailing is not required. This comb creates less tension on the hair while cutting, creating a softer or more diffused edge. The finishing trimmer is used for outlining perimeter areas in the nape, the sides, and especially around the ears. This is typically smaller and more lightweight, and has a smaller cutting blade. The motorized clippers are larger and heavier and accommodate different sizes of cutting blades, from very coarse to very fine. In the photo are two fine-cutting blades, designated as #000 and #1. These clippers are often used for overall cutting and length removal.

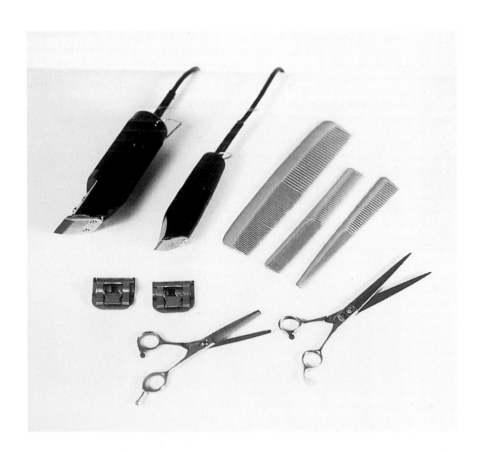

David Raccuglia

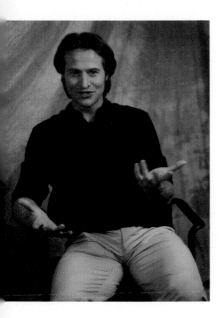

David Raccuglia, founder of American Crew (hair and grooming products for men) and the author of the men's haircutting education in this program, was inspired by Bob DeAngelo, a barber in his hometown of LaSalle, Illinois. Impressed by this man's skillful blending of fashion and grooming, David attended a nearby barber-college and then went on for graduate education at a nationally known advanced cosmetology education center in Chicago.

From there David became a member of the international artistic team of a world-famous education company that was known for its hip trend-setting styles in the late '70s. David became renowned for his ability to create cutting-edge looks for men. He went on to found his own education company and then, with several colleagues, he opened an upscale salon in suburban Chicago.

Throughout his climb up the ladder of success, however, David was continually disappointed at the lack of professional products for men. His research revealed that men comprised 50 percent of the adult population but only 28 percent of salon clients nationally. Here was a huge untapped market with unlimited profit potential, and David tapped it by creating American Crew, a line of high quality professional grooming products for men, backed up by outstanding marketing and educational support. Today, American Crew products are considered the gold standard in grooming for men.

As a role model for young students, David conveys his passion for his craft: "It's very important that the student understand the history of men's haircutting and the origin of its time-honored techniques. Although the principles of men's and women's haircutting are the same, there are important differences in both terminology and tools. The stylist who masters these nuances will build a profitable men's hair-care business."

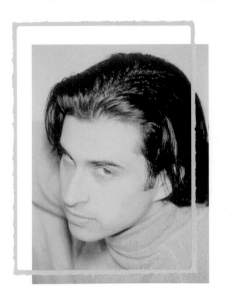

Long Layer

Overview

With this first men's haircut, you will learn how to create designs by producing a more squared shape. As you remember from the women's haircutting part of this program, shapes for females are more rounded and curved. Men's shapes generally have more defini and squared weight areas.

The procedures you'll use with men's cuts come from classical men's barbering techniques, and they'll serve you well in the salon. For example, with this long layer haircut, you will learn how and why to hold your hands in certain positions as you work around the head. Holding the hair straight out will allow you to achieve the desired layered effect while keeping longer lengths. At the same time you are creating a definite style and design for the male client, not just removing uneven ends. Another example is cutting in the palm your hand; this allows you to better see what you're cutting, as well as creating a flatter surface to cut on for more control.

Another method introduced with this haircut is cutting the sideburn area with a scissor-over-comb technique. In this technique, you use the comb to hold the hair in place while you use the tips of your scissors to remove the lengths. This requires a steady hand and close attention to what you're doing. For men's designs, sideburns play a key role in the total look.

Men's haircutting techniques use scissors with longer cutting blades. These allow you to remove more hair at a time, and are also necessary for the fine tapering techniques often used in the nape are of shorter haircuts. The haircutting comb has both fine-spaced and wide-spaced teeth, which are used for shorter and longer lengths of hair. The spacing of the teeth will adjust the tension for cutting.

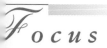

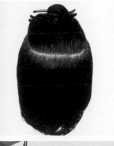

Even Proportions—Be certain there are evenly proportioned areas for cutting. Here, the hair is parted from the recession area upward from the eyes around the crown area. This will ensure a balanced form.

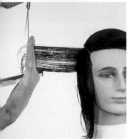

Consistent Tension/Holding Position—Maintain even tension for precision results. Comb and hold the hair straight out from the head. Maintain consistent holding positions throughout the cutting process for an evenly balanced cut when you are finished.

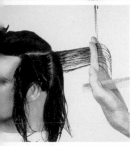

Hand Cutting Position—With palms facing out and fingers pointing up, you have greater control, allowing you to see more clearly what you are cutting. You also have a flatter surface to cut against.

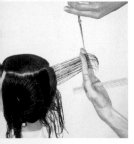

Head Position—Move the head and angle it as needed to ensure that the section of hair you're holding is straight out. Generally, you will move the head forward, back, and to either side to allow you to cut more accurately and comfortably. Remember to maintain a hand position throughout a given area so that you don't distort the line or shape as it's developing.

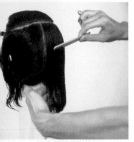

Begin the Cut—Generally, you'll begin a haircut at a central area of the head to establish balance and symmetry. The center back of the head is a neutral position and the hair is often the thickest in this area. By starting here, you are able to establish better control.

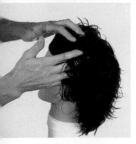

Finishing—Styling should be kept natural with a center or side part, depending on the hair's texture. This allows for easier maintenance and works well for a range of finishes and looks.

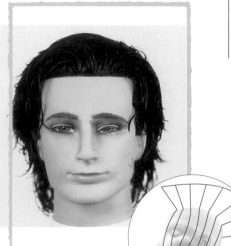

Apply
Long Layer

With your clients, these technical steps will follow consultation and shampoo.

This long layered silhouette provides textural movement and dimension. The layers begin at the nose level and progress to the collar-length perimeter.

1. Begin this haircut by parting off the lower section from the top section using a horseshoe-shaped parting.

2. Use the recession areas at the front hairline and the crown as your guidelines.

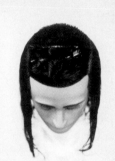

3. Take a vertical section that moves from the top of the back area to the center of the nape. This section, when cut, will be your traveling guide for the entire haircut. Use small sections throughout the cut to ensure an even length balance.

4. Comb the section straight out from the back of the head. Establish the length to be removed and cut your traveling guide.

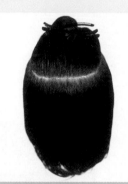
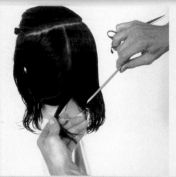
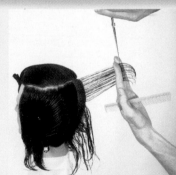

5. Cut from the top of the section to the bottom, working toward the nape of the neck.

6. Continue parting vertical sections, holding them straight out from the side of the head and cutting vertically, as you work around the head. Use the traveling guide as you cut, until you reach the front hairline.

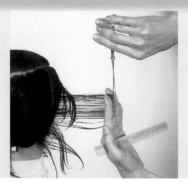
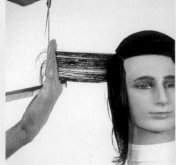

7. Return to the center back of the head and pick up your initial guide. Use it to cut the opposite side in the same manner, taking small sections and working toward the opposite side of the head. Again, stop when you reach the hairline.

8. To cut the sideburn, comb and clip the hair above it out of the way, exposing the sideburn section. Establish the desired length and cut. Then use a scissor-over-comb technique to remove excess fullness from the sideburn.

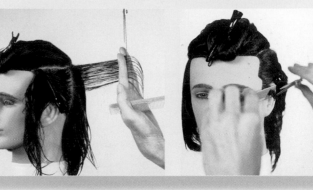
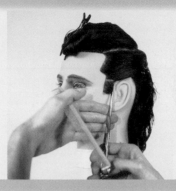
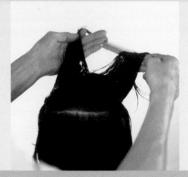

9. Detail the perimeter of the sideburn using a freehand technique. Use your opposite hand to stabilize as you cut.

10. Unclip the hair on the top. Take a center part that moves from the back of the head to the front.

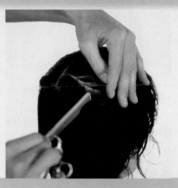
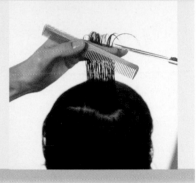

11. To cut the top section, take a horizontal parting at the back of the section that moves from the center to the right side of the head.

12. Use the previously cut exterior as your guide. Be certain to hold the hair straight out from the head as you cut out and, in this instance, parallel to the head.

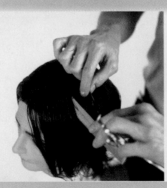
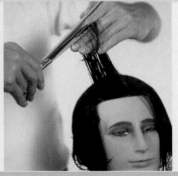

13. Work toward the front, horizontally parting out small sections and cutting to the established length. Notice that each section of hair is directed straight out from the head. Be certain not to overdirect any of your partings.

14. When you reach the front hairline, move to the back of the section and cut the left side of the top, using the same technique.

15., 16. For a natural finished look apply the desired liquid styling product, then finger style the hair.

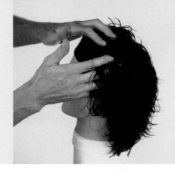
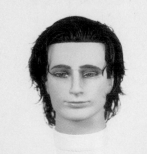

R eflect

E xplore

Apply this technique to different lengths, colors, and cuts for almost endless possibilities.

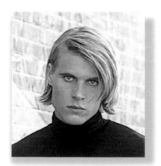

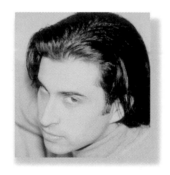

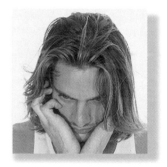

Referrals

*ccept the challenges,
o that you may feel
e exhilaration of
ictory.*

neral George S. Patton

The success of the average salon depends on its satisfied clients telling others about their experiences at it. This category of marketing is called "word-of-mouth referral." Successful salons increase the number of referrals their clients make by reminding them how important their recommendation is, and rewarding them when they do refer someone to the salon.

Let's face it: Our clients like us, but they aren't thinking of us every minute. Unless someone asks them, "Who does your hair?" they aren't spending all their time trying to drum up new business for the salon. That is, not unless the salon makes it worth their while.

Some salons give their clients a "Referral Card," which is often simply a business card on one side that, on the opposite side, says:

> Thank you for your referral. When a new client presents this card on his/her first visit, the client whose name appears below will receive a free haircut the next time they visit.
>
> _____
> Name of Client

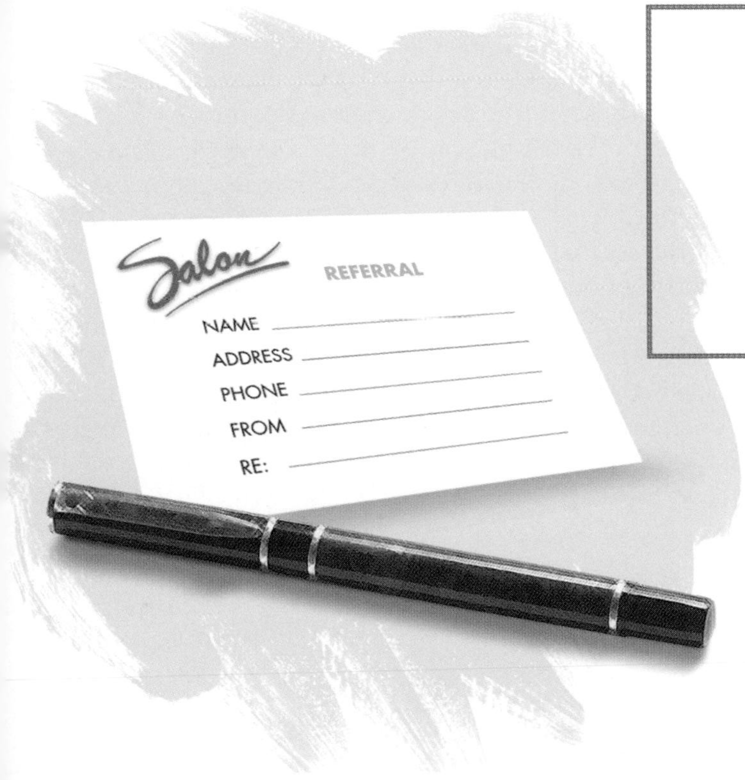

Salon REFERRAL

NAME _____
ADDRESS _____
PHONE _____
FROM _____
RE: _____

These cards are kept on the reception desk where clients can see them, and the stylists explain the referral reward program to their clients. When a new client presents a referral card, it is filed under the referring client's name or attached to the client card so that, the next time he's in the salon, he can be properly thanked and rewarded for his referral.

The rewards can vary—from a percentage off a service to dollars off retail products. To guarantee success, however, the program must be regularly communicated to all clients—and the rewards must be worthwhile.

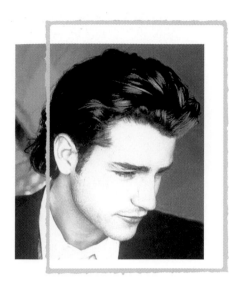

Layered Shape

medium length

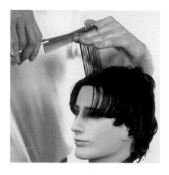

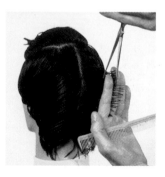

Overview

This haircut begins with the longer-length haircut you just created. You will not be removing a great deal of length—just enough to create a medium-length layered shape. You will establish a long length guide using facial features as reference points. By holding the hair in a vertical position when you cut and not moving it away from its parting, you have greater control, because you have a more accurate length to work with. Since this is a traveling guide, pay clo attention to the sizes of sections that you take. For accuracy, part ou smaller or medium-sized sections, 1/4 to 1/2 inch and use the portion of your cutting comb that has wider-spaced teeth. You will cut on th the back and inside of your hand. You'll be creating a squared shape to accentuate and complement the male head shape. Avoid creating a curved or rounded shape as you cut by keeping the head in an upright position.

Connect

Angular Shape

The male head is more angular than the female head because it has more pronounced flat areas and is not as curved in the crown or at the back. The facial shape and features, such as a squared jawline, may be more angular as well.

Evenly Proportioned Sections

If the sections of hair you take are too wide, your fingers will not have as much control holding them and the resulting lengths will be uneven.

Sideburns

The detailing of the sideburns is a critical part of the haircut because these lengths must blend in a progressive or gradual manner.

Focus

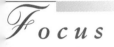

Even Tension—If the hair is combed evenly, smoothly, and with even tension, lengths will be balanced.

Section Width—Cut sections no more than 1/2 inch (1.25 cm) wide. If the sections are too thick, the ends of the lengths will be uneven when you release them. Too wide a section is too thick and too hard to control.

Guides—Traveling guides are used through the external and internal areas of this cut. For symmetry, first cut the section at the center back of the head, which determines your traveling guide.

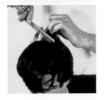
Connect the Sections—Connect the top with the sides and back. Here is the combining point and area of blending for two different parts of the head—the flatter to the more curved areas.

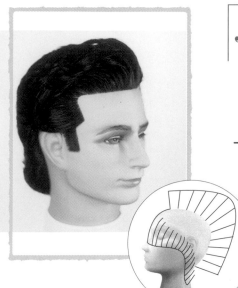

Apply
Layered Shape
medium length

With your clients, these technical steps will follow consultation an shampoo.

The layered effect in this shape is created by cutting the entire perimeter to a mid-length traveling guide. This blends with the interior lengths that are cut to build weight around the crest area.

1. Establish the length for the cut by using a reference point on the face. Once established, this length will be the guide for the remainder of the cut.

2. Take a vertical section through the center top of the head. Hold the hair straight out and cut parallel to the head.

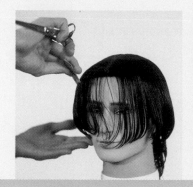
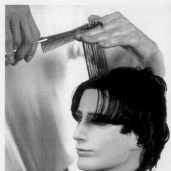

3. Use this length as a guide and continue cutting the center section, working toward the crown following the curvature of the head.

4. Now, section off the top of the head from the crown to both recession areas at the front hair-line.

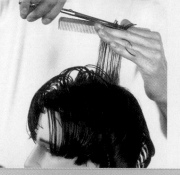
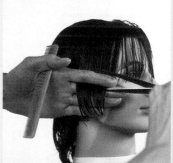

5., Moving to the back, vertically part down the center and continue establishing the length from the crown to the nape of the neck by cutting vertically. This will be your guide for the entire back section.

6. Continue through the back using this technique.

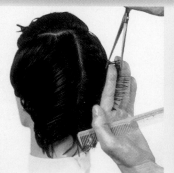
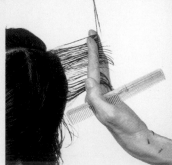

7. Work from the center back to the front hairline, continuing to cut vertical sections to your traveling guide

8. The completed side should blend neatly. Cross-check horizontally where needed.

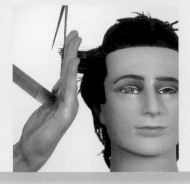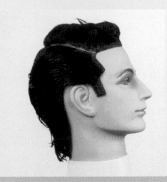

9. Return to the guide at the center back and cut the left side all the way to the front hairline, continuing to use the same technique.

10. Moving to the top section, unclip the hair and comb it forward. Take a horizontal parting across the top, at the back of the section.

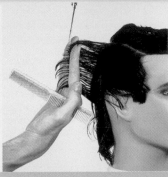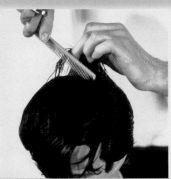

11. Comb and hold the hair straight out from the top of the head and cut, using the previously cut section from the top center as your guide.

12. Continue cutting the top section, taking small partings as you move from the crown to the front hairline. To ensure the desired layered effect, use consistency in the holding, cutting, and scissor positions. Upon finishing the cut, comb through the lengths to check the cut response. Cross-check vertically as needed.

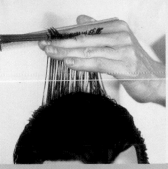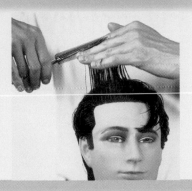

13. The backswept lengths are easily achieved in this haircut with the internal layers that flow over the perimeter graduation.

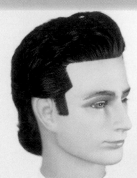

Reflect

Explore

Apply this technique to different lengths, colors, and cuts for almost endless possibilities.

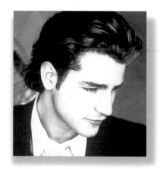 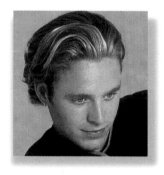

Marketing
Made
Simple

*M*arketing is a word used to describe all the activities performed by a business to attract customers and earn income, or revenue. Under the category of "marketing" come all of the following:

- ◆ **The name, logo, and physical image of the company**
- ◆ **The stationery, envelopes, business cards, brochures, flyers, postcards, and other printed materials**
- ◆ **Signs on the building and windows**
- ◆ **Newspaper and magazine advertising**
- ◆ **Radio advertising**
- ◆ **Billboard advertising**
- ◆ **Television advertising**
- ◆ **Promotional events**
- ◆ **Public relations (such as sponsoring a sports team or a theatrical performance)**
- ◆ **Referrals from existing customers**

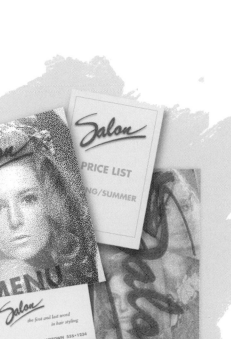

For a variety of reasons, many salons do not spend as much time or money on marketing as other businesses do. They rely instead on clients telling their friends about the salon, or on the fact that they have a good location, to attract enough clients to keep the chairs filled and the stylists busy. If you are working in such a salon, and there are not enough new clients coming through the door and being assigned to you to keep you busy, there are some things you can do on your own to make things happen. It's called "self-marketing," and it requires some time and creativity on your part.

Some of the suggestions that follow involve your contacting clients on your own, which means you need access to the clients' mailing addresses and phone numbers. Some salon owners will not want you to have this information, however, because they consider the clients to be the property of the salon; any attempt by employees to contact clients independently could be seen as a way of "stealing" business. Before you print business cards of your own, or send birthday cards to your clients, or offer any "specials"—even if you do these things on your own time and at your own expense—be sure you discuss your ideas with the salon owner. Explain that you're trying to keep busy and at the same time attract new business to the salon. The salon owner may like your ideas so much, that she may implement them salonwide. "Nothing ventured, nothing gained," as the saying goes.

Understanding
Clients
and
Dollars

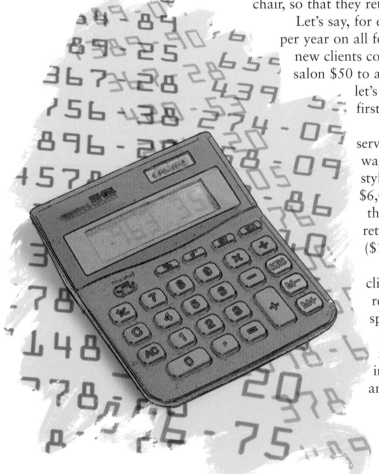

One of the most important factors in your success as a stylist—as well as in a salon's overall success—is the number of clients who remain with the salon over a period of time. This important measure of success is called the salon's client retention rate. Here we'll demonstrate what it costs to attract clients. This might help you understand how important it is to provide satisfying service to the clients already in your chair, so that they return over the long term.

Let's say, for example, that your salon spends $10,000 per year on all forms of marketing and, as a result, 200 new clients come in. $10,000/200= $50. It costs your salon $50 to attract each new client in that year. Now let's say each new client spends $30 on her first visit. 200 x $30= $6,000.

The salon now must pay the stylists who service those clients. Some salons pay hourly wages, some weekly salaries, but most pay stylists 50 percent of their service sales. $6,000 - $3,000 commission = $3,000. If those clients are not satisfied and do not return to your salon, it has lost $7,000 ($10,000 marketing cost - $3,000 = $7,000

In fact, it takes about three visits by a client, on average, before the salon ever realizes a profit from her. If it continues to spend more to attract clients than it makes on them, the result is . . . no salon. And no job. So all in all, satisfying and retaining clients is the best way to run a salon—and build a career.

Client
Retention

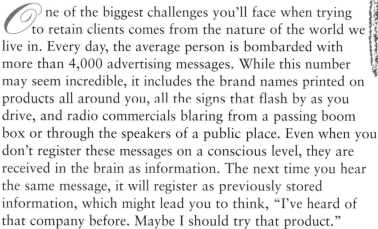

One of the biggest challenges you'll face when trying to retain clients comes from the nature of the world we live in. Every day, the average person is bombarded with more than 4,000 advertising messages. While this number may seem incredible, it includes the brand names printed on products all around you, all the signs that flash by as you drive, and radio commercials blaring from a passing boom box or through the speakers of a public place. Even when you don't register these messages on a conscious level, they are received in the brain as information. The next time you hear the same message, it will register as previously stored information, which might lead you to think, "I've heard of that company before. Maybe I should try that product."

That recognition from repeated messages is just what advertisers count on. That's why successful companies continue to advertise, even when you would think they could save their money because everyone in the world is already aware of their existence. Take McDonald's hamburgers, for example. Do you think you'll ever forget that there's a company called McDonald's that sells paper-wrapped sandwiches from little square buildings with golden arches? Didn't think so! Yet it continues to increase its advertising budget (currently in the billions) every year. That's because it's competing with everyone else who sells paper-wrapped sandwiches, and there's a new kid on the block every day.

Since the average salon client visits the salon only every four to six weeks (on average, eight times per year), there's an excellent chance that, sometime in the interval between visits, she will hear or see another salon's promotional message. Unless she's completely satisfied with every visit to your salon, she's vulnerable to the messages your competitors send.

That is why you must ensure satisfaction with your services when your client is in the salon. Make sure the memory of the service and attention you gave the client are so pleasing that she won't say "yes" to any other salon's offer!

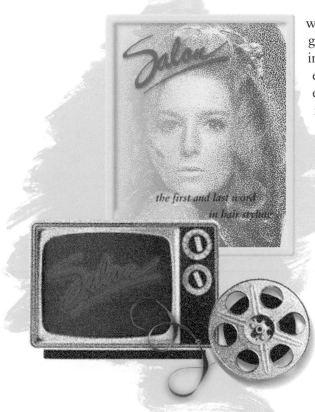

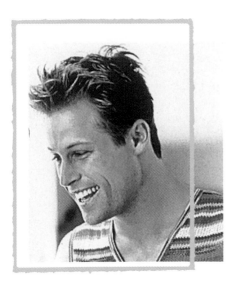

Short Layer

Overview

You are now preparing to cut to a shorter length. As with the two previous haircuts, you will begin by establishing the traveling length guide. Begin at the back of the head and work your way toward the face. Since you are cutting the lengths shorter, your hands will be closer to the head. Note that you will want to avoid resting your hands against the head as you cut, so that you are able to control the cutting angles. When you hold the sections straight out relative to the head area being cut don't overdirect them forward or back. By holding them straight out, the accuracy of your cutting will remain constant.

Connect
Layers

A short layered haircut emphasizes the ends of the hair as they progressively lie upon one another.

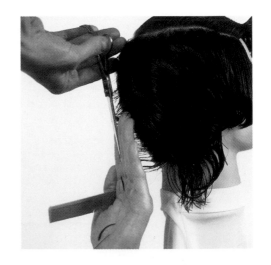

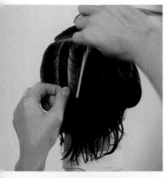

Evenly Balanced Lengths—To ensure even lengths, take sections of even or equal size. Think of the sections you take as being the space needed for the "shingle"—in this case length of hair—to occupy.

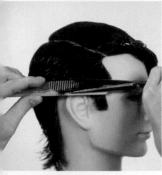

Comb Position for Scissor-over-comb—Hold the comb upside down and control short lengths of hair with its teeth. The comb should be exactly parallel to the horizon to ensure the evenness and balance of the cutting in this area, which will be fully exposed.

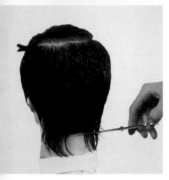

Controlling Length—Be certain to establish a length that balances with the overall perimeter of the haircut. The length of the nape area is very important for blending the back to the sides to the front in a proportionate way.

Luck is what happens when preparation meets opportunity.

Elmer Letterman

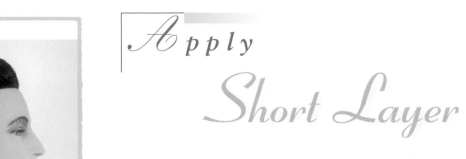

Apply *Short Layer*

With your clients, these technical steps will follow the consultation and shampoo.

This silhouette provides a closely tapered perimeter hairline to combine with the short internal layers.

1. Sectioning off the top, start at the round of the head in the back and working toward the recession area on both sides at the front. At the back, take a 1/2" vertical section down the center back, all the way to the nape.

2. Hold the section straight out from the back of the head and cut vertically from the top to the nape. This will be your traveling guide for the rest of the haircut. Starting next to the guide section, work vertically, taking 1/2" sections as you move around the back area of the head.

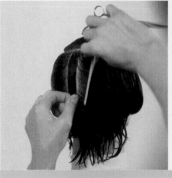

3. Leave the sideburn section free for now.

4. Return to the center back to cut the opposite side of the head. Pick up the traveling guide, sweep it over to each new section being cut. Make sure that the traveling guide is visible at all times. Work around the head toward the front hairline.

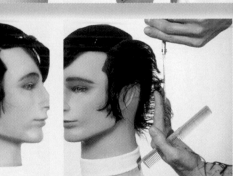

5. Establish the length of the sideburn.

6. Use a scissor-over-comb technique to remove bulk around the ear. This will create a nice clean look all around the ear. Cut both sideburns in the same manner.

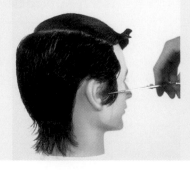
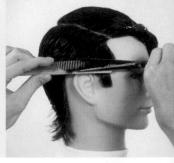

7. Establish the length at the nape of the neck and cut both sides of the nape horizontally.

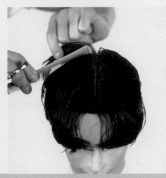

8. To complete the cut, move to the top area, which was previously sectioned out. Take a horizontal parting that moves from the center of the back of the section to the right side of the head.

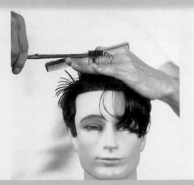

9. Use the previously cut lengths from the crest area as a guide, making certain to hold the hair straight out from the curve of the head. Cut parallel to the curve of the head.

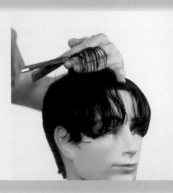

10. Continue cutting small, horizontal sections to the guide as you work toward the front hairline. Be certain not to overdirect any of your partings. When you reach the front hairline, repeat the cutting technique on the left side of the top section.

11. The lengths of the finished haircut blend perfectly when the hair is combed back. The finished style highlights the precise layers created in this shape.

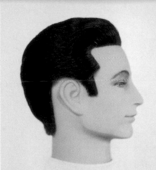

You have to expect things of yourself before you can do them.

Michael Jordan

Explore

Apply this technique to different lengths, colors, and textures for almost endless possibilities.

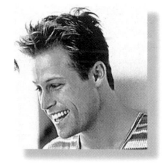

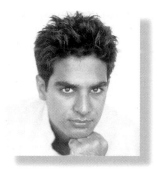

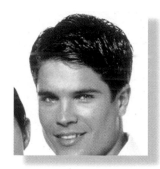

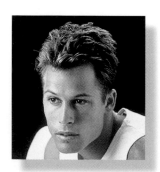

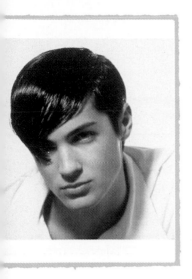

Long Graduation

Overview

This long graduation cut creates more fullness than you've created in the previous two haircuts, because you use no close tapering or fade techniques. Working with your scissors, you will create a graduation of balanced lengths throughout. Note that the techniques used in this graduation cut will remove considerable bulk, even though the finished look sports a full amount of volume. The main key to this haircut is using exact elevation angles.

Connect

Graduation

This haircut emphasizes graduation, which relates to ages, or degrees, of lengths. The lengths become shorter or longer in barely perceptible stages to produce the finished design. The look is unified by emphasis on longer lengths at the front half of the head.

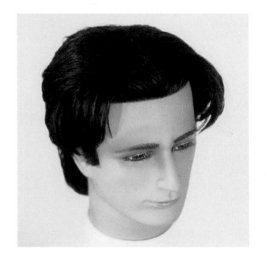

Focus

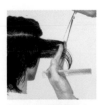

Even Tension—Maintain evenly balanced tension.

Pre-determined Length—With this technique you can freehand and detail a desired length before creating the graduated effect.

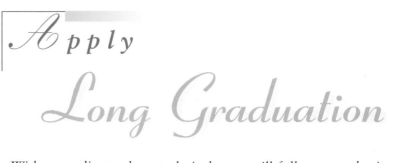

Apply
Long Graduation

With your clients, these technical steps will follow consultation and shampoo.

The long graduation is the classic silhouette for the male client who desires longer hair. Lengths graduate upward toward the crest area where a concentration of weight is located.

1. Part off a section at the round of the head, as shown. Clip this top section out of the way.

2. Comb the hair straight down and cut a blunt perimeter line around the head. The comb is used to control the lengths and create the cut line. Make certain you have a clean, balanced perimeter length all around the head.

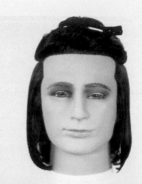
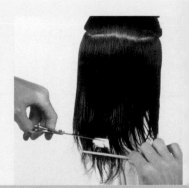

3. Move to the back and take a vertical section down the center of the head. Elevate and hold the hair straight out from the back of the head and cut in, diagonally, using the perimeter as your guide.

4. Continue cutting vertical sections, working from the center of the back toward the front. Return to the center back and continue working through the opposite side. Cut all the way to the front hairline.

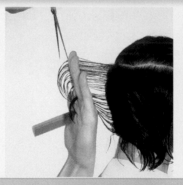
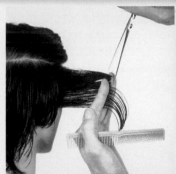

5. Clean up the sideburn as needed.

6. Unclip the top section and part horizontally through the side, moving from the back to the front hairline.

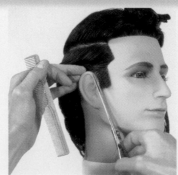
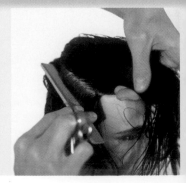

7. Using the previously cut exterior length as your guide, direct the hair straight out from the curve of the head and cut to the guide. Use this procedure from the back of the section all the way through to the sides. Continue cutting small sections until you run out of hair.

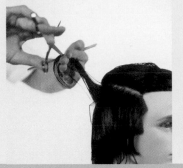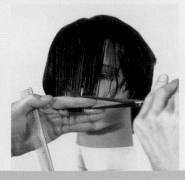

8. Comb the hair down in the front and cut to the lipline to refine the front perimeter line.

9. The hair has been styled to accentuate the graduated effect. This graduation may be adapted according to the clients needs and desires.

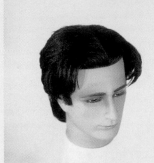

Magic is believing in yourself, if you can do that, you can make anything happen.

Foka Gomez

Reflect

<table>
<tr><td></td><td></td><td></td></tr>
<tr><td></td><td></td><td></td></tr>
<tr><td></td><td></td><td></td></tr>
</table>

Explore

Apply this technique to different lengths, colors, and textures for almost endless possibilities.

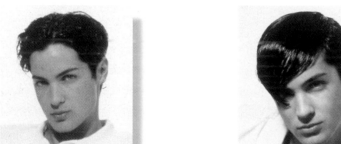

Retailing

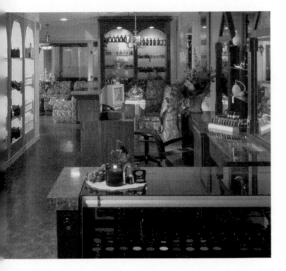

We've talked about retailing already. It's crucial to the salon's success to develop a retailing program. Simply put, it's a great way to generate profits that can be used for critical salon activities such as marketing, education, and the like.

And we've discussed the importance of making retail recommendations to the client. An important part of the professional stylist's job is educating clients about the appropriate retail products to use. This benefits the client because it helps him sort through all the competing product claims and, relying on the advice of someone he trusts who knows his hair, make the appropriate selection of products to use at home.

Now let's talk about the benefits you will realize in your career as a hairstylist if you pay attention to retailing:

◆ **First of all, there's money. Most salons pay a commission to the stylist (usually 10 percent of the retail price) on all salon products purchased during a service visit. Some salons even make sure the stylist receives a commission when the client stops in between service visits to buy products. Figure it out: If each of your clients spends just $10 per visit on products, and you service 50 clients a week, that's an extra $50 a week in your paycheck—or another $2,500 a year. Why, you can make a car down payment just from your retail commissions!**

◆ **Client loyalty is another important result of educating clients about proper home care of hair. When you help clients look good all the time, not just on the day they visit the salon, you increase their trust in you and their loyalty to you.**

◆ **And don't forget a satisfied client will refer other clients—increasing your commissions even further!**

◆ **By educating and advising your clients about the right retail products to use, and helping them make their selections on each visit, you will further your own career.**

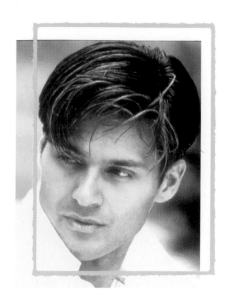

Medium Graduated Taper

Overview

This design emphasizes volume in the crown area, with a more closely tapered look on the sides and in the back. New to you with this haircut will be parting the hair horizontally, elevating it at a consistent angle throughout the crest area of the head, and creating a balanced form. Along with cutting with your fingers in a vertical position, you will also hold your hands and fingers in horizontal positions. You'll see results of these techniques in the weight line that you create around the crest area.

Connect
Removing Weight While Keeping Length

Cutting the hair to a stable guide at the crest area is a technique that allows for blending throughout the different areas of the head as you are cutting. To ensure a consistent length, check at the back of the head for any hair that needs to be blended.

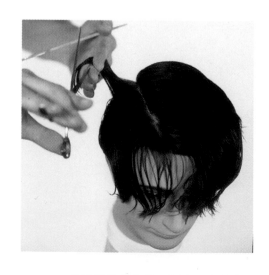

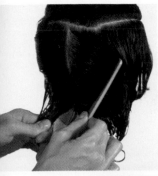

Even Proportions—Be sure to take a small-enough section to allow you to direct the hair straight out from the base section. Taking too large a section will create overdirection and unevenness in the haircut.

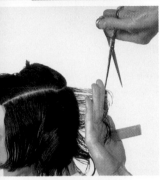

Starting to Cut—Starting in the back will ensure a long length related to the nape neckline. Determine that length with your first section.

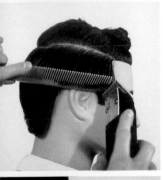

Low Taper—Use a very low taper around the hairline. Maintaining the low angle here will allow for enough length to be combed back, but without a buildup of weight.

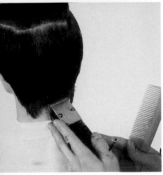

Clipper Rocking Technique—Both hands hold the clipper and rock it outward in an arcing pattern.

> ***You can't stop the waves,***
> ***but you can learn to surf.***
>
> *Jon Kabat-Zinn*

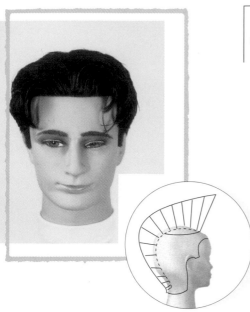

Apply

Medium Graduated Taper

With your clients, these technical steps will follow consultation and shampoo.

This silhouette is extremely popular with the male clientele. Longer graduated interval lengths contrast with the short tapered exterior lengths. This is a truly versatile shape that can be styled in a number of ways.

1. Part off a section at the round of the head, using the points of recession at the front hairline and the crown of the head as guidelines.

2. Begin by taking a vertical parting at the center of the back of the head from the crown to the nape.

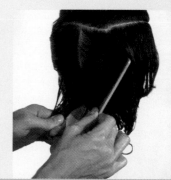

3. Hold each section out from the head and cut in diagonally. This will be your guide for the entire perimeter area. Continue taking vertical partings and cutting to the traveling guide, as you work toward the front. Repeat on both sides.

4. Move to the nape and use your comb to hold the hair, resting it against the head at an angle. Cut the hair at the neckline. Work across the comb to cut, then blend upward with a freehand clipper technique using a light and meticulous touch.

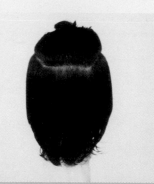

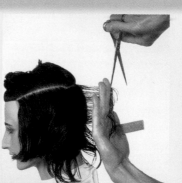

5. To finish the bottom of the hairline, cut freehand, using a clipper rocking technique.

6. To graduate short lengths around the ear, rest the base of the comb on an angle from the hairline outward. Run the clipper lengthwise along the comb.

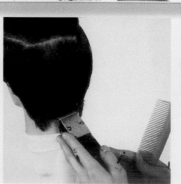

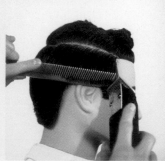

7. Hold the blade of the clippers at an angle as you trim around the ear.

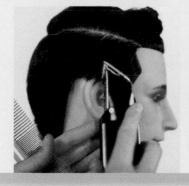

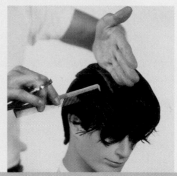

8. Comb the interior hair forward and down. To cut the top, take a horizontal parting, as you move from the back to the front. The partings should be small enough to ensure an even length throughout the top.

9. Using the length from the crest as your stable guide, comb the section of hair up to the guide which should be held straight out from the head.

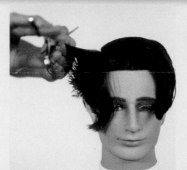

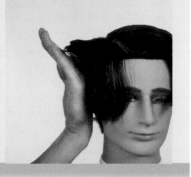

10. Notice the graduated angle as well as the diminished weight at the crest from using the outlined cutting technique.

11. Continue taking horizontal partings and directing the hair out from the crest area and cutting. Work from the perimeter of the top section to the center and from back to front. Hold the hair straight out from the crest of the head. This becomes increasingly important as you move toward the front hairline.

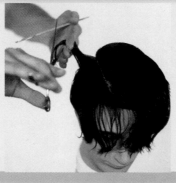

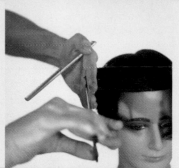

12. Upon completing this area, repeat the process in the opposite top side area.

13. Blend the lengths at the back of the head by directing the hair back to the graduated exterior guide. The elevation or holding position used here is consistent with the method used for the sides.

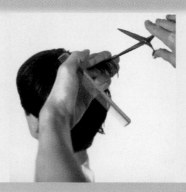

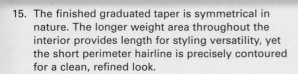

14. Comb the hair around the face forward, and cut the entire front hairline section, blending it to create a clean line at the front.

15. The finished graduated taper is symmetrical in nature. The longer weight area throughout the interior provides length for styling versatility, yet the short perimeter hairline is precisely contoured for a clean, refined look.

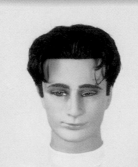

Reflect

Explore

Apply this technique to different lengths, colors, and textures for almost endless possibilities.

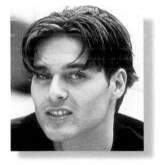

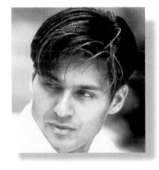

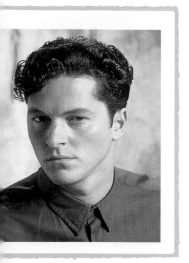

Graduated Taper

Overview

This design uses the technique of graduation on shorter lengths than the previous haircut and involves cutting with a combination of scissors and clippers. Clippers are frequently used for cutting men's hair because they allow for quick cutting and close cropping of the hair around the sides, the ears, and in the nape. They also work well in the clipper-over-comb technique, which is highly controlled.

Since you can remove a large amount of hair with the clipper blades, you will need to gain expertise through continued practice so that you do not remove too much when you cut. You can return to any area of the head in order to remove more length, if need be.

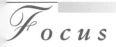

Focus

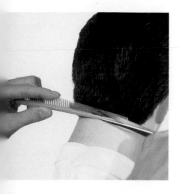

Comb Positions—The angle of the comb is very important. If you angle it toward the head, hair gets shorter; if you angle it away, hair gets longer. Resting the base of the comb against the head provides stability. The purpose of re-cutting with the scissor-over-comb technique is to fine-tune the tapering. Tapering is done from the bottom of the hairline to approximately one inch (2.5 cm) up from hairline.

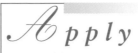

Apply

layers over short

Graduated Taper

With your clients, these technical steps will follow consultation and shampoo.

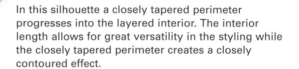

In this silhouette a closely tapered perimeter progresses into the layered interior. The interior length allows for great versatility in the styling while the closely tapered perimeter creates a closely contoured effect.

1. Section off the hair at the round of the head, using the recession areas at the front and the crown of the head as guidelines.

2. Start at the front temple on one side of the head, taking a 1/2" (1.25 cm) vertical section. This will be cut to become your traveling guide. Direct the lengths straight out from the side of the head and position the fingers diagonally. Cut in diagonally to create the desired length. Continue taking vertical partings as you work your way back.

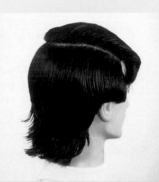
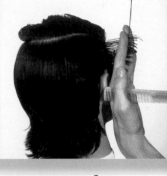

3. Once you pass the ear, extend the guide from the top to the nape of the neck as you move around the head.

4. Cut to your traveling guide, continuing to hold the hair straight out as you go. Work all the way around to the temple area on the opposite side.

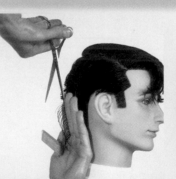
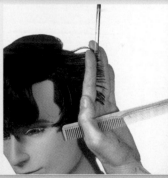

5. Change to the clippers and begin cutting at the center of the nape with the blade resting against the head. Notice how the two hands are holding the clippers for steadiness and balance. As you move up into the hairline, slowly rock the clippers away from the round of the head. Repeat the cutting technique throughout the entire nape area.

6. Taper the sides next. Blend freehand at the lower hairline area, then use a comb to pick up the hair behind the ear and cut. Notice that the previously cut hair in the comb acts as your guide. The comb and scissors must move together.

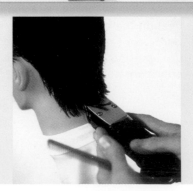
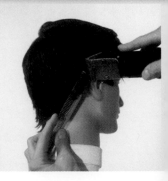

7. Holding the clippers at an angle, continue to cut the outline around the ear. This will create a nice, smooth line around the ear. Notice the angle of the blades against the head.

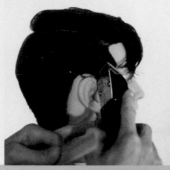 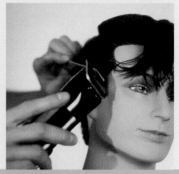

8. With the comb held at an angle and the base of the comb resting against the head, cut the hair by moving the clippers across the comb. Your previously cut vertical sections will be your guide for the angle at which you should hold the comb.

9. Refine the neckline and entire perimeter using the barbering comb or a tapering comb. The taper comb will create the closest possible degrees of taper around the perimeter, given the narrowness of the comb and the narrow-spaced teeth.

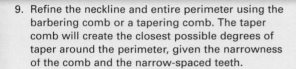 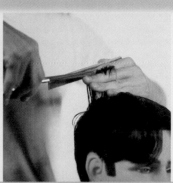

10. Starting at the back top of the head, cut the top section. Take a horizontal parting that moves from the center to the right side of the head. Using the previously cut vertical section as your guide, hold the hair straight out from the head, then cut toward the center top.

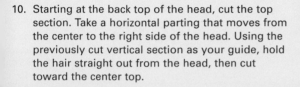 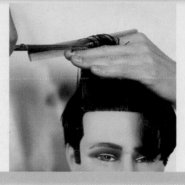 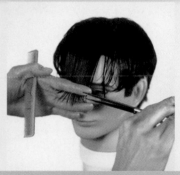

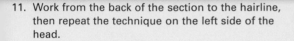

11. Work from the back of the section to the hairline, then repeat the technique on the left side of the head.

12. Comb the hair down onto the face and connect the front section of the fringe across the front. Be sure to cut the hair line in front of the temple to blend in with the fringe.

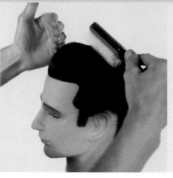 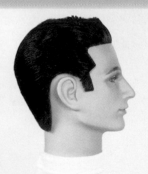

13. Add the finishing touch. Brush and place the lengths of hair for a well balanced shape. If desired, mist through the top area with a light hold finishing spray.

14. This sophisticated style is a perennial favorite among male clients. It is neat, controlled and well groomed in its' expression.

Reflect

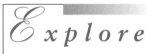

Explore

Apply this technique to different lengths, colors, and textures for almost endless possibilities.

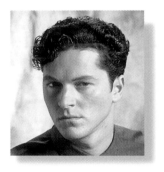

The Art of Commerce

Style

The hand is the cutting edge of the mind.

Jacob Bronowski

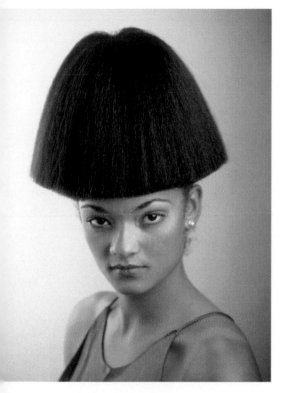

Now that you will be working on paying clients, a new element enters the picture. Until now, you have been absorbed with the artistic side of hair design. There's also a business, or commercial, side. Stylists who can balance both the needs of business and the demands of art will be the most successful.

Sometimes, art and commerce conflict with one another. Imagine for a moment you're working in a salon. You just learned a great new haircutting technique at a workshop, and you're dying to try it out. A client walks in whose hair and face shape would be perfectly suited to this particular cut. But what if that haircut doesn't suit the client's lifestyle and self-image? If you cut hair for the sake of design alone, without taking into consideration the needs of the client who will wear the design, then you could lose the client. Lose too many clients, and you have no career.

Stylists love to attend hair fashion shows and expos and to enter competitions, because that's where they can truly explore their artistic potential. If you need to flex your artistic muscle, that's the place to do it. But you'll also hear and read several phrases throughout this book and in other hairstyling publications: commercially viable, salon acceptable, and market reality. The commercially successful hair designer is the one whose designs make sense for the person who wears the hair.

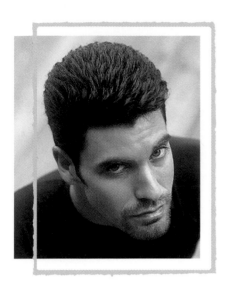

Classic Taper

Overview

This classic, tapered haircut brings you to another level of expertise as you learn how to apply the razor within men's cutting. As you've seen so far, each cutting tool is chosen to produce exact results. Although the razor is not used throughout this entire haircut, it will create finely detailed transitions between areas around the perimeter hairline, as well as blending the ends through the interior.. Working with the razor will give you new options for future haircutting and personalizing haircuts for clients with many kinds of hair types. Working with scissors, clippers, and a razor helps you create a popular, yet timeless look that will always be in demand.

Connect
Cutting Position

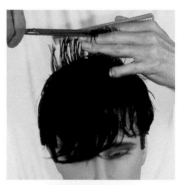

Note how the comb is held exactly in a horizontal position. to illustrate the angle at which you will cut the hair through the crown and top of the head.

Horizontal Line

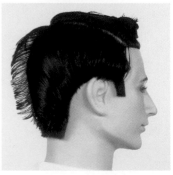

The strength of this haircut largely depends on how well you are able to create a horizontal line at the top of the head. Remember that a horizontal line is parallel to the horizon line, and is cut in this instance to build weight from the top outward toward the crest area.

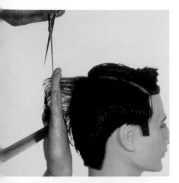

Hand Position—For this cut the back of the hand should be toward the head.

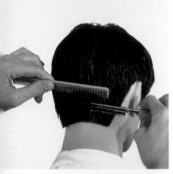

Remove Weight/Blend Ends—Use the razor to remove excess bulk and weight while establishing a strong natural shape. A more contoured, well blended effect will be achieved, particularly on very short, heavily layered shapes. Be certain to work in a precise, balanced way in the areas you're contour tapering with the razor.

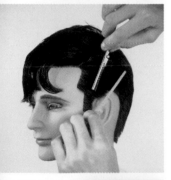

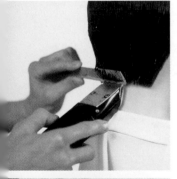

Head Position—Use the head to establish stability and maintain even graduation. Maintain the same head position within a given technique or area, but do position the head for your comfort as well as the clients.

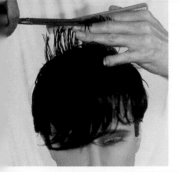

Balance—Clean, small partings will allow you to maintain an even length throughout the top.

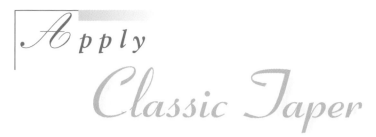

Apply
Classic Taper

With your clients, these technical steps will follow consultation and shampoo.

This shape features a dynamic tapered perimeter that progresses into the squared silhouette in the interior. The weight area in this cut is around the crest area.

1. Part off a section at the round of the head, using the recession areas at the front hairline and the crown of the head as guidelines.

2. Part a vertical section that moves down the center back to the nape of the neck. Direct and hold lengths straight out from the back of the head. Cut to the fingers which are held in a precise, vertical position. Cut the vertical section all the way down to the nape. The shape as influenced by the cutting position will feature a weight buildup around the crest area.

3. Continue to take vertical partings as you move toward the side; cut from the top of the parting all the way to the nape.

4. Take small, clean sections to ensure an even length throughout the exterior area.

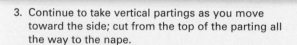

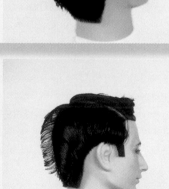
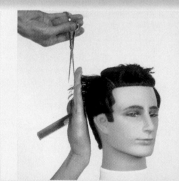

5. When you reach the front hairline, return to the center back and use the same technique to cut the opposite side of the head.

6. Moving to the back nape area, use a clippers-over-comb technique, and cut in a low taper. Place the base of the cutting comb against the hairline area, angling the comb out, as clippering lengths creates a smooth, even tapered closeness between the hairline and vertically cut hair.

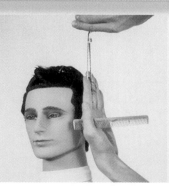
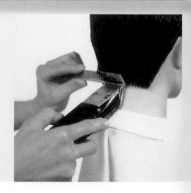

7. Continue this tapering technique all the way around the perimeter to the front of the head.

8. Next, angle the clippers around the ear to make a cleanly cut line around it.

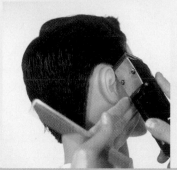
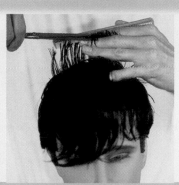

9. Moving to the top crown area, comb and hold the hair straight up from the top of the head for cutting horizontally. This will ensure a square shape. Using the previously cut exterior lengths as your guide, take horizontal sections across the top of the head and cut horizontally to the guide.

10. Continue working toward the front until all the hair is cut. Direct and hold the lengths straight up from the top of the head and cut to the horizontal traveling guide.

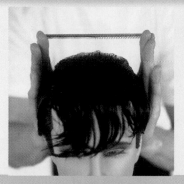
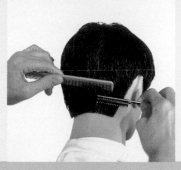

11. Use the razor with a guard on and the blade against the hair to blend the transition area. The comb and razor rotate to control and cut the hair.

12. Use the comb to control the hair and hold the blade at a medium angle as you run it through the hair to reduce any weight buildup. Work down toward the nape.

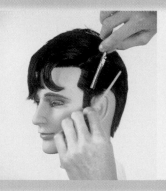
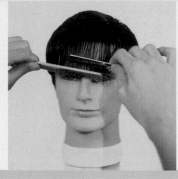

13. Repeat the razoring technique all around the perimeter, maintaining an even amount of pressure and a consistent angle. A light touch is to be used with this technique to avoid removing too much hair. Use light strokes while personalizing the area around the ear.

14. Use extra caution as you remove excess weight in the front fringe area. By removing weight here, you'll have more control in styling the hair.

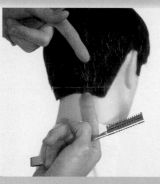
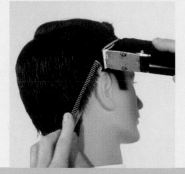

15. Notice the clean lines in the finished look.

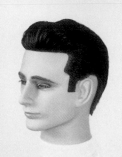

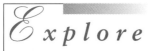

Reflect

Explore

Apply this technique to different lengths, colors, and textures for almost endless possibilities.

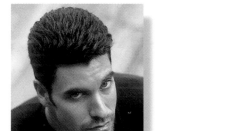

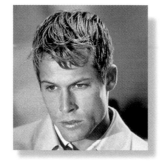

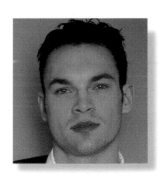

Exploring Your
Marketplace

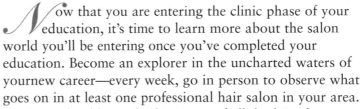

All your experiences are stepping stones to a greater good.

Louise Hay

Now that you are entering the clinic phase of your education, it's time to learn more about the salon world you'll be entering once you've completed your education. Become an explorer in the uncharted waters of your new career—every week, go in person to observe what goes on in at least one professional hair salon in your area.

How should you do this? First of all, look in the telephone directory and make a list of names, addresses, and phone numbers. This is your "target list." Visit your list of salons one by one.

You can go "incognito" if you wish. Simply pretend that you are stopping in to look for a certain retail product, or ask the receptionist for a pamphlet that lists the salon's services and prices. But a preferred method, one that will help you make contacts for future jobs, is to call the salon owner or manager in advance. Tell her that you are a student trying to learn more about salons in your area; ask if you can come in and observe for a half hour.

Consider this a business appointment. It is. Dress as you would for a job interview. (If you're not sure how to do this, see the *Clinic Success Journal*.) Make sure your hair and (if applicable) makeup reflect your professional standards. Be polite and stay out of the way of people while they are working. If you get a chance when stylists are not with clients, then you may ask any questions you have.

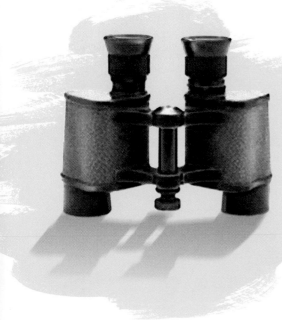

Record your observations. In a simple notebook, using a separate page for each salon you visit, make notes about new things you discovered. Keep records of the names of people you meet, for future use. Write a brief summary of your impressions of each salon. Note its strengths and weaknesses. Describe the kinds of clients you saw. You can refer back to these notes when the time comes to secure that first job. You'll be ahead of the game, because you'll already know where to look. Happy hunting!

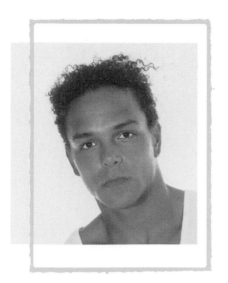

High Taper

Overview

This highly tapered men's haircut uses very short graduation cutting techniques in order to create a "fade" look. This means that the hair is very closely cut, with the scalp showing in the perimeter areas. At the same time, the overall finish of this cut shows smooth transitions from very short to somewhat longer lengths in the crown for styling freedom. Here the focus is on using scissors, clippers, and both types of cutting combs in order to produce specific results. With each haircut, you are seeing how you need accuracy and increased skill to produce these carefully planned and cut designs. With shorter length of hair, the planning of the haircut and the application of the techniques becomes very important. The balance of the shape and how well it complements the client's head shape and facial features are really the keys to the success of your efforts. With your increasing experience, your eye will tell you if a cut is proportionate for the client.

Connect
Comb Technique

Keep the comb moving vertically straight upward in relation to the head to allow you to create a square look. If you follow the round of the head, you will end up with a round finished look.

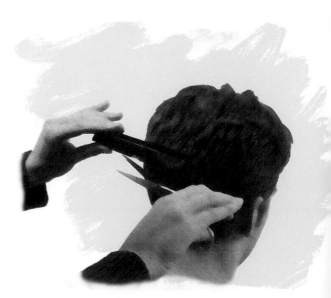

Clipper Technique

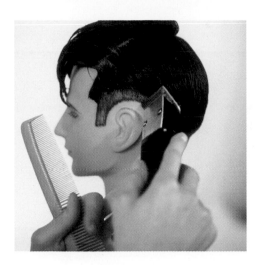

Use a freehand arcing or rocking motion with the clippers that will allow you to get very close to the scalp around the perimeter hairline. As you slowly increase the distance away from the scalp and the round of the head, a smooth, high degree of graduation results. Some clippers may allow for guard attachments that will automatically distance the initial placement of the clipper 5mm away from the scalp. Be guided by your instructor as to the guard attachment variables.

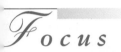 *ocus*

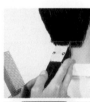 **Blade**—The blade on the clippers is a #1 (1mm).

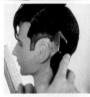 **Guide**—Your first finished section will serve as your visual guide for the entire perimeter of the haircut.

 Comb—Use the comb to work straight upward from the side of the head.

 Scissor-Over-Comb Technique—When you're using a scissor-over-comb technique, it is important to only move your thumb as you close the blades. Finishing with a scissor-over-comb technique will refine the closeness of the shape and balance any irregularities in the haircut.

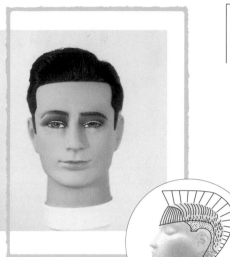

$\mathcal{A}pply$

$\mathcal{H}igh\ \mathcal{T}aper$

With your clients, these technical steps will follow consultation and shampoo.

The dramatic "fade" around the perimeter can be progressive and edgy or classic in nature. The tight perimeter progresses into the longer internal lengths.

1. Part off a section at the round of the head, using the recession areas and the crown as guidelines. Moving to the nape of the neck start cutting in the middle using the clippers. Move up against the head and slowly rock the clippers away from the round of the head. This section will be your guide for the entire perimeter.

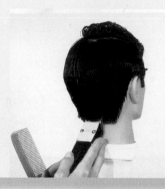
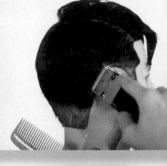

2. Work from the center of the nape to the side. When you reach the side perimeter, move the clippers parallel to the hairline while cutting.

3. Now cut the other side, restarting at the center nape and working toward the front of the head. Be certain to maintain an even amount of pressure while working with the clippers. Cut each section to the same length as the previous one, before you move onto another section.

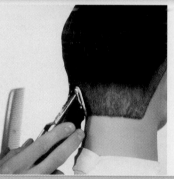
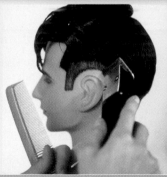

4. When the perimeter hairline is complete, hold the clippers at an angle and cut a clean line around the ear. This makes a smooth finish around the hairline. Repeat on the other side.

5., 6. Using a larger cutting comb and scissors, start at the center nape of the neck and continue to cut the hair to the established perimeter length. Be certain to work consistently from section to section, up to the top crown area of the head. Work straight upward through the back of the head using the scissor-over-comb technique.

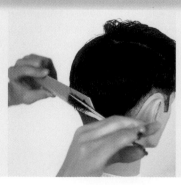
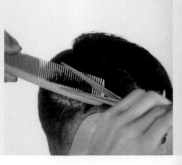

7. Continue working to the front of the head, using the previously cut hair as a guide. Complete one side, then cut the opposite side, starting at the center nape and working toward the front.

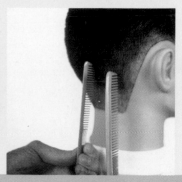
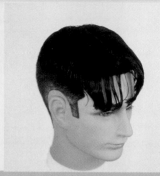

8. Use the tapering comb to finish the hairline at the back and sides. The length of hair you're removing in this process is very small, but it will make the finished results perfect. This type of comb makes it very easy to work closely around the perimeter hairline.

9. Taper in this transition area all the way around the perimeter hairline.

10. Comb the top forward and divide the top section in half by taking a center parting that moves down the middle of the head.

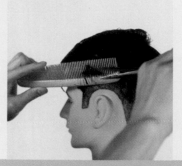
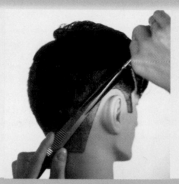

11., 12. Moving to the crown, take a horizontal parting that moves from the center to the right side of the head. Using the exterior cut section as your guide, cut the hair, working toward the center top of the head. Continue cutting small partings as you work toward the front of the head. Direct lengths straight out and cut diagonally to the traveling guide. After you cut your last section at the recession area, shift the final partings back to this guide.

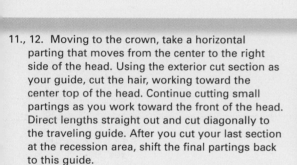
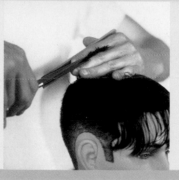
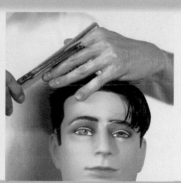

13. Repeat the procedure on the opposite side of the head. Using the first guide established at the crown and the perimeter guide on the side, cut the hair between the two guides. Work from the back of the section toward the hairline, remembering to shift the final partings.

14. When you've completed the second side, comb the front fringe lengths forward and cut the hair from the shorter sides straight across the front. To finish, apply the appropriate product and syle into the desired shape.

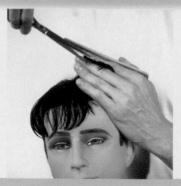
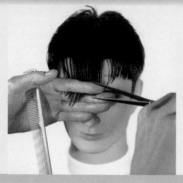

15. Here, the hair is styled asymmetrically.

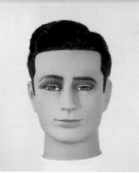

Apply this technique to different lengths, colors, and textures for almost endless possibilities.

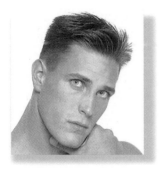

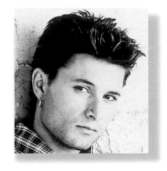

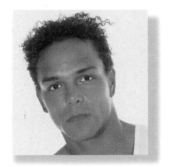

Connecting with Clients

When you have the opportunity in the coming weeks and months to work with real clients in the clinic or models for competition work, do your best to make a connection with each and every one. Take advantage of each opportunity you're given to practice your professional communication and rapport-building skills.

With each client, follow the four steps of consultation: connection, direction, execution, and extension. Smile and make eye contact when you greet each client. Introduce yourself. Even if you are not given time to sit down and consult with each client, once he's in your chair, ask open-ended questions to learn more about him—his job, his lifestyle, and what type of image he wants to project. Educate and inform about home care and maintenance. Create a service plan for each client. Follow up with retail recommendations and remind him about the home care tips you discussed. Escort him to the desk and thank him warmly.

After each client visit, make notes in your *Clinic Success Journal* about what did and didn't work, and what you might have done differently. If you gave a client a new chemical service, make a note to call him in a few days and see how he likes it. Make the time with every client count. The skills you build today will serve you well throughout your career.

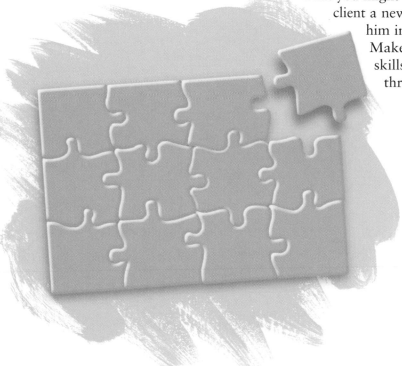

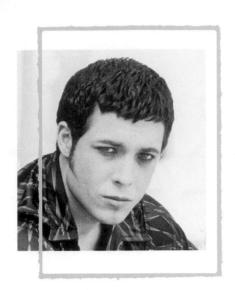

Short Brush Cut

Overview

With this short men's haircut, you will learn the shortest graduation technique, which produces shorter lengths at the nape progressing to longer lengths at the top of the head. This is a versatile and popular design, because it allows the comfort and ease of short hair while at the same time offering a longer length interior.

You'll want to fine-tune your scissor-over-comb coordination, which you'll need to master for this haircutting technique. There are fewer partings, so you must have extra control as you cut in a freehand style. You'll use the scissor-over-comb technique both to create a finely tapered effect throughout the exterior area of the head, and to hold longer internal lengths out from the head to cut. Thus, this one technique produces a pair of distinct effects seen in the contrasting lengths of hair. The combination of haircutting techniques and shapes created opens new possibilities for designing as you master your skills.

Connect
Graduation

Graduation will be created by working at an angle from the close perimeter upward. The longest lengths are at the top of the head. These lengths change gradually in small degrees from the perimeter to the top of the head to create a weight buildup.

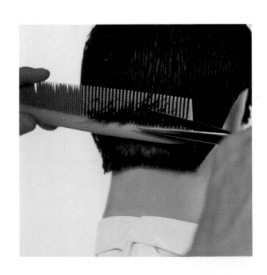

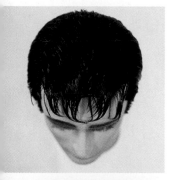

Visual Check—A visual check of hair texture, density, and growth patterns, as well as the head's bone structure and the scalp will tell you how short you want to cut the hair. The thicker the hair, the closer you can go, the finer the longer.

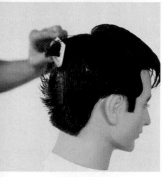

Comb Position—The angle of your comb should move up and out with the head shape through the exterior area. The comb moves outward at the crest area to add length and weight. The comb will follow the head shape through the interior from the crest to the top of the head.

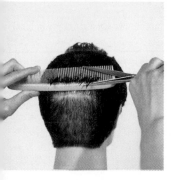

Graduation—You are creating graduation at the exterior area, which is shorter at the perimeter hairline area and gets slightly and progressively longer as you work up the head shape.

A goal is a dream with a deadline.

Napoleon Hill

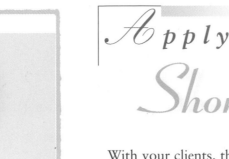

Apply
Short Brush Cut

With your clients, these technical steps will follow consultation and shampoo.

This short dynamic shape features closely graduated lengths through the interior that progress into longer interval lengths that echo the curve of the head.

1. Use a pie-shaped parting to section off the top, from the center crown to the front recession area on both sides.

2. Note the combing and holding of the large-toothed cutting comb for working upward through the back area.

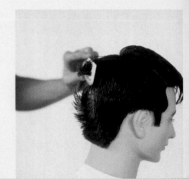

3. Begin cutting at the center of the nape of the neck, using a scissors-over-comb technique.

4. Continue with your scissors-over-comb cutting until the hair is the length that you want. Do not move onto the next section until you have established the desired length and the hair is even, this will be your guide for the entire cut. Once the length is established, work toward the right side and continue using a scissors-over-comb technique. Complete the entire side, making certain that there are no lines of unevenness in the hair.

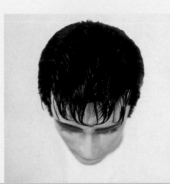

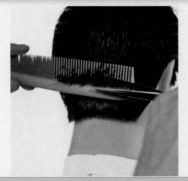

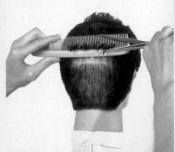

5. Return to the center of the nape and use the previously established length as your guide. Feed the hair through the base of your comb and cut the hair precisely when it passes through the base.

6. It is very important to hold the still blade stationary and at the base of the comb when you cut. (Use your thumb to move the cutting blade only.) Work toward the left and complete the side as before.

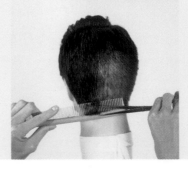

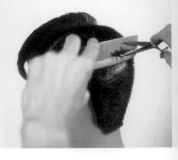

7. Use a barbering or taper comb to create the final details of the finished taper. When you're cutting with a taper comb, use the same procedure and technique that you used with the large-toothed comb.

8. The taper comb allows you to get the hair shorter and closer at the lower part of the perimeter hairline and makes cutting the nape, the sideburns, and the ear area easier.

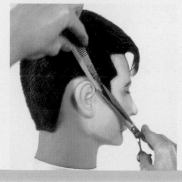
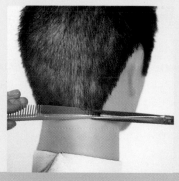

9. To detail around the sideburns, use a freehand technique and the blade tips of your scissors.

10. Using your large-toothed cutting comb, begin cutting through the crest area and top, using a scissor-over-comb technique. First, comb the hair up from the side until you see the guide from the perimeter hairline feed into the base of the comb. As you continue to work upward toward the center top, use the previously cut section as your guide.

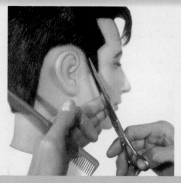
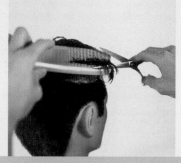

11. Incorporate the front with the length on the sides. Work from one side upward through the center top, and repeat on opposite side.

12. Move to the front hairline and work toward the crown, using the same cutting technique to blend the entire top.

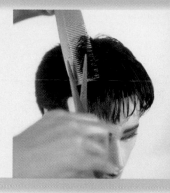
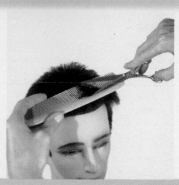

13. In the finished, short brush cut, all the hair blends evenly. This cut is styled here for a more accentuated and piecy texture effect.

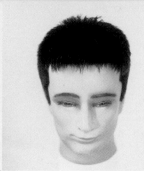

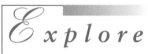

Reflect

Explore

Apply this technique to different lengths, colors, and textures for almost endless possibilities.

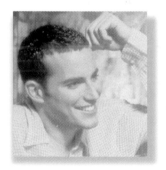

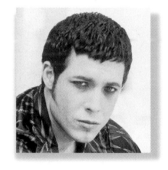

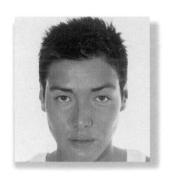

Cooperating with Coworkers and Supervisors

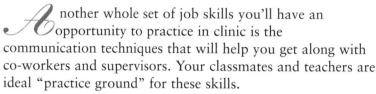

Diversity: the art of thinking independently together.

Malcolm Forbes

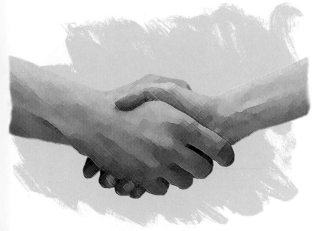

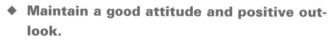

Another whole set of job skills you'll have an opportunity to practice in clinic is the communication techniques that will help you get along with co-workers and supervisors. Your classmates and teachers are ideal "practice ground" for these skills.

Have you ever heard the old saying "Familiarity breeds contempt"? In short, this means that the closer you are to someone, the easier it is to come into conflict. If you grew up with brothers and sisters, you probably understand what that means. Anytime you live in close quarters day after day with people, get to know their personalities and habits, and come to be comfortable or "familiar" with them, the potential for disagreement increases.

Disagreements between co-workers can make the workplace unpleasant for everyone. In service businesses such as salons, the clients sense the tension, too. That's why it's especially important to remember your communication skills when dealing with co-workers and supervisors. Remember and practice the communication clues and techniques that will help you do your part to maintain harmony in the workplace:

- ◆ Maintain a good attitude and positive outlook.
- ◆ Avoid negative people.
- ◆ Offer to help coworkers when you have the time.
- ◆ Turn "downtime" into productive time.
- ◆ Avoid "you" messages when criticizing or disagreeing.
- ◆ Don't take criticism personally. Take it professionally.

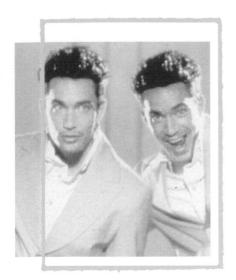

Contemporary
Taper

Overview

In this cut, you will use your tapering techniques to fashion a medium-length look that sports volume, versatility, and finishing options. Paying close attention to detail work throughout this haircut results in a smooth finish that is sure to please. A closely tapered neckline progresses to increasingly longer lengths through the interior for volume and height. You will create this design by using your scissors and clippers with a variety of techniques to both remove length and create detailed work.

Connect
Taper

The tapered haircut allows you to carefully remove length and bulk, yet retain the desired length for a range of styling options.

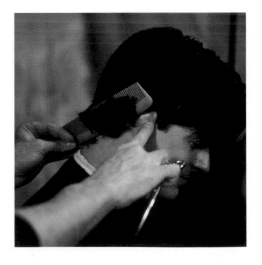

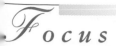

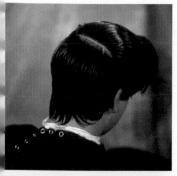

Hair Growth—Natural hair growth patterns may also determine your length.

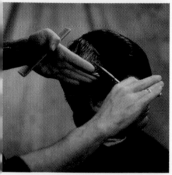

Guide—Make certain you follow your guide and that it is visible at all times.

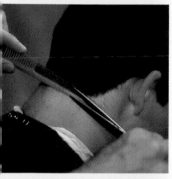

Even Angle—Maintain an even angle when you work around the nape area.

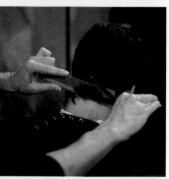

Movement—Maintain an even flow of movement with the your scissors and comb.

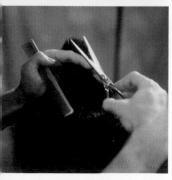

Finger Position for Blending—Notice how the fingers are rounded blending through the center top.

$\mathcal{A}$pply
$\mathcal{C}$ontemporary $\mathcal{T}$aper

With your clients, these technical steps will follow consultation and shampoo.

This cut is close and sculptured around the perimeter hairline progressing to longer lengths through the interior.

1. Part off a section at the round of the head, using the recession areas at the front hairline and the crown as your guidelines.

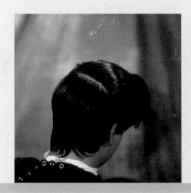
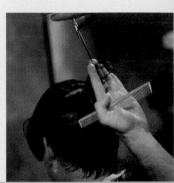

2. Begin at the center back, just below the sectioned-off crown area. Take a vertical section, shift the hair diagonally up and out from the head, and cut vertically. Be sure to maintain consistency in the holding and cutting positions along with even tension when working toward the sides. Repeat on the opposite back side of the head.

3. At the crown, release a diagonal section and cut to the guide length. Continue to release diagonal settings, direct lengths straight out from the side of the head, and cut. Bring the hair straight out from the side of the head and angle the fingers slightly to the line that increases in length from the crest area. Angle the fingers diagonally for cutting toward the front hairline. Use this technique to the center top.

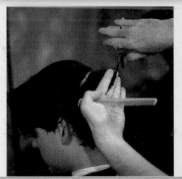
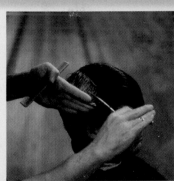

4. Repeat this procedure on the opposite side of the head.

5. At the center crown area, check and blend the lengths from the two panels that were cut through the top.

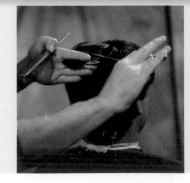
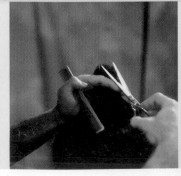

6. Take horizontal sections across the top of the head. Hold the hair straight out and round off any unevenness through the center as you work toward the front hairline.

7. Use a scissor-over-comb technique to remove any bulk and weight around the ear. Notice the angle at which the comb is held.

8. Refine the line around the ear, using your scissors in a freehand technique as you outline the ear.

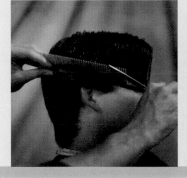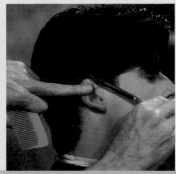

9. Use a scissor-over-comb technique to taper the perimeter sides, toward the nape. This ensures a smooth, clean look. It is very important to move your scissors and the comb in unison. Note how the ear is held out of the way.

10. Again, refine and detail the perimeter line.

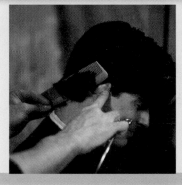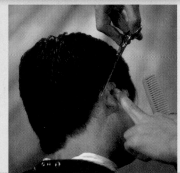

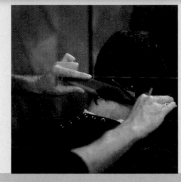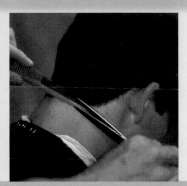

11. When both perimeter sides are complete, remove bulk at the nape, with your scissors and a comb.

12. Detail and refine the taper of the nape, using a small barbering comb. Note the fine detailing that you can achieve.

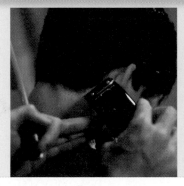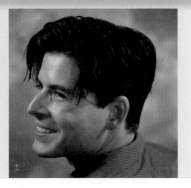

13. To complete the haircut, use a clipper to refine any extra hair around the neck and sides.

14. In the finished look, there is enough length in front for a variety of styling options.

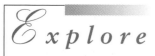

Reflect

Explore

Apply this technique to different lengths, colors, and cuts for almost endless possibilities.

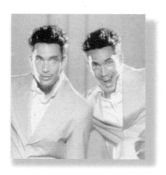

Building Your
Portfolio

Another tip for using your clinic time wisely is to start building a portfolio of your work. Just as art students keep samples of what they consider to be their best work, you too can keep samples of your achievements to show prospective employers.

No, you cannot keep every mannequin head you cut and style. But you can take photographs of your best and keep them attractively displayed in a three-ring binder. If you don't already have one, purchase an inexpensive "point and shoot" 35-millimeter camera for taking close-up color portraits of your work.

Choose the best photos, and keep them in a photo album dedicated to your work; or mount them with glue on white 8 1/2 by 11 inch cardboard. Put these into clear plastic, three-hole-punched sheet protectors. All of these items are available at office supply stores and stationery stores.

If you compete while a student, photograph your finished mannequins and models. If your instructors will permit you, ask your clients if you can take their photographs before and after. Create a collection that represents the full range of your skills. Include photos that depict daytime, evening, men's, and women's looks that feature your cutting, styling, coloring, and texturing abilities.

When you apply for a job, the salon owner or manager typically will ask you to demonstrate your skills. Usually, you're required to bring someone with you and cut and style that person's hair. With a portfolio, you can show so much more.

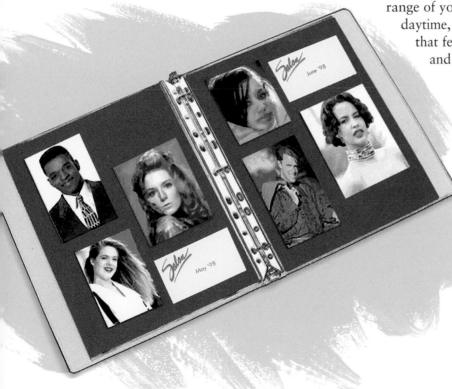

*C*ongratulations! You've accomplished an important goal, and you're about to enter the next phase of your career education. You've studied and learned the "theory" of hair and beauty in classroom and workshop, and now you will try your new skills and knowledge in a vitally important part of your education—your clinic practice.

The amount of time spent performing services on the clinic floor by cosmetology students varies from state to state and, sometimes, from school to school, depending on each school's curriculum. Clinic practice was created to give students as much practical knowledge of their craft as possible.

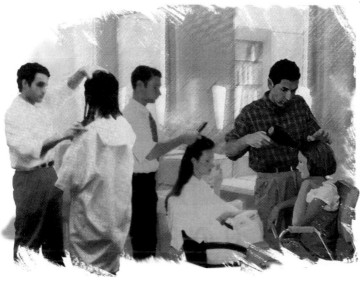

What is important for you to do, however, is to use this period wisely. Treat the work you do in the clinic as if you were getting paid for it. Treat the clients like real clients—they are! They are paying for your services. Practice all the skills you've learned—in both technical and business and communication subjects—while there are still instructors and others nearby to advise and guide you. Look for the challenges that will help you grow as a stylist and as a professional. Don't be afraid to try.

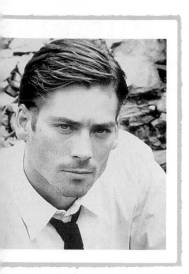

Gentleman's Taper

Overview

This shorter tapered look is ideal for the well-groomed businessman, who prefers shorter lengths but still wants enough length for styling choices. This look converts easily from a recreational to a professional setting, for an always-groomed image. It would work well for several different face shapes and hair textures, including naturally curly and wavy hair. Note that no area is cut too short or extreme; instead the look projects a well-designed image, a result of precision cutting based on the understanding of cutting techniques.

Focus

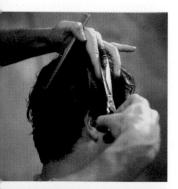

Even Tension—Maintain even tension and consistent sectioning throughout the cut.

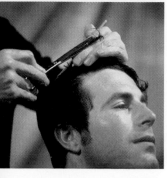

Length Retention—Front hairline lengths are shifted back to create a length increase around the recession areas for detailing the front fringe lengths.

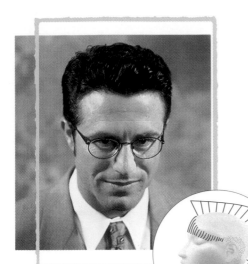

Apply *Gentleman's Taper*

With your clients, these technical steps will follow consultation and shampoo.

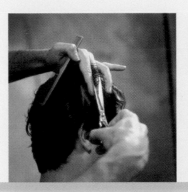

This heavily layered and tapered cut features a slight elongation through the top and around the fringe area for adaptability.

1. Establish a section at the round of the head, using the recession areas at the front hairline and the crown of the head as your guidelines. Start above the ear. Take a vertical section, hold the hair straight out from the head, and cut.

2. Work from the ear to the front hairline, shifting the last section at the front hairline back to slightly increase the length. This will allow extra length to personalize the fringe area, particularly when the front hairline is receding.

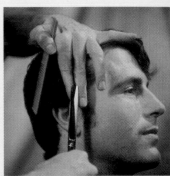

3. Vertically part out sections, hold straight out from the head. Cut parallel to the head. Move to the panel above the ear, and cut to blend with the previously cut section. Continue through the center back. Repeat on the other side.

4. Take horizontal sections through the interior from the center top to the outside of the panel. Direct these lengths straight up and cut. Work forward through this panel, releasing the horizontal sections and cutting to the traveling guide. Use pivotal partings through the crown area cutting to the established length guide.

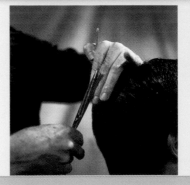
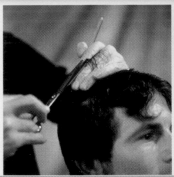

5. Direct front lengths back to create increased lengths. Repeat the techniques on the other side of the head, then work through the center top to blend away the weight corner created. Note the curved finger position.

6. Use a cutting comb to taper the sides and back. Be careful not to cut into the previously cut length. Taper both sides, then continue, tapering the entire nape area.

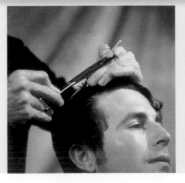
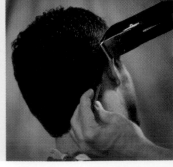

7. To create a smooth transition all around the hairline, refine and detail the cut, using a scissor-over-comb technique. Then style the hair into place.

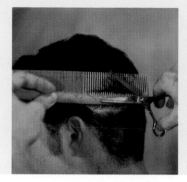
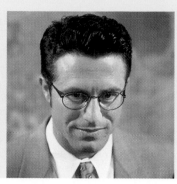

8. The finished classic taper is a perfect business look.

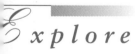 *Reflect*

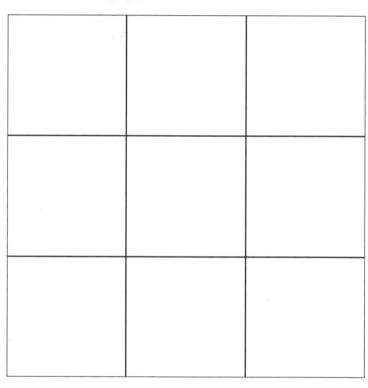

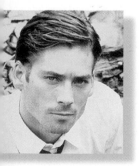 *Explore*

Apply this technique to different lengths, colors, and cuts for almost endless possibilities.

*C*onsultation, to be successful, does not just happen once—on the first client visit. It is as important a part of each client visit as is the technical service.

To be sure, client consultations after the first visit don't need to last as long as the first consultation, but a truly professional designer will know to ask a returning client more than "Same as last time?" Let's look in on a stylist consulting a client who has returned for her second visit:

STYLIST: "Hi, John, it's so good to see you again. How did that shampoo and conditioner you purchased last time work out?"

CLIENT: "I really liked it. And I'm glad you asked. Please remind me that I need more before I leave. It almost slipped my mind."

STYLIST: "Okay, I'll make a note of it. I'm sure that its special formulation for color-treated hair helped maintain the color for six weeks. And by the way, how do you like that new color?"

CLIENT: "I love it! I got a lot of compliments."

STYLIST: "Good! The condition of your hair is very good, as well. And it looks like the length is right where we want it for the style we discussed last time. I have the picture right here from the book we looked at before. Is this still the look you're aiming for?"

CLIENT: (looking impressed) "Why, yes it is. How good of you to remember."

STYLIST: "May I offer you coffee? I see by the card that you like yours with cream, no sugar."

CLIENT: (laughing) "Wow! I bet you know more about me than the FBI!"

STYLIST: (smiling and making eye contact) "Well, maybe just the important stuff."

Your Clinic
Success
Journal

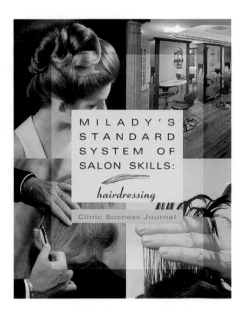

o much is about to happen. As you take all the knowledge and information you've been given, and through practice, practice, practice transform that knowledge into design skills that are uniquely yours, there will be questions and exclamations, doubts and concerns, complaints and celebrations.

Keep track of it all by taking notes in your *Clinic Success Journal*. Use it to record the goals you've set, and track your progress toward those goals. It can be a self-evaluation tool that helps you:

- ◆ **Refine your consulting skills**
- ◆ **Improve your speed and productivity**
- ◆ **Keep retailing records**
- ◆ **Keep client retention records and**
- ◆ **Write yourself a weekly "paycheck"**

Write yourself a paycheck? That's right. Well, not one that you can cash, but one that helps you measure your progress. With each mannequin or client you style, keep track of the service and what price the client would have paid in a salon. If you do that, you'll notice something happening week after week. You're accomplishing more . . . and you're earning more. Success is within your reach.

Throughout the *Clinic Success Journal* you've received with this course, you'll find simple exercises, checklists, and motivating ideas to help you practice what you've learned until you're comfortable with your skills and abilities. We're with you all the way. To the top.

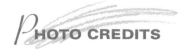

PHOTO CREDITS

Thanks to the following for their photos:

▶ PIERO SALON, Santa Monica, CA, *Photos:* Kelly Taggart for Purely Visual Productions

▶ GENE JUAREZ SALON AND SPA, Seattle, WA, *Photo:* Chris Webber

▶ THE FORUM INTERNATIONAL SALON, Sarasota, FL

▶ ZANO SALON AND SPA, Naperville, IL

▶ ULTA 3, Romeoville, IL

▶ JCPENNEY STYLING SALONS, Plano, TX

▶ KIMBERLEY'S A DAY SPA, Latham, NY

WOMEN'S HAIRCUTTING

P. 26	Alberto-Culver/TRESemme, *Hair:* Luciano Santini & Joe Tristino, *Photo:* Gianni Ugolini & Patrick O'Neil	
P. 26	Hair by Wella	
P. 26	*Hair:* Team Anasazi, *Makeup:* Brett Jackson, *Photo:* Nesti Mendoza	
P. 27	John Paul Mitchell Systems, *Hair:* Suzanne Chadwick, *Photo:* Alberto Tolot	
P. 27	*Hair:* Team Anasazi, *Makeup:* Brett Jackson, *Photo:* Nesti Mendoza	
P. 27	ARTec Systems Group Inc., *Hair:* Jamie & Vincent Mazzei	
P. 28	Sculpt Salon, *Hair:* George Alderete, *Makeup:* Rose Marie, *Production:* Purely Visual, *Photo:* Taggart/Winterhalter	
P. 30	Hair by Wella	
P. 30	John Paul Mitchell Systems, *Hair:* Pamela Perettie, *Photo:* Michael James Slattery	
P. 32	*Hair:* Team Anasazi, *Makeup:* Brett Jackson, *Photo:* Nesti Mendoza	
P. 32	*Hair:* Team Anasazi, *Makeup:* Brett Jackson, *Photo:* Nesti Mendoza	
P. 32	John Paul Mitchell Systems, *Hair:* John & Suzanne Chadwick, *Photo:* Alberto Tolot	
P. 33	*Hair:* Jamie & Vincent Mazzei of the ARTec Global Design Team, ARTec Systems Group Inc.	
P. 33	*Hair:* Team Anasazi, *Makeup:* Brett Jackson, *Photo:* Nesti Mendoza	
P. 33	John Paul Mitchell Systems, *Hair:* Suzanne Chadwick & Richard Dalton, *Photo:* John Niero	
P. 34	John Paul Mitchell Systems, *Hair:* John Chadwick, *Photo:* Alberto Tolot	
P. 34	John Paul Mitchell Systems, *Hair:* Jeanne Braa & Stephanie Kocielski, *Photo:* Alberto Tolot	
P. 34	John Paul Mitchell Systems, *Hair:* Suzanne Chadwick & Richard Dalton, *Photo:* John Niero	
P. 35	John Paul Mitchell Systems,	

Hair: Suzanne Chadwick & Richard Dalton, *Photo:* John Niero

P. 37	ARTec Systems Group Inc., *Hair:* Jamie & Vincent Mazzei
P. 37	Primo Hair Design, *Hair:* Ivani Lamani, *Makeup:* Lisa Tully, *Production:* Purely Visual, *Photo:* Taggart/Winterhalter
P. 38	ARTec Systems Group Inc., *Hair:* Jamie & Vincent Mazzei
P. 39	Pon International, *Hair:* Pon Saradeth, *Makeup:* Rose Marie, *Production:* Purely Visual, *Photo:* Winterhalter
P. 39	Hair by Wella
P. 39	*Hair:* Team Anasazi, *Makeup:* Brett Jackson, *Photo:* Nesti Mendoza
P. 39	John Paul Mitchell Systems, *Hair:* Jeanne Braa, *Photo:* Alberto Tolot
P. 65	John Paul Mitchell Systems, *Hair:* John Chadwick, *Photo:* Alberto Tolot
P. 65	Hair by Wella
P. 65	*Hair:* Brian and Sandra Smith, *Makeup:* Rose Marie, *Wardrobe:* Victor Paul, *Production:* Purely Visual, *Photo:* Taggart/Winterhalter
P. 65	*Hair:* Team Anasazi, *Makeup:* Brett Jackson, *Photo:* Nesti Tricoci
P. 65	Mario Tricoci Hair Salons & Day Spas
P. 72	Gebhart Int'l., *Hair:* Dennis & Sylvia Gebhart, *Makeup:* Rose Marie, *Production:* Purely Visual, *Photo:* Winterhalter
P. 72	Salon JKL, *Hair:* Janie Koger-LaPrairie & Ken LaPrairie, *Makeup:* Glenn Mosely, *Production:* Purely Visual, *Photo:* Winterhalter
P. 78	John Paul Mitchell Systems, *Hair:* Suzanne Chadwick, *Photo:* Alberto Tolot
P. 78	ARTec Systems Group Inc., *Hair:* Jamie & Vincent Mazzei
P. 78	Salon Norman Dee, *Hair:* Dee Levin
P. 98	*Hair:* Brian & Sandra Smith, *Makeup:* Rose Marie, *Wardrobe:* Victor Paul, *Photo:* Taggart/Winterhalter, *Production:* Purely Visual

P. 98	Paris Parker Salon & Spa, *Hair:* Jennifer Northey, *Makeup:* Ade Solorzano, *Photo:* Taggart/ Winterhalter for Purely Visual
P. 98	*Hair:* Brian & Sandra Smith, *Mal* Rose Marie, *Wardrobe:* Victor *Photo:* Taggart/Winterhalter, *Production:* Purely Visual
P. 98	Pon International, *Hair:* Pon Sara *Makeup:* Rose Marie, *Photo:* Winterhalter, *Production:* Purely V
P. 113	Hair by Wella
P. 113	John Paul Mitchell Systems, *Ha* Suzanne Chadwick & Richard Da *Photo:* John Niero
P. 113	*Hair:* Team Anasazi, *Makeup:* Johnson, *Photo:* Nesti Mendoza
P. 113	*Hair:* Lea Jurno, Yellow Strawb Paris, *Colorist:* Flo Briggs, Yello Strawberry USA, *Photo:* Tom Ca
P. 126	John Paul Mitchell Systems, *Ha* Suzanne Chadwick & Richard Da *Photo:* John Niero
P. 126	Evolution Hair Design, *Hair:* M Putnam, *Makeup:* Tanja Weller *Photo:* Rudy Hernandez
P. 138	Clairol Professional, *Hair:* Vict DiSanto, *Colorist:* Jessica Skoy, *Makeup:* Brian Duprey, *Photo Sty* Athena Dugan, *Photo:* Eric Von Loc
P. 138	Hair by Wella
P. 138	John Paul Mitchell Systems, *Ha* People & Schumacher, *Photo:* Andreas Elsner
P. 138	Evolution Hair Design, *Hair &* *Photo:* Mark Putnam
P. 145	Team Anasazi, *Makeup:* Brett Jackson, *Photo:* Nesti Mendoza
P. 145	Team Anasazi, *Makeup:* Brett Jackson, *Photo:* Nesti Mendoza
P. 145	Mario Tricoci Hair Salons & D Spas, *Hair:* Mario Tricoci, *Make* Shawn Miselli
P. 145	Model's Workshop, *Hair &* Mak Christine Merle, *Photo:* Ricardo Ra

Glossary/Index

A

accelerating machine, is used to reduce the processing time for lightening and tinting the hair. The machine accelerates the molecular movement of the chemicals in the color so that they work much faster.

acid, an aqueous (water-based) solution having a pH less than 7.0 on the pH scale. The opposite is alkaline.

acids, are compounds of hydrogen, a nonmetal, and sometimes oxygen that release hydrogen in a solution.

H

T